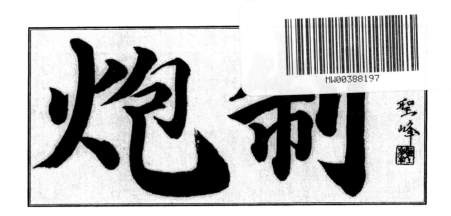

An Introduction to the

Use of Processed Chinese Medicinals

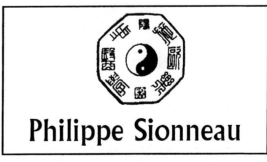

Philippe Sionneau

Translated by Bob Flaws

Blue Poppy Press

Published by:

BLUE POPPY PRESS
A Division of Blue Poppy Enterprises, Inc.
5441 Western Ave., Suite 2
BOULDER, CO 80301

First Edition, April, 1995
Second Printing, May, 2003
Third Printing, November, 2003
Fourth Printing, May, 2005
Fifth Printing, April, 2006
Sixth Printing, May, 2007

ISBN 0-936185-62-7
LC 94-74294

COPYRIGHT 1995 © BLUE POPPY PRESS

All rights reserved. No part of this book may be reproduced, stored in a retrieval system, transcribed in any form or by any means, electronic, mechanical, photocopy, recording, or any other means, or translated into any language without the prior written permission of the publisher.

DISCLAIMER: The information in this book is given in good faith. However, the author and the publishers cannot be held responsible for any error or omission. The publishers will not accept liabilities for any injuries or damages caused to the reader that may result from the reader's acting upon or using the content contained in this book. The publishers make this information available to English language readers for research and scholarly purposes only.

The publishers do not advocate nor endorse self-medication by laypersons. Chinese medicine is a professional medicine. Laypersons interested in availing themselves of the treatments described in this book should seek out a qualified professional practitioner of Chinese medicine.

COMP Designation: Connotative translation

Printed at National Hirschfeld, Denver, CO
on acid-free paper
Cover design by Eric J. Brearton

10 9 8 7 6

Dedication

I dedicate this work to my master and friend, Pierre Henri Meunier, who enlightened my conscience on humanity and medicine.

> *Medicine does not reside with he who chooses humanity but with he who chooses God. He who understands the heart of the doctor pays no attention to grades, schools, pomp, titles, letters, or degrees but pays attention to those who are suffering and providing them with a remedy. Know that those who are blessed and none others, those who have been chosen by God and not those who have been chosen by men have discovered whatever medical truths have arrived at our ears. Also, it is necessary for us to glorify the safeguarding of this truth of the blessed and not that of the gossips of the great schools.*

Paracelsus (1493-1541 CE)

Acknowledgments

This publication has seen the light of day thanks to the kindness of several persons.

I must first thank Celeste DaSilva Santos who was charged with the delicate task of designing the pages of the text [French edition]. Without her counsel and diligence it would have been difficult to manage this project.

I must also doff my hat to Thierry Riesser who, in the face of the inertia of the big houses of specialized editions, proposed to me without hesitation to take on the publication and distribution of this book. I am happy to have had the confidence of such a person. Within his hands, I rested assured of the birth of this book.

A thousand *mercis* must also go to Pierre Henri Meunier, Bruno Lazzari, and Catherine Azali for their support and precious aid, not the least of which was their rereading and correction of my handwritten manuscript.

In addition, I render homage to my professors and friends at the Hubei College of TCM and in particular to Hao Jian-xin, Zhou Zhen-xiang, and Li Jia-fa for their inestimable teachings on the Chinese materia medica with which they were so prodigal to me. And a wink of the eye goes to my accomplice Lu Gang for his devotion.

Finally, I testify my recognition of Wu Kai-jian, Director of the Foreign Affairs Office of the Hubei College of TCM, and of Zhang Liu-tong, President of the Hubei College of TCM, who allowed me to study with such good teachers and practitioners and in the best possible conditions within their institution. Thanks to their confidence and cordiality, I had the privilege of tasting the authentic flavor of Chinese medicine.

Translator's Preface

This book is a translation of Philippe Sionneau's *Utilisation Clinique de la Pharmacopee Chinoise, [Vol.] I: Les Substances Medicinales Preparees*, So Dai Editions, Paris, 1994, minus the very first section of his introduction and a number of quotations by Pierre Streckx towards the end of the introduction. We did not feel that these were as appropriate for our readership as perhaps for M. Sionneau's French audience. In terms of the Council of Oriental Medical Publishers' system of designation, I believe this work should be classified as a connotative translation. By this I mean that I did not try to translate each and every word to its closest standard English equivalent. Rather, my intention has been to translate this book so that its Chinese medical terminology would be the same as in other Blue Poppy Press books and as in the books of other Chinese medical publishers using the same standard translational terminology. That means that I first translated this text into everyday English and then back into Chinese. From there I retranslated it using Nigel Wiseman's *Glossary of Chinese Medical Terms and Acupuncture Points* published by Paradigm Publications, Brookline, MA.

Other ways in which this English language edition differs from its French original is that many of the Latin pharmacological names are different from those given by M. Sionneau. In some cases this means only that the author was constrained to only use the first part of a binomial name because of lack of space in his tables. In other cases, an actual different Latin name is used. When such a different name has been used, it is in order to remain consistent with other Blue Poppy Press books and the majority of other English language books on Chinese herbal medicine. We have also reversed the order of presentation of medicinals' identification so that the Latin comes first followed by the Pinyin in parentheses. In no case have we changed the Pinyin identifications given by M. Sionneau.

In addition, we have changed the page design of this English language edition. The French edition was done in the form of tabular boxes. Although that format provides a certain graphic simplicity, we did not feel it fit our English language translation nor the importance of the information contained in this book. Therefore, we have designed the pages similar to the most popular and authoritative English language *ben cao* to which we hope this book will be a complement and extension.

As an extension of the page design changes we have instituted and in the interest of conserving paper, we have combined some of M. Sionneau's short paragraphs as long as their subject matter was continuous and we have taken some of the author's lists and turned them into punctuated sentences. Further, in a few instances, we have broken M. Sionneau's long and elegant French sentences into shorter ones characteristic of easily understandable English. We have also removed the parentheses from a number of parenthetical phrases and removed a number of etc.'s in order to make the English read more felicitously.

As not only translator of this book but also publisher of Blue Poppy Press, I have long wished to issue a good English language *pao zhi* book. After studying *pao zhi* at the Shanghai College of TCM, I returned to the United States and began using prepared and processed Chinese medicinals in my clinic's pharmacy. My experience is that using specifically processed ingredients to enhance certain of their effects does achieve increased therapeutic efficacy. However, all the Chinese books I own on *pao zhi* are so large that the thought of translating any one of them seemed overwhelming. When I saw Philippe Sionneau's French *pao zhi* book, I realized that he had already culled the best and most useful information on the most commonly used Chinese medicinals and had arranged this in an easy to access order.

Therefore, it did not seem so difficult to translate his more manageably sized book from French.

Although *pao zhi* can and is studied in China as a subject in its own right, I hope that this book finds its place as a textbook in Western TCM colleges' materia medica classes. *Pao zhi* is an important refinement to the prescription and use of Chinese medicinals. Thus the appearance of this book not only fulfills one of my own longstanding desires but signals another step forward in the understanding and practice of TCM in the West.

Bob Flaws, Dipl. Ac., Dipl. C.H., FNAAOM
Boulder, CO
November 16, 1994

Preface

Pao zhi, also known as *xiu zhi*, refers to the traditional techniques for processing and preparing Chinese medicinal substances. These techniques are based on the theory of Traditional Chinese Medicine (TCM) and on traditional Chinese pharmacology and are adapted to clinical use, the methods of prescription, and to the nature the medicinal substances themselves.

These methods of preparation have their origins in the remote history of our primitive society and were born along with the discovery and application of these medicinal substances. The most ancient document on such methods of preparation is found in the *Huang Di Nei Jing Su Wen (The Yellow Emperor's Internal Classic: Simple Questions)*. During the North & South Dynasties period, *Lei Xue-neng* wrote the *Lei Gong Pao Zhi Lun (Lei's Treatise on the Preparation of Medicinal Substances)* which was the first treatise of its type. During the Ming Dynasty more than a thousand years later, *Niao Xi's Principal Methods of Preparation* gave a description of 17 of Lei's specific techniques, such as *zhi fa* (mix-frying with auxiliary liquids), *chao fa* (stir-frying), *wei fa* (roasting under cinders), and *duan fa* (calcining). Thus, as the result of thousands of years of development plus the work of our contemporaries in the standardization of the methods of preparation of medicinal substances and modern clinical re-

search, the domain of *pao zhi* today is vast and profound. In fact, this subject has become one of the fundamental departments of traditional pharmacology as taught in TCM colleges and is the object of specialized study.

These processes of preparation of medicinal substances are intimately linked to the clinical practice of TCM and rightly so. This includes not only those processes which reduce or eliminate toxicity or the side effects of medicinal substances, change or moderate their properties, modify their tropism, or reinforce their action, but also those which render them more pure and facilitate their use, storage, and absorption. In order to insure a good therapeutic effect, medicinal substances must be prepared after their collection and before their use in clinic. Thus one can say that, in terms of TCM, without preparation there would be no complete use of medicinal substances.

Philippe Sionneau has taken great pains to introduce this knowledge of the relationship between the preparation and clinical use of medicinal substances to the Western world. His book, *[Pao Zhi, An Introduction to Processing Chinese Medicinals to Enhance Their Therapeutic Effect]* is destined to play an important role in the spread and development of TCM. Therefore, I am very happy to have been asked to write this preface.

Prof. Zhang Liu-tong
President, Hubei College of TCM
Wuhan, Wuchang, PRChina
April 21, 1994

Author's Foreword

My objective has not been to make a work on the techniques and processes of preparation of Chinese medicinals for the sake of those preparing such medicinals working in pharmacies. Rather this book is meant to help clarify for the practitioner the clinical use of prepared medicinals.

It is theoretically possible today to import almost all of the prepared Chinese medicinals discussed in this book. Therefore it is necessary to hope that the importers specializing in Chinese herbal medicine will rapidly make an effort to regularly furnish the majority of such prepared medicinals since these products are the indispensable foundation of the correct application of the Chinese materia medica. Persons who wish to specifically study in detail the techniques of preparation should travel for instruction to China where several colleges offer courses for the training of traditional Chinese pharmacy workers.

The main intention of this book is also not to put forward a classical materia medica. Numerous serious reference texts exist in French, English, German, Dutch, etc. which have already laid the basis of that knowledge. Hence, I have purposely omitted the precise classical instructions on these medicinals' production, their time of harvesting, their botanical name, their channel tropisms, their contraindications, and the precautions of the use of medicinal substances which figure so largely in the Western literature to date. This has allowed me to concentrate solely on previously unpublished, practical information.

All of the information in this work has been taken from the Chinese medical literature and from teachings received at the Hubei College and Hospital of TCM (PRChina).

Because my search for perfection is constant, I welcome all suggestions and (constructive) criticism concerning the different aspects of this book.

Philippe Sionneau
La Fagua, France
April 3, 1994

Contents

Introduction

What Constitutes a Medicinal Substance in TCM?

Each remedy's particular therapeutic specificity essentially depends upon two characteristics:

The first characteristic is the specific part of the substance used. That is to say that the grain, the flower, or the root of a certain plant, the carapax or plastron of a certain turtle each represent a distinct medicinal. Thus the Lotus provides different medicinal substances depending upon which part is used. The node of the rhizome provides Nodus Nelumbinis Nuciferae (*Ou Jie*). The grain of the seed provides Semen Nelumbinis Nuciferae (*Lian Zi*), while the germ of the seed provides Plumula Nelumbinis Nuciferae (*Lian Xin*). The stamen of the flower provides Stamen Nelumbinis Nuciferae (*Lian Xu*), and the leaves provide Folium Nelumbinis Nuciferae (*He Ye*).

Hence one can see that the same plant represents in fact five different medicinal substances. But even more, the same part of the plant, root, stalk, flower, etc., may also offer numerous specific remedies. This is the case of the fruit of the Mandarin Orange (*Citrus Reticulata Blanco*), which produces six individual medicinals whose actions and indications are distinct:

1. Pericarpium Citri Reticulatae (*Ju Pi*): This is the skin of the entire fruit. It rectifies and harmonizes the center and fortifies the spleen, dries dampness and transforms phlegm.

2. Exocarpium Rubrum Citri Reticulatae (*Ju Hong*): This is the external, reddish-orange part of the skin of the fruit. It rectifies the lung qi, resolves the exterior and scatters cold, dries dampness and transforms phlegm.

3. Exocarpium Album Citri Reticulatae (*Ju Bai*): This is the internal, whitish part of the skin of this fruit. It moderately rectifies the middle and lung qi, moderately dries dampness, and is pre-

scribed in case of yin vacuity with simultaneous dampness.

4. Fasciculus Vascularis Citri Reticulatae (*Ju Luo*): These are the whitish filaments which are located on the flesh and between the sections of the fruit. These free and quicken the network vessels, move the qi and blood, and transform phlegm.

5. Semen Citri Reticulatae (*Ju He*): These are the seeds inside the fruit. They rectify the qi of the liver and kidney channels, scatter nodulations, and stop pain.

6. Pericarpium Viridis Citri Reticulatae (*Qing Pi*): This is the entire fruit when it is small or the skin of the fruit when it is large. In both cases it is still immature. It drains the liver, breaks qi stagnation, disperses stagnant food, and strongly dispels accumulations.

The second characteristic is the specific type of preparation used. This means that the same medicinal processed by a different method of preparation may be considered as if a different medicinal substance entirely. For instance, Rhizoma Pinelliae Ternatae (*Ban Xia*) is a generic term which actually covers several different medicinals:

1. Uncooked Rhizoma Pinelliae Ternatae (*Sheng Ban Xia*): This is the base preparation, which is toxic and only used in external applications. It disperses swelling, stops pain, outthrusts pus as in the case of abscesses, inflammation, nodulation, etc.

2. Clear Rhizoma Pinelliae Ternatae (*Qing Ban Xia*): This is prepared with the aid of an Alumen (*Bai Fan*) solution. It dries dampness and transforms phlegm.

3. Ginger-processed] Rhizoma Pinelliae Ternatae (*Jiang Ban Xia*): This is prepared with the aid of ginger juice. It warms the center, transforms phlegm, downbears counterflow qi, and stops vomiting.

4. Lime-processed Rhizoma Pinelliae Ternatae (*Fa Ban Xia*): This is prepared with the aid of lime. It dries dampness, transforms phlegm, and fortifies the function of the spleen.

5. Fermented Rhizoma Pinelliae Ternatae (*Ban Xia Qu*): This transforms phlegm, stimulates the digestion, and disperses food stagnation.

Thus, one can see from the above that this concept of the preparation of medicinal substances has been elaborated down the centuries giving birth to a veritable pharmaceutical alchemy which transforms a simply empirical phytotherapy into an energetic pharmacology. These methods of preparation rely upon complex, precise, and codified techniques, which require the competence of a specialist to provide. In China today, the trade of a Chinese pharmacologist requires several years of study at a TCM college.

As an extension of this, when one wishes to specify a particular remedy within the Chinese materia medica, one must specify the particular method of preparation of the particular medicinal substance, be it animal, vegetable, or mineral. If as a practitioner one does not take both of these two characteristics into account when using the Chinese materia medica, it will considerably reduce one's efficacy. Unfortunately, these two aspects are often overlooked by Western authors writing on the Chinese materia medica, and this forcefully diminishes the potency of our therapeutic acts as practitioners of TCM.

The Utilization of Prepared Substances: An Absolute Necessity

Except in rare cases or when one chooses to use the fresh plant (most often in replete heat patterns), one should use various transformations of basic TCM medicinals for the most of the ingredients in any formula. Although certain medicinals only require elementary treatment, such as washing, drying, or chopping, most often one uses medicinals which have been subjected to elaborate and sometimes complex methods of preparation.

Non-usage of such prepared medicinals makes up a large part of our deficiency as TCM practitioners in the West. For the most part up till now, we Westerners have only been attentive to this issue in rare cases and only tend to make the distinction between such medicinals as uncooked Radix Glycyrrhizae (*Sheng Gan Cao*) and mix-fried Radix Glycyrrhizae (*Zhi Gan Cao*), uncooked Radix Rehmanniae (*Sheng Di Huang*) and prepared Radix Rehmanniae (*Shu Di Huang*), and Rhizoma Arisaematis (*Tian Nan Xing*) and bile[-processed] Rhizoma Arisaematis (*Dan Nan Xing*) but not between others!

We know that the actions and indications of individual substances are totally distinct and that one cannot use one in place of the other. Then why should we not make the same distinction between uncooked Rhizoma Atractylodis Macrocephalae (*Sheng Bai Zhu*) and stir-fried Rhizoma Atractylodis Macrocephalae (*Chao Bai Zhu*) or between uncooked Radix Bupleuri (*Sheng Chai Hu*) and stir-fried Radix Bupleuri (*Chao Chai Hu*)? After all, this is the same problem, the same dialectic, the same law, the same necessity. Is it logical and appropriate to prescribe a remedy that precipitates heat and frees the stools when one wishes to nourish yin and liver/kidney essence? Yet this is exactly what we are doing when we prescribe Radix Polygoni Multiflori (*He Shou Wu*) in place of processed Radix Polygoni Multiflori (*Zhi He Shou Wu*). The systematic prescription of herbs (or concentrated powders) which are not prepared completely disturbs the action of those remedies, often in important ways, and this can bring damage to our patients. Below is a comparison of the functions of the ingredients in *Bu Zhong Yi Qi Tang* (Supplement the Center & Boost the Qi Decoction) when one uses prepared ingredients and non-prepared ingredients.

Bu Zhong Yi Qi Tang	
Non-prepared Ingredients	**Prepared Ingredients**
Uncooked Radix Astragali Membranacei (*Sheng Huang Qi*) Secures the exterior, disinhibits urination, disperses swelling + **Uncooked Radix Codonopsis Pilosulae (*Dang Shen*)** Supplements the qi, engenders fluids + **Uncooked Rhizoma Atractylodis Macrocephalae (*Sheng Bai Zhu*)** Secures the exterior, disinhibits urination, fortifies the spleen & dries dampness + **Uncooked Radix Glycyrrhizae (*Sheng Gan Cao*)** Clears heat, resolves toxins + **Uncooked Radix Angelicae Sinensis (*Sheng Dang Gui*)** Moistens the intestines, frees the stools + **Uncooked Pericarpium Citri Reticulatae (*Sheng Chen Pi*)** Dries dampness, transforms phlegm + **Uncooked Rhizoma Cimicifugae (*Sheng Sheng Ma*) & Uncooked Radix Bupleuri (*Sheng Chai Hu*)** Clear heat, resolve the exterior, resolve toxins **In sum:** Secures the exterior Disinhibits urination Frees the stool Clears heat and resolves toxins Dries dampness	**Honey mix-fried Radix Astragali Membranacei (*Mi Zhi Huang Qi*)** Supplements the center, boosts the qi, upbears the qi + **Honey mix-fried Radix Codonopsis Pilosulae (*Mi Zhi Dang Shen*)** Supplements the center, boosts the qi + **Stir-fried Rhizoma Atractylodis Macrocephalae (*Chao Bai Zhu*)** Fortifies the spleen, dries dampness, promotes the function of transformation + **Mix-fried Radix Glycyrrhizae (*Zhi Gan Cao*)** Supplements the center, harmonizes the stomach + **Wine stir-fried Radix Angelicae Sinensis (*Jiu Chao Dang Gui*)** Supplements & quickens the blood, harmonizes the constructive qi + **Stir-fried Pericarpium Citri Reticulatae (*Chao Chen Pi*)** Rectifies the qi, harmonizes the stomach + **Honey mix-fried Rhizoma Cimicifugae (*Mi Zhi Sheng Ma*) & stir-fried Radix Bupleuri (*Chao Chai Hu*)** Upbear the qi **In sum:** Supplements the center Boosts the qi Upbears the qi
CONCLUSION	
This formula superimposes different types of incongruous actions. Its supplementation is weak, and to this is added a draining, heat-clearing effect. Its action of upbearing the qi has disappeared completely. The ascending property is annulled and loses its place to descending, centripetal properties. The nature of this decoction tends to be cooling. It does not correspond at all to the traditional functions of *Bu Zhong Yi Qi Tang*.	This formula is harmonious. It combines qi supplements of a warm nature with plants which upbear the qi. It is benefitted by substances which rectify the qi (*Chen Pi*) and the blood (*Dang Gui*). All in all, it corresponds exactly to the traditional functions of *Bu Zhong Yi Qi Tang*.

This example well demonstrates that success in treatment depends equally on the choice of the proper preparation as on the choice of medicinal substances themselves. Thus the prescription should mention not only the names of the herbs but also their respective method of preparation.

Continuing Our Apprenticeship: An Ethical Obligation

One should not think that using such prepared remedies is only an "extra" employed by TCM fanatics. On the contrary, it is one of the fundamental characteristics of this science. It is that which distinguishes it from some simple phytotherapy and makes it into a veritable energetic pharmacology. The prescription of prepared medicinals composes an integral part of traditional Chinese therapeutic strategy. To forget this fundamental facet damages the enormous efficiency of the Chinese materia medica and can even render it dangerous. Each type of preparation of the same medicinal represents a specific action and specific indications. To systematically use the uncooked (*sheng*) form of any TCM medicinal reduces the potential of these medicinal substances from 25-80%.

To date, Western language works on Chinese herbal medicine have only given scanty practical information on this subject and have not insisted enough on this capital aspect of the Chinese materia medica. Thus the objective of this work is to fill this gap and to offer a highly practical tool for application in daily clinical practice.

It is clear that we in the West are as yet far from penetrating the arcana of TCM such as this aspect of the Chinese materia medica. Therefore, we must have humility in order to recognize our large lacunae. If we collectively wish to bring this art to its culmination in the West, we are obligated to continue our research and apprenticeship. This possibility is within our reach. Everything depends on our determination, our degree of awakening to this problem, and our vigilance in confronting our privileged teachers, or, in other words, the Chinese who tend to offer a simplified teaching to Westerners.

Without doubt, TCM is a subtle science, complex and difficult to access. However, when mastered, it is revealed to be a system of considerable efficacy permitting the solution of numerous problems which our modern Western medicine cannot solve.

Methods of Preparing
the Chinese Materia Medica

Introduction

Pao zhi is a general term for defining a group of methods of preparing the ingredients of the Chinese materia medica. These processes are guided by the theory of TCM and that of the materia medica or *ben cao*. They are adapted to the exigencies of clinical practice, to pharmaceutical necessities, and to the nature itself of these remedies. Even if some of these medicinals are used in crude form, the majority are submitted to some special transformation in order to fully profit from their qualities and specific advantages. During the preparation of these medicinal substances, all of the operations, such as the length and degree of cooking and the selection of adjuvants, exercise a direct influence on the nature and efficacy of these medicinals. This is based on the traditional saying, "If it is not cooked enough, it is difficult to obtain the best efficacy, while if it is cooked too long, its efficacy is lost."

Thus, the terms uncooked (*sheng*) and prepared (*shu*) in TCM pharmacology are used in a precise way for differentiating the character of medicinals. *Sheng* does not mean crude or fresh, nor does it mean not prepared as one reads commonly in the Western literature. *Sheng* is itself a method of preparation, commonly the most elementary one, but also sometimes very elaborate. Its characteristic is that it is *not* made through the intervention of fire or cooking. This mode is opposed to *shu,* which always uses heat or cooking.

For example, uncooked Massa Medica Fermentata (*Sheng Shen Qu*) is a fermentation which is made from not less than six ingredients in its most simple form and by a complex process. However, it is never cooked at any moment. On the contrary, if it is fried, one obtains the remedy called prepared Massa Medica Fermentata (*Shu Shen Qu*) or, more precisely as we will see below, stir-fried Massa Medica Fermentata (*Chao Shen Qu*).

In addition, these methods of preparation permit the control of toxic ingredients or those having a drastic action, thus ensuring the safety of the sick.

In sum, these methods of transformation are an indispensable link between medicinal substances and their clinical use, guaranteeing their efficacy and safety of treatment.

I. The Objectives of Preparation

The various methods of preparation permit one to modify or control the nature and functions of the remedies, thus adapting them to the needs of the medical practice and pharmacy. The principal objectives of these transformations are the following:

A. Lessening toxicity, moderating drastic action, diminishing side effects _____

Certain medicinal substances which are very effective and very useful may sometimes be toxic and cause side effects. Therefore they are altered in order to make them safer for the sick. In order to eliminate or reduce their toxicity and side effects without affecting the beneficial action of these medicaments, one can use certain methods of transformation.

For instance, Radix Aconiti Kusnezofii (*Cao Wu Tou*) is cooked in steam or boiled with Radix Glycyrrhizae (*Gan Cao*) and Semen Sojae Hispidae (*Hei Dou*). Uncooked Rhizoma Pinelliae Ternatae (*Sheng Ban Xia*) and uncooked Rhizoma Arisaematis (*Sheng Tian Nan Xing*) are prepared with uncooked Rhizoma Zingiberis (*Sheng Jiang*) and Alumen (*Ming Fan*). The oil from the grains of Semen Crotoni Tiglii (*Ba Dou*) should be extracted, while Flos Daphnis Genkwae (*Yuan Hua*) is prepared in vinegar, and Resina Olibani (*Ru Xiang*) and Resina Myrrhae (*Mo Yao*) are fried.

B. Modifying the energetic properties (flavor, nature, action) _____

Almost all of the components of the Chinese materia medica have a particular nature (cold, cool, warm, or hot) and one or more specific flavors (sour, bitter, salty, sweet, or acrid). Various processes of preparation can modify the nature and flavor of ingredients and, therefore, their action according to clinical needs. The functions and indications of very numerous remedies depend directly on their mode of transformation.

For instance, Radix Rehmanniae (*Di Huang*) in its uncooked form (*sheng*) possesses a cold nature and cools the blood. However, in its prepared form (*shu*), its nature is warm and it nourishes the blood. Uncooked Pollen Typhae (*Sheng Pu Huang*) quickens the blood and dispels stasis, but carbonized Pollen Typhae (*Pu Huang Tan*) stops bleeding. Uncooked Rhizoma Zingiberis (*Sheng Jiang*) is very acrid, slightly warm, and possesses a dispersing, centrifugal function, while roasted Rhizoma Zingiberis (*Wei Jiang*) cinders is less acrid and is warm and bitter, and, for this reason, its dispersing function is replaced by a centripetal function (thanks to the bitter flavor). It is also more warming. Radix Polygoni Multiflori (*He Shou Wu*) in its uncooked form (*sheng*) has a neutral nature, its bitter flavor predominates over its sweet flavor, and it clears heat and frees the stools. In its prepared form (*shu*), its nature is warm, its sweet flavor predominates over its bitter flavor, and it supplements the liver and kidneys, blood and essence.

C. Reinforcing therapeutic effects _____

The therapeutic power of certain medicinals can be stimulated with the aid of certain processes. For instance, Flos Tussilaginis Farfarae (*Kuan Dong Hua*) is mix-fried (*mi zhi*) in honey in order to fortify its moistening of the lungs and ability to stop cough. Rhizoma Corydalis Yanhusuo (*Yan Hu Suo*) is stir-fried in vinegar (*cu chao*) in order to fortify its stopping pain. Rhizoma Atractylodis Macrocephalae (*Bai Zhu*) is stir-fried in medicinal earth (*tu chao*) in order to fortify its supplementation of the spleen and stopping diarrhea, while Radix Bupleuri (*Chai Hu*) is stir-fried in vinegar (*cu chao*) in order to fortify its action on the liver and dispersing of stagnant liver qi.

D. Modifying the tropism

The Chinese materia medica uses the theory of the channels and network vessels (*jing luo*) and of the viscera and bowels (*zang fu*) for determining the tropism of medicinals and their energetic movement (upbearing, downbearing, exiting, or entering). Various processes of preparation are able to modify these tropisms and energetic movements.

For instance, the tropism of Radix Et Rhizoma Rhei (*Da Huang*) is fundamentally for the lower burner and possesses a downbearing property.

However, when prepared in rice wine (*jiu zhi*), its action can be upborne to the upper body in order to precipitate upper burner fire. When Radix Bupleuri (*Chai Hu*) and Rhizoma Cyperi Rotundi (*Xiang Fu*) are prepared in rice vinegar (*cu*), their action is directed at the liver channel. And when prepared with salt (*yan*), the actions of Cortex Phellodendri (*Huang Bai*) and Fructus Gardeniae Jasminoidis (*Shan Zhi Zi*) are focused on the kidneys.

E. Dissipating disagreeable odors and flavors

In order to facilitate patients' taking of these remedies, certain substances which have a disagreeable odor or taste are treated. For instance, Zaocys Dhumnades (*Wu Shao She*) is treated in rice wine (*jiu*). Feces Trogopterori Seu Pteromi (*Wu Ling Zhi*) is treated in vinegar (*cu*). Bombyx Batryticatus (*Jiang Can*) is treated in wheat bran (*fu*). Corium Erinacei (*Ci Wei Pi*) is treated in Talcum (*Hua Shi*). And Herba Sargassii (*Hai Zao*) is treated in clear water.

F. Facilitating storage, pharmaceutical production, and assimilation

In order to extract the principal active ingredients and ensure their best assimilation and in order to facilitate pharmaceutical production as powders, pills, compressed tablets, etc., certain herbs are cut (sliced, shaved, chopped), while certain minerals, shells, and animal carapaces are pulverized. In addition, in order to aid storage and to prevent moisture, numerous medicinals are dried.

G. Washing and eliminating foreign, non-medicinal substances

As a preamble to all other complex transformations, crude remedies are subjected to some elementary preparations such as washing, scraping, and cutting, in order to insure a certain degree of purity so as to render them suitable for consumption. For instance, earth and sand are removed from roots and rhizomes. The hairs of Folium Eriobotryae Japonicae (*Pi Pa Ye*) are brushed off and eliminated. The heads and feet of Periostracum Cicadae (*Chan Tui*) are eliminated. The heart of Radix Polygalae Tenuifoliae (*Yuan Zhi*), that is to say the center of the root, is removed, while Herba Sargassii (*Hai Zao*) and Herba Cistanchis (*Rou Cong Rong*) are rinsed in abundant clear water in order to get rid of their disagreeable odor.

II. Methods of Preparation

Although a certain number of medicinal substances demand only an elementary method of preparation, such as washing, cutting, and drying, a number of others require more elaborate procedures. These procedures are very numerous, certain of them being specific for a particular medicinal. The most common are presented below.

A. Simple preparations

These types of preparation encompass the most basic processes, such as washing, pulverization, cutting, and defatting.

Washing

In reality, this procedure is integral to the methods of selection, harvesting, culling, sifting, scraping, brushing, washing in water, etc. The goal is the disappearance of all dust, earth, sand, foreign substances, and the non-medicinal parts of the principal material, thus rendering them pure and appropriate for consumption. For instance, one eliminates the stalks and leaves of Flos Albizziae Julibrissinis (*He Huan Hua*) and keeps the flowers, and one scrapes the pith of Cortex Magnoliae Officinalis (*Hou Po*) and of Cortex Cinnamomi (*Rou Gui*). See the examples in paragraph G. in section I above.

Pulverization

This process includes crushing, pounding, trituration, etc. The goal of these procedures is to meet the needs of pharmaceutical production as in the making of granules, pills, and compressed tablets. This also results in the increase of the surface of these medicinals in order to increase the extraction and assimilation of their active principles. For instance, Concha Ostreae (*Mu Li*) and Os Draconis (*Long Gu*) are reduced to a fine powder for decocting. Cornu Rhinocerotis (*Xi Jiao*) and Cornu Antelopis (*Ling Yang Jiao*) are ground into flakes for decocting or are ground into powder for the manufacture of certain pharmaceuticals. [However, these last two ingredients are from endangered species and should no longer be used in TCM.] In addition, the great majority of grains and seeds are crushed just before decoction for the same reason. However, after this operation, these herbs should be rapidly consumed so that they do not [go stale and] lose their quality.

Cutting

This process includes the cutting of plants into slices or pieces. Its objective is to facilitate the extraction of their active principles during decoction, to promote their drying and thus storage of such medicinals, and to enable the easy weighing of medicinals. The ingredients of the Chinese materia medica are cut in different sizes and precise thicknesses in agreement with their features and clinical utilization.

For instance, Rhizoma Gastrodiae Elatae (*Tian Ma*) and Semen Arecae Catechu (*Bing Lang*) are cut into fine slices, while Rhizoma Alismatis (*Ze Xie*) and Rhizoma Atractylodis Macrocephalae (*Bai Zhu*) are cut into thicker slices. Radix Astragali Membranacei (*Huang Qi*) and Caulis Millettiae Seu Spatholobi (*Ji Xue Teng*) are cut obliquely. Radix Albus Paeoniae Lactiflorae (*Bai Shao Yao*) and Radix Glycyrrhizae (*Gan Cao*) are cut vertically. Cortex Cinnamomi (*Rou Gui*) and Cortex Magnoliae Officinalis (*Hou Po*) are cut diametrically in keeping with the circular shape of their skin. Cortex Radicis Mori Albi (*Sang Bai Pi*) and Folium Eriobotryae Japonicae (*Pi Pa Ye*) are cut in such manner as to give them a filiform shape, while Rhizoma Imperatae Cylindricae (*Bai Mao Gen*) and Herba Ephedrae (*Ma Huang*) are cut into segments, Sclerotium Poriae Cocos (*Fu Ling*) and Radix Puerariae (*Ge Gen*) are cut into large cubes, and Cornu Parvum Cervi (*Lu Rong*) is cut into fine slices.

Defatting

This process is far less common than the three preceding ones. It is used for a limited number of substances. It permits one to eliminate the oily matter from certain grains and seeds. The most commonly used method is the following: The grains are first dried in the sun. Then their husks are removed in order to recover the seeds. These latter are reduced to a paste. This paste is placed in fine pouches between two paper blotters. All this is exposed to the sun or pressed mechanically so that the paper absorbs the maximum amount of oil. This operation is repeated until there are no more traces of oil on the paper.

The objectives of this process are to: 1) lessen toxicity, such as with Semen Crotonis Tiglii (*Ba Dou*) and Fructus Euphorbiae Lathyridis (*Qian Jin Zi*), and 2) moderate drastic action, such as with Semen Crotonis Tiglii (*Ba Dou*), Fructus Euphorbiae Lathyridis (*Qian Jin Zi*), and Semen Biotae Orientalis (*Bai Zi Ren*). The latter is defatted when one wishes to quiet the spirit without causing diarrhea.

One should note that *Xi Gua Shuang* or so-called Watermelon Frost (Fructus Praeparatus Citrulli Vulgaris) is made by a different type of process. One first hollows out an opening in the fruit. One adds a small amount of Mirabilitum (*Mang Xiao*) and then the hole is filled in again. The Mirabilitum produces a fine white frost on the surface of the fruit, which is used in the production of certain pharmaceuticals.

B. Preparations made with the help of water (*Shui Zhi*)

These procedures use water and sometimes other liquids to transform various remedies. The objectives of this method of processing are to 1) eliminate foreign objects and impurities, 2) eliminate disagreeable odors and tastes, 3) soften the plants in order to facilitate their cutting, 4) lessen their toxicity or side effects, and 5) refine certain minerals. The most commonly used of these methods are the following:

Rinsing and washing (*Piao Xi*)

The herbs are rinsed or washed repeatedly in an abundant quantity of clear water. The objectives of this method are to 1) eliminate foreign objects and impurities, such as with Rhizoma Phragmitis Communis (*Lu Gen*) and Rhizoma Anemarrhenae (*Zhi Mu*); 2) remove salt, such as with Thallus Algae (*Kun Bu*) and Herba Sargassii (*Hai Zao*); and 3) lessen disagreeable odors and tastes, such as with Placenta Hominis (*Zi He Che*) and Herba Cistanchis (*Rou Cong Rong*). These materials are not left to soak in the water too long so that their medicinal actions are not lessened. This method is not suitable for certain flowers, which are too fragile and which may easily lose their active principles in water.

Moistening (*Men Run*)

This refers to the production of a progressive penetration of moistness from the exterior to the interior of an herb. For this, different methods are used: moistening by spraying, by percolation, by washing, by soaking, by dampening, by steeping, by covering with a damp tissue, etc. Particular attention is necessary to control the temperature of the water and the temperature of the humidification so as to avoid fermentation and mildew.

Examples of plants which often receive this treatment are Herba Schizonepetae Tenuifoliae (*Jing Jie*), Herba Menthae (*Bo He*), Cortex Magnoliae Officinalis (*Hou Po*), Semen Arecae Catechu (*Bing Lang*), Rhizoma Gastrodiae Elatae (*Tian Ma*), and Radix Et Rhizoma Rhei (*Da Huang*).

Soaking (*Jin Pao*)

Some medicinals are soaked in clear water or in an aqueous solution. Steeping or short soaking is reserved for the most fragile of materials whose active substances disappear rapidly in water. Soaking (for a long time) has the following objectives: 1) to facilitate the cutting of remedies, such as with Semen Arecae Catechu (*Bing Lang*) and Cortex Magnoliae Officinalis (*Hou Po*); 2) to lessen toxicity, such as with Rhizoma Arisaematis (*Tian Nan Xing*) and Rhizoma Pinelliae Ternatae (*Ban Xia*), which are soaked in an Alumen (*Ming Fan*) solution; and 3) to eliminate non-medicinal parts, such as with Semen Pruni Armeniacae (*Xing Ren*) and Semen Pruni Persicae (*Tao Ren*), which are soaked in water in order to remove their non-medicinal skins. How long a medicinal is soaked depends on the texture of the remedy, the amount of humidity in the air, and the climate.

Aqueous trituration (*Shui Fei*)

This refers to the triturating of certain minerals and shells in water. The original material is first pounded grossly and then deposited in a mortar filled with water. The substance is then pestled until one obtains fine particles in suspension on the surface of the water. This fine powder is sal-vaged. One continues to forcefully pound the material, which remains in the bottom of the mortar until a new suspension is produced, which is drawn off in the same manner. This operation is repeated several times until all that remains is a very little residue. Finally, the fine powder is dried. This process is used for hard materials which are insoluble in water such as minerals, shells, and animal products.

The objectives of this procedure are to: 1) facilitate the extraction and assimilation of active principles, such as from Cinnabar (*Zhu Sha*) and Talcum (*Hua Shi*); 2) lessen the irritating effect of certain remedies when one uses them topically, such as Smithsonitum (*Lu Gan Shi*) and Realgar (*Xiong Huang*); and 3) facilitate the production of certain pharmaceutical specialties, such as powders, compressed tablets, and pills.

C. Preparations made with the aid of fire (*Huo Zhi*)

These processes introduce the heat of cooking. The materials treated with this general method are first exposed directly or indirectly to fire in order to make them yellow, brown, carbonized, or calcined with the goal of obtaining a precise modification in the character of such remedies.

Stir-frying (*Chao Fa*)

The medicinal substances treated with this method are fried while being constantly stirred. One is trying to obtain a certain degree of frying by the aid of certain types of fire, such as a low, moderate, or high fire, and sometimes with the aid of certain additional adjuvants.

1. Stir-frying without additional adjuvants (*Qing Chao*)

The medicinals are deposited in a wok and are stir-fried until dry without any additional adjuvants. There are three degrees of frying in this process:

a) Stir-frying till yellow (*Chao Huang*)

The remedy is stir-fried with the aid of a low or moderate fire until one obtains a yellowish color and a burnt aroma. The objectives of this method are to: 1) Reinforce an action. For instance, Semen Nelumbinis Nuciferae (*Lian Zi*) becomes more aromatic and astringent. This makes it more powerful for supplementing the spleen and for stopping diarrhea or for supplementing the kidneys and securing the essence. 2) Lessen toxicity as, for instance, with Semen Pharbitidis (*Qian Niu Zi*). 3) Moderate an action, such as the acrid flavor and dispersing action of Fructus Viticis (*Man Jing Zi*).

b) Stir-frying till scorched (*Chao Jiao*)

The remedy is stir-fried with the aid of a moderate fire until one obtains a brown color similar to coffee and a burnt aroma. The objectives of this method are to: 1) Lessen toxicity or side effects. For instance, the toxicity of Fructus Meliae

Toosendan (*Chuan Lian Zi*) is reduced and, in addition, its bitter flavor and cold nature are diminished, thus avoiding damage to the stomach. 2) Strengthen an action. For instance, stir-fried till scorched Massa Medica Fermentata (*Shen Qu*) is better able to supplement the spleen and disperse food stagnation, while stir-fried till scorched Fructus Crataegi (*Shan Zha*) is better able to eliminate abdominal distention and to stop diarrhea and dysentery.

c) Stir-frying till carbonized (*Chao Tan*)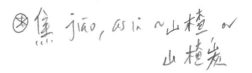

The remedy is stir-fried with the aid of a powerful fire until it becomes black on the outside and brown on the inside. The objective of this method is to reinforce ingredients' hemostatic action. This is based on the saying, "When blood sees black, (bleeding) is stopped." Ingredients processed in this way for this purposes include: Cortex Eucommiae Ulmoidis (*Du Zhong*), Radix Et Rhizoma Rhei (*Da Huang*), Folium Artemisiae Argyii (*Ai Ye*), Herba Cirsii Japonici (*Da Ji*), and Herba Cephalanoploris Segeti (*Xiao Ji*).

However, modern research has shown that this process destroys or strongly attenuates the hemostatic effect of certain plants which are traditionally prepared in this manner, such as Cacumen Biotae Orientalis (*Ce Bai Ye*), Rhizoma Imperatae Cylindricae (*Bai Mao Gen*), and Radix Sanguisorbae (*Di Yu*).

One should note that medicinals should not be completely carbonized or else they will lose their medicinal properties. It is necessary, therefore, that one perfectly master this mode of transformation.

2. Stir-frying with additional adjuvants

A certain number of adjuvants are used in the preparation of numerous medicinals in order to modify their nature, change their tropism, reinforce an action, or lessen their toxicity or side effects. These adjuvants can be either liquids or solids.

Solid adjuvants:

Wheat bran (*Fu*): This is sweet, bland, and neutral. It lessens certain drastic actions, protects the stomach, supplements the spleen, harmonizes the middle burner, and deodorizes.

Rice (*Mi*): This is sweet and neutral. It eliminates dampness and reinforces an anti-diarrhea action. It supplements the spleen and qi, harmonizes the stomach, eliminates vexation, stops sweating, and lessens toxicity.

Terra Flava Usta (*Fu Long Gan*): This is acrid and warm. It harmonizes and warms the middle burner and stops diarrhea.

Powdered Concha Cyclinae (*Hai Ge Ke Fen*): This is salty and cold. It eliminates dampness and oily materials, clears heat, transforms phlegm, and softens the hard.

Powdered Alumen (*Bai Fan*): This is sour and cold. It lessens toxicity, eliminates phlegm, expels parasites, dries dampness, and reinforces any astringing effect.

Other adjuvants are sometimes used, such as salt (*Yan*) and Talcum (*Hua Shi*).

Liquid adjuvants:

Honey (*Feng Mi*): This is sweet and cool when it is crude and warm when it is cooked. It calms spasms and stops pain, moistens dryness, stops cough, supplements the middle burner, lessens toxicity, and harmonizes medicinals.

Rice vinegar (*Cu*): This is bitter, sour, and warm. It directs therapeutic effects to the liver, rectifies the qi, quickens the blood and stops pain, lessens toxicity, reinforces astringent actions, and deodorizes.

Rice wine (*Mi Jiu*): This is sweet, acrid, and very hot. It frees the flow of the channels and quickens the network vessels, moderates a cold nature,

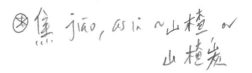 焦 jiāo, as in ~山楂 or 山楂炭

directs therapeutic effects to the upper body, and deodorizes.

Salt water (*Yan Shui*): This is salty and cold. It directs therapeutic effects to the kidneys, softens the hard, clears heat and cools the blood, and supplements yin and downbears vacuity fire.

Ginger juice (*Jiang Zhi*): This is acrid and warm. It stops vomiting, expels phlegm, warms the middle burner, resolves the exterior, lessens toxicity, and reduces the cold nature.

Animal fat (*You*) (lamb, goat, beef, pork): This promotes penetration of the bones and supplements the spleen and kidneys.

Licorice solution (*Gan Cao Tang*): This is sweet and neutral. It harmonizes the center, calms spasms, moistens the lungs, supplements the spleen, lessens toxicity, and harmonizes medicinals.

Black soybean juice (*Hei Dou Zhi*): This is sweet and neutral. It quickens the blood, disinhibits urination, supplements the liver and kidneys, nourishes the blood and dispels wind, and lessens toxicity.

Bile (*Dan*) beef, pork, or goat): This clears liver heat, brightens the eyes, rectifies the gallbladder, frees the stool, resolves toxins, disperses swelling, and moistens dryness.

Other adjuvant liquids are traditionally used but only seldom these days, such as milk, infant's urine, rice rinsing water, etc.

3. Stir-frying with solid adjuvants

This method consists of the following processes:

a) Stir-frying with wheat bran (*Fu Chao*): The wok is first preheated with a strong fire. Then the wheat bran is sprinkled into it. When smoke appears, the medicinals are added and stir-fried until their surface becomes yellowish. At that moment,

the cooking is stopped and the surplus of the wheat bran is separated from the plants. The objectives of this method are to: 1) reinforce the action of supplementing the spleen, such as with Rhizoma Atractylodis Macrocephalae (*Bai Zhu*) and Radix Dioscoreae Oppositae (*Shan Yao*); 2) moderate drastic action, such as with Fructus Immaturus Citri Seu Ponciri (*Zhi Shi*) and Rhizoma Atractylodis (*Cang Zhu*); or 3) eliminate disagreeable odors, such as with Bombyx Batryticatus (*Jiang Can*).

b) Stir-frying with rice (*Mi Chao*): The wok is first preheated. The rice is then put in and stir-fried. When an aromatic odor appears, the medicinal substances are added. The cooking is stopped when the rice and the plants have become brown. At that moment, the cooking is halted and the rice and the medicinals are separated. The objectives of this method are to: 1) reduce toxicity, such as with Huechys Sanguinea (*Hong Niang Zi*) and Mylabris (*Ban Mao*), and 2) reinforce the action of supplementing the spleen for stopping diarrhea, such as with Radix Codonopsis Pilosulae (*Dang Shen*).

c) Stir-frying with medicinal earth (*Tu Chao*): The wok is first preheated on a strong fire. The earth is put in and stir-fried. The plants are then added and fried just until they are coated in a fine layer of earth and until one smells a burnt odor. At this moment, the fire is extinguished and the surplus earth eliminated.

The earth used is Terra Flava Usta (*Zao Xin Tu* a.k.a. *Fu Long Gan*), which is itself a medicinal substance. It warms the middle burner, fortifies the spleen, and stops diarrhea by its astringent property. It is a naturally occurring earth, which is used in China for the manufacture of traditional ovens. After having been used in this way for a number of years, it is recollected. The high temperatures have made it alkaline and permit one to obtain from it, most notably, zinc oxide.

The objective of this method is to reinforce the supplementing action on the spleen for stopping diarrhea, such as with Rhizoma Atractylodis Macrocephalae (*Bai Zhu*) and Radix Dioscoreae Oppositae (*Shan Yao*).

d) Stir-frying with sand (*Sha Chao*): The sand is heated over an open fire. The medicinals are then added and fried until they become friable and swell up. At that moment, the cooking is stopped and the sand is removed. The objectives of this method are to: 1) reduce toxicity, such as with Semen Strychnotis (*Ma Qian Zi*); 2) facilitate pulverization, such as with Squama Manitis Pentadactylis (*Chuan Shan Jia*) and Os Tigridis (*Hu Gu*); and 3) eliminate disagreeable tastes and odors, such as with Corium Erinacei (*Ci Wei Pi*).

e) Stir-frying with powdered Concha Cyclinae (*Ge Fen Chao*): The powdered shell, Concha Cyclinae (*Hai Ge Ke*), is stir-fried over a moderate fire. The medicinals are then added and fried until they become soft and swell up. At that moment, the cooking is stopped and the excess powder eliminated. This adjuvant is a weak one for conducting heat. Therefore, it reduces the risk of carbonization of the original materials. The objectives of this method are to: 1) reduce the fatty nature of certain remedies; 2) lessen disagreeable odors and tastes; and 3) reinforce the heat-clearing action and the transformation of phlegm. Gelatinum Corii Asini (*E Jiao*) is often prepared with this process.

f) Stir-frying with Talcum (*Hua Shi*): The Talcum is stir-fried over a moderate fire. The medicinals are then added and fried just until they become brown. At this moment, the cooking is stopped and the surplus Talcum eliminated. Talcum is a mineral substance which conducts heat weakly. Thus it reduces the risk of carbonizing the original materials. The objectives of this method are to: 1) reduce toxicity, such as with Corium Erinacei (*Ci Wei Pi*) and Hirudo (*Shui Zhi*); 2) eliminate disagreeable tastes and odors, such as with Corium Erinacei (*Ci Wei Pi*) and Hirudo (*Shui Zhi*); and 3) facilitate pulverization and decoction, such as with Penis Canidis (*Huang Gou Shen*).

4. Stir-frying with liquid adjuvants

In this process, the medicinal substances are stir-fried with liquid adjuvants so that the latter penetrate to their interior, cover them, or attach to their surface. The objectives of this method are to: 1) change their nature and flavors, 2) modify their tropism, 3) reinforce an action, or 4) reduce toxicity.

a) Mix-frying with honey (*Mi Zhi*): The honey is first cooked over a low fire (20-40 parts to 100 parts of the herbs). The medicinal substances are then added and stir-fried until the honey is no longer sticky to the touch. The objectives of this method are to: 1) reinforce the supplementation action on the spleen and qi, such as with Radix Codonopsis Pilosulae (*Dang Shen*), Radix Glycyrrhizae (*Gan Cao*), and Radix Astragali Membranacei (*Huang Qi*); 2) attenuate strong flavors, such as with Fructus Aristolochiae (*Ma Dou Ling*), which possesses a powerfully bitter flavor and which can occasionally cause nausea and vomiting. Treated in honey, it advantageously stops cough without causing vomiting; 3) reinforce the moistening action on the lungs for stopping cough, such as with Flos Tussilaginis Farfarae (*Kuan Dong Hua*), Folium Eriobotryae Japonicae (*Pi Pa Ye*), Radix Stemonae (*Bai Bu*), and Radix Asteris Tatarici (*Zi Wan*); 4) moderate a drastic action. For instance, the powerful sudorific action of Herba Ephedrae (*Ma Huang*) is reduced in order to promote its antitussive and anti-asthma action.

b) Mix-frying with rice vinegar (*Cu Zhi*): The medicinals are stir-fried in 15 parts vinegar to 100 parts plants. The plants are soaked in the vinegar until it is all absorbed. Then they are fried over a low fire until they obtain a golden color and burnt aroma. However, shells, carapaces, and resins are fried over a low fire while the vinegar is added progressively until it is completely absorbed and the medicinal substances also have a golden color and a burnt aroma. The objectives of this method are to: 1) direct the action of the remedy to the liver, such as with Radix Bupleuri (*Chai Hu*), Rhizoma Cyperi Rotundi (*Xiang Fu*), and Pericarpium Viridis Citri Reticulatae (*Qing Pi*); 2) reinforce the action of quickening the blood in order to stop pain, such as with Rhizoma Corydalis Yanhusuo (*Yan Hu Suo*), Feces Trogopterori Seu Pteromi (*Wu Ling Zhi*), Rhizoma Sparganii (*San Leng*), Resina Myrrhae (*Mo Yao*), and Resina Olibani (*Ru Xiang*); 3) lessen toxicity, such as with Flos Daphnis Genkwae (*Yuan Hua*), Radix Euphorbiae Kansui (*Gan Sui*), and Radix Euphorbiae Pekinensis (*Jing Da Ji*); and 4) eliminate disagreeable tastes and odors, such as with Feces Trogopterori Seu Pteromi (*Wu Ling Zhi*), Resina Myrrhae (*Mo Yao*), and Resina Olibani (*Ru Xiang*).

c) Mix-frying with wine (*Jiu Zhi*): The medicinals are stir-fried over a low fire with wine (10-20 parts or even 30-50 parts per 100 parts plants) until they are dry or become slightly yellowish but still an aromatic odor of alcohol persists. The color of the remedies should not change nor should they smell burnt. Yellow wine (*Huang Jiu*) made from rice or millet is the most often used, while white alcohol (*Bai Jiu*) made from sorghum is less often used. The objectives of this method are to: 1) reinforce the action of freeing the flow of the channels and quickening the blood in the network vessels, such as with Radix Angelicae Sinensis (*Dang Gui*), Radix Ligustici Wallichii (*Chuan Xiong*), and Radix Cyathulae (*Chuan Niu Xi*); 2) moderate the cold nature of certain materials and to guide their action to the upper part of the body, such as with Radix Et Rhizoma Rhei (*Da Huang*), Rhizoma Coptidis Chinensis (*Huang Lian*) and Radix Scutellariae Baicalensis (*Huang Qin*); and 3) to eliminate disagreeable tastes and odors, such as with Agkistrodon Seu Bungarus (*Bai Hua She*) and Zaocys Dhumnades (*Wu Shao She*).

d) Mix-fried with a salt solution (*Yan Zhi*): The medicinal substances are moistened in a 2-3% salt-water solution and then they are fried over a low fire until they are dry. The objectives of this method are to: 1) guide the action of the remedies to the kidneys and to reinforce the supplementing action on the kidneys, such as with Fructus Psoraleae Corylifoliae (*Bu Gu Zhi*), Cortex Eucommiae Ulmoidis (*Du Zhong*), and Radix Morindae Officinalis (*Ba Ji Tian*); 2) reinforce the supplementing yin action and downbearing of vacuity fire of the kidneys, such as with Rhizoma Anemarrhenae (*Zhi Mu*) and Cortex Phellodendri (*Huang Bai*); 3) promote the softening action on nodulations in the treatment of *shan*, such as with Fructus Foeniculi Vulgaris (*Xiao Hui Xiang*), Semen Citri Reticulati (*Ju He*), and Semen Litchi Chinensis (*Li Zhi He*); and 4) stimulate the diuretic action, such as with Semen Plantaginis (*Che Qian Zi*).

e) Mix-frying with ginger juice (*Jiang Zhi Zhi*): The medicinals are moistened with ginger juice and then stir-fried over a low fire until they are dry and aromatic. The objectives of this method are to: 1) reinforce the anti-emetic action, such as with Rhizoma Pinelliae Ternatae (*Ban Xia*) and Fructus Amomi (*Sha Ren*); 2) lessen the cold nature, such as with Rhizoma Coptidis Chinensis (*Huang Lian*) and Caulis In Taeniis Bambusae (*Zhu Ru*); and 3) reduce toxicity, such as with Rhizoma Arisaematis (*Tian Nan Xing*), Rhizoma Typhonii (*Bai Fu Zi*), and Rhizoma Pinelliae Ternatae (*Ban Xia*).

f) Mix-frying with oil (*You Zhi*): The medicinals are stir-fried with oil or fat (beef, pork, or sesame). The objectives of this method are to: 1) render the ingredients friable in order to facilitate their pulverization, such as with Os Tigridis (*Hu Gu*) and Gecko (*Ge Jie*); 2) reduce their toxicity, such as with Semen Strychnotis (*Ma Qian Zi*); and 3) reinforce a particular action. For instance, Herba Epimedii (*Yin Yang Huo*) treated with mutton fat is more powerful for supplementing kidney yang.

Calcination (*Duan Fa*)

The objective of this method is to directly or indirectly calcine various medicinal substances with a strong fire and at a high temperature (300-700°). This method may be classified in two groups:

1. Open calcination (*Ming Duan*)

In this process, the medicinals are calcined directly over a fire or in an unbreakable earth receptacle. The objectives of this method are to: 1) render minerals, shells, and other hard substances friable in order to promote their pulverization, such as with Fluoritum (*Zi Shi Ying*), Hematitum (*Dai Zhe Shi*), and Concha Haliotidis (*Shi Jue Ming*); and 2) reinforce their astringent action, such as with Os Draconis (*Long Gu*), Concha Ostreae (*Mu Li*), and Hallyositum (*Chi Shi Zhi*).

2. Sealed pot calcination (*An Duan*)

In this process, the medicinal materials are calcined in a receptacle without oxygen. This process is used for fragile substances which would otherwise be completely consumed by the open calcination method. The objectives of this method are to: 1) reinforce the hemostatic action, such as with carbonized Folium Et Petiolus Trachycarpi (*Zong Lu Tan*) and Crinis Carbonisatus (*Xue Yu Tan*), and 2) reduce toxicity, such as with Lacca Sinica Exiccata (*Gan Qi*) and Nidus Vespae (*Lu Feng Fang*).

Roasting (*Wei Fa*)

The plants are enveloped in wet paper or in a paste of rice flower, wheat bran, or Talcum (*Hua Shi*). They are then plunged under live coals until their envelope becomes brownish and crackly.

Once they have cooled, they are removed from their envelope. The objectives of this method are to: 1) partially remove fatty materials, such as with Semen Myristicae Fragrantis (*Rou Dou Kou*); 2) lessen a drastic action or side effect, such as with Radix Euphorbiae Kansui (*Gan Sui*); and 3) reinforce an astringent effect, such as with Fructus Terminaliae Chebulae (*He Zi*) and Radix Puerariae (*Ge Gen*) and especially to stop diarrhea, such as with Radix Saussureae Seu Vladimiriae (*Mu Xiang*).

Blast-frying (*Pao Fa*)

The original materials are fried over an open fire, and stirred without stopping until they become brown, burnt, swollen, and crusty but not carbonized. The objectives of this method are to: 1) lessen toxicity, such as with Radix Praeparatus Aconiti Carmichaeli (*Tian Xiong*) and Radix Lateralis Praeparatus Aconiti Carmichaeli (*Fu Zi*); and 2) modify a medicinal's nature, such as with blast-fried Rhizoma Zingiberis (*Pao Jiang*).

Baking (*Hong*) or stone-baking (*Bei*)

This refers to drying over a low fire (*bei*) certain insects, such as Hirudo (*Shui Zhi*) and Tabanus (*Meng Chong*), or over a very low fire (*hong*) certain flowers, such as Flos Chrysanthemi Morifolii (*Ju Hua*) and Flos Lonicerae Japonicae (*Jin Yin Hua*). The objective of this method is to permit the slow, progressive drying of certain substances in order to facilitate their storage and pulverization, but without a strong heat which would otherwise destroy their active properties.

D. Combined Water & Fire Processes

These processes are made by the intervention of heat and certain liquids. They are represented by the following methods:

Steaming (*Zheng Fa*)

The materials are placed in a receptacle and are cooked in steam or pressure cooked. The objectives of this method are to: 1) modify a nature or action, such as with processed Radix Polygoni Multiflori (*Zhi He Shou Wu*). (For this, one frequently adds to the water an adjuvant for reinforcing the transformation of the ingredient, such as rice wine in the case of Radix Rehmanniae (*Di Huang*) or a decoction of Semen Glycinis Hispidae (*Hei Dou*) in the case of *He Shou Wu.*); 2) lessen a drastic action or side effect, such as with Radix Et Rhizoma Rhei (*Da Huang*) or Rhizoma Polygonati (*Huang Jing*); and 3) facilitate preservation, cutting, and storage, such as with Radix Scutellariae Baicalensis (*Huang Qin*) and Ootheca Mantidis (*Sang Piao Xiao*).

Preparing or boiling (*Zhu Fa*)

The medicinal substances are boiled in water or in an herbal decoction. The objectives of this method are to: 1) Reinforce an action. For instance, Rhizoma Typhonii (*Bai Fu Zi*) is boiled in an Alumen (*Bai Fan*) decoction, Rhizoma Curcumae Zedoariae (*E Zhu*) is boiled in vinegar water, and Radix Polygalae Tenuifoliae (*Yuan Zhi*) is boiled in a decoction of licorice; and 2) lessen toxicity. For instance, Radix Aconiti Carmichaeli (*Chuan Wu Tou*) and Radix Aconiti Kusnezofii (*Cao Wu Tou*) are boiled in water, Rhizoma Pinelliae Ternatae (*Ban Xia*) is boiled in water and ginger juice, while Flos Daphnis Genkwae (*Yuan Hua*) is boiled in vinegar water.

Scalding (*Dan Fa*)

The remedies are plunged into boiling water. This has the effect of stopping the boiling for a moment. The plants are then removed when the water comes to a new boil. The objectives of this method are to: 1) eliminate the non-medicinal parts, such as with Semen Pruni Armeniacae (*Xing Ren*) and Semen Pruni Persicae (*Tao Ren*); and 2) facilitate drying and preservation, such as with Semen Dolichoris Lablab (*Bai Bian Dou*) and Tuber Asparagi Cochinensis (*Tian Men Dong*).

Dip-calcining (*Cui Fa*)

The original materials are heated till red hot and are then dipped while hot into a liquid (clear water or vinegar). The operation is repeated several times. This procedure is used for minerals, shells, carapaces, and scales. The objective of this method is to render the material friable in order to facilitate pulverization. This then permits better assimilation of the active principles, such as with Haematitum (*Dai Zhe Shi*), Magnetitum (*Ci Shi*), Plastrum Testudinis (*Gui Ban*), Squama Manitis Pentadactylis (*Chuan Shan Jia*), and Pyritum (*Zi Ran Tong*).

Distilling (*Zheng Lu*)

Certain aromatic plants are distilled slowly in steam to capture their essential oils, such as Flos Caryophylli (*Ding Xiang*), Herba Menthae (*Bo He*), Flos Lonicerae Japonicae (*Jin Yin Hua*), and Herba Agastachi Seu Pogostemi (*Huo Xiang*).

E. Fermentation & Germination

Fermentation (*Fa Jiao Fa*)

The ingredients are exposed to a certain humidity (30-37%) until they ferment. The objective of this method is to transform the nature of the remedy and to confer new actions and indications, such as with fermented Rhizoma Pinelliae Ternatae (*Ban Xia Qu*), Semen Praeparatum Sojae (*Dan Dou Chi*), and Massa Medica Fermentata (*Shen Qu*).

Germination (*Fa Ya Fa*)

The grains or seeds of certain plants are exposed to a certain humidity (watered 2-3 times per day) and a certain temperature (18-25°C) until they germinate. The objective of this method is to transform the nature of the remedy and to confer new actions and indications, such as with Fructus Germinatus Oryzae (*Gu Ya*), Fructus Germinatus Hordei Vulgaris (*Mai Ya*), and Semen Germinatum Glycinis (*Da Dou Huang Juan*).

F. Other Processes

We have discussed the most common processes above. However, many others are used to a lesser extent and are sometimes limited to only one or two substances. Some of these are complex, such as the transformation of Rhizoma Pinelliae Ternatae (*Ban Xia*), Rhizoma Typhonii (*Bai Fu Zi*), and Rhizoma Arisaematis (*Tian Nan Xing*). Others are simple, such as Sclerotium Pararadicis Poriae Cocos (*Fu Shen*), Medulla Junci Effusi (*Deng Xin Cao*), Tuber Asparagi Cochinensis (*Tian Men Dong*), Tuber Ophiopogonis Japonicae (*Mai Men Dong*), and Radix Polygalae Tenuifoliae (*Yuan Zhi*), which are all mixed with Cinnabar (*Zhu Sha*) powder.

About Using This Book

In the following chapters 1 through 21 which describe individual prepared medicinals, each entry for a specific method of preparation includes a list of indications and typical combinations. Please note that each number listed under the subheading **"Indications "** has a corresponding number listed under the subheading **"Typical Combinations"** to which it is directly related.

1
Warm, Acrid Exterior-resolving Medicinals

Semen Praeparatum Sojae *(Dan Dou Chi)*

Clear *(Qing)*[1]

Names: *Qing Dou Chi, Dan Dou Chi, Chao Dou Chi*[2], *Sheng Dou Chi*[3]

Flavors & nature: Acrid, bitter, and sweet; cold

Functions: Clears heat, resolves vexation

Indications: Vexation following a warm disease with chest oppression, insomnia, agitation, easy anger, a sensation of discomfort...

Typical combinations: With stir-fried Fructus Gardeniae Jasminoidis (*Chao Zhi Zi*) as in *Zhi Zi Chi Tang* (Gardenia & Prepared Soybean Decoction [441])

Dosage: 6-15g and up to 50g in severe cases

Notes: 1. *Qing (Dan) Dou Chi* is a fermented product made from Semen Glycinis Hispidae (*Hei Dou*) as the base and using Folium Mori Albi (*Sang Ye*) and Herba Artemisiae Apiaceae (*Qing Hao*). *Qing Dou Chi* possesses the properties of resolving the exterior and inducing a light perspiration (however much less forcefully than *Wen Dou Chi* below).
2. In order to lessen the above actions and to accentuate its principal functions, one should use stir-fried or *Chao Qing Dou Chi*. Stir-fried *Qing Dou Chi* is then much less acrid and cool.
3. If one wishes to use *Qing Dou Chi* nevertheless in order to resolve the exterior and clear heat, one should prescribe *Sheng Qing Dou Chi* or uncooked *Qing Dou Chi*.

Warm *(Wen)*[1]

Names: *Wen Dou Chi, Dan Dou Chi, Sheng Dou Chi*[2]

Flavors & nature: Acrid, sweet, and slightly bitter; warm

Functions: Resolves exterior, induces perspiration

Indications: Colds and flu due to 1) external wind (*i.e.*, an early stage affection by wind cold or wind heat); 2) wind cold; or 3) wind heat[3]

Typical combinations:

1. With Bulbus Allii Fistulosi (*Cong Bai*) as in *Cong Chi Tang* (Allium Fistulosum & Prepared Soybean Decoction [I; 56])

2. With uncooked Herba Ephedrae (*Sheng Ma Huang*) and Bulbus Allii Fistulosi (*Cong Bai*) in *Cong Chi Tang* (Allium Fistulosum & Prepared Soybean Decoction [II; 57])

3. With Herba Menthae Haplocalycis (*Bo He*) and uncooked Fructus Forsythiae Suspensae (*Sheng Lian Qiao*) in *Cong Chi Jie Geng Tang* (Allium Fistulosum, Prepared Soybean & Platycodon Decoction [55])

Dosage: 6-15g and up to 30g in severe cases

Notes: 1. *Wen (Dan) Dou Chi* is a fermented product made from a base of Semen Glycinis Hispidae (*Hei Dou*) and using Herba Ephedrae (*Ma Huang*). Folium Perillae Frutescentis (*Zi Su Ye*), Herba Eupatorii (*Pei Lan*), Herba Agastachis Seu Pogostemi (*Huo

Semen Praeparatum Sojae continued . . .

Xiang), Herba Artemisiae Apiaceae (*Qing Hao*), Folium Nelumbinis Nuciferae (*He Ye*), and Herba Polygoni Lapathifolii (*La Liao Cao*).
2. One does not have to further process *Wen Dou Chi* to enable it to increase its dispersing action. In that case, one should simply prescribe *Sheng Wen Dou Chi*.
3. Even though *Wen Dou Chi*'s nature is warm, it may be used in the treatment of wind heat affections. The remedies which disperse wind heat are less powerful sudorifics than those which disperse wind cold. It is, therefore, interesting that one should add *Wen Dou Chi* to a formula which treats wind heat if one wants to accentuate diaphoresis. In this case, its warm nature is controlled by other cooling herbs. This is the case in *Yin Qiao San* (Lonicera & Forsythia Powder).

Radix Ledebouriellae Sesloidis (Fang Feng)

——————————— Uncooked (Sheng)[1] ———————————

Names: *Fang Feng, Qing Fang Feng, Guan Fang Feng*

Flavors & nature: Acrid, sweet; slightly warm

Functions: Dispels wind and resolves the exterior

Indications:

1. Colds and flu due to wind cold with aversion to cold, fever, headache, nasal congestion, cough, itching of the throat...

2. Exterior invasion of wind dampness with aversion to wind, fever, heavy body, joint pains...

3. Headache due to external wind

Typical combinations:

1. With uncooked Herba Schizonepetae Tenuifoliae (*Sheng Jing Jie*) and uncooked Radix Platycodi Grandiflori (*Sheng Jie Geng*) as in *Jing Fang Bai Du San* (Schizonepeta & Ledebouriella Vanquish Toxins Powder [183])

2. With Radix Et Rhizoma Notopterygii (*Qiang Huo*) and Radix Angelicae Pubescentis (*Du Huo*) as in *Qiang Huo Sheng Shi Tang* (Notopterygium Overcome Dampness Decoction [247])

3. With Radix Angelicae Dahuricae (*Bai Zhi*) and uncooked Radix Ligustici Wallichii (*Sheng Chuan Xiong*) as in *Fang Feng Chong He Tang* (Ledebouriella Harmonious Flow Decoction [103])

Dosage: 5-15g and up to 30g for severe cases

Note: 1. The word *sheng* is translated by Nigel Wiseman in his *Glossary of Chinese Medical Terms and Acupuncture Points* as crude and unprocessed. However, this does not necessarily mean uncooked or fresh. As pointed out previously, *sheng* as a modifier of medicinal ingredients means uncooked.

——————————— Stir-fried [till] Yellow (Chao Huang) ———————————

Names: *Chao Fang Feng*

Flavors & nature: Sweet and slightly acrid; slightly warm

Functions: Dispels wind, frees *bi*, stops convulsions, relaxes contracture

Indications:

1. Rheumatic complaints[1] due to wind dampness with pain in the joints and tendons, restricted mobility, swelling of the hands and feet...

2. Tetany[1] due to wind toxins with trismus, opisthotonus, convulsions...

Radix Ledebouriellae Sesloidis continued. . .

Typical combinations:

1. With Rhizoma Curcumae (*Jiang Huang*) and Radix Et Rhizoma Notopterygii (*Qiang Huo*) as in *Juan Bi Tang* (Alleviate *Bi* Decoction [192]) or with Radix Gentianae Macrophyllae (*Qin Jiao*), Radix Angelicae Pubescentis (*Du Huo*), and Ramulus Cinnamomi (*Gui Zhi*) as in *Fang Feng Tang* (Ledebouriellae Decoction [103a])

2. With uncooked Rhizoma Arisaematis (*Sheng Tian Nan Xing*) and uncooked Rhizoma Typhonii (*Sheng Bai Fu Zi*) as in *Yu Zhen Tang* (True Jade Decoction [422])

Dosage: 5-10g and up to 30g in severe cases

Note: 1. In clinical practice for the treatment of these two conditions, stir-fried Ledebouriella is often replaced by uncooked Ledebouriella without diminishing the action of this medicinal. On the other hand, stir-fried Ledebouriella reduces this medicinal's sudorific action when necessary.

_____ **Stir-fried [till] Carbonized (*Chao Tan*)** _____

Names: *Fang Feng Tan*

Flavors & nature: Sweet and slightly astringent; slightly warm

Functions: Stops bleeding and diarrhea

Indications:

1. Bloody stools (*e.g.* hemorrhoids) with discharge of red blood before defecation due to affection of the intestines by wind heat (*i.e., chang feng bian xue*)

2. Diarrhea due to spleen vacuity or disharmony of the liver and spleen

Typical combinations:

1. With uncooked Cacumen Biotae Orientalis (*Sheng Ce Bai Ye*), uncooked Radix Sanguisorbae (*Sheng Di Yu*), and carbonized Fructus Immaturus Sophorae Japonicae (*Huai Jiao Tan*)

2. With stir-fried Rhizoma Atractylodis Macrocephalae (*Chao Bai Zhu*), stir-fried Pericarpium Citri Reticulatae (*Chao Chen Pi*), and stir-fried Radix Albus Paeoniae Lactiflorae (*Chao Bai Shao Yao*) as in *Tong Xie Yao Fang* (Painful Diarrhea Essential Formula [333])

Dosage: 5-8g

Ramulus Cinnamomi (*Gui Zhi*)

_____ **Uncooked (*Sheng*)** _____

Names: *Gui Zhi, Chuan Gui Zhi*

Flavors & nature: Acrid and sweet; warm

Functions: Scatters cold, resolves the exterior

Indications:

1. Common cold and flu due to wind cold of either A) the vacuity type with disharmony of defensive and constructive, aversion to wind, perspiration,

fever, a floating (*fu*) and relaxed/retarded (*huan*) pulse or B) the repletion type with aversion to cold, no perspiration, fever, headache, joint stiffness, a floating (*fu*), tight (*jin*) pulse...

2. Rheumatic complaints due to A) wind, cold, and dampness with pain of the joints and tendons, restricted mobility, etc. or B) damp cold transforming into heat with painful, hot, swollen joints...

Ramulus Cinnamomi continued . . .

Typical combinations:

1. A) With uncooked Radix Albus Paeoniae Lactiflorae (*Sheng Bai Shao Yao*) as in *Gui Zhi Tang* (Cinnamon Twig Decoction [129])
B) With uncooked Herba Ephedrae (*Sheng Ma Huang*) as in *Ma Huang Tang* (Ephedra Decoction [215])

2. A) With Radix Lateralis Praeparatus Aconiti Carmichaeli (*Fu Zi*) as in *Gui Zhi Fu Zi Tang* (Cinnamon Twig & Aconite Decoction [124])
B) With uncooked Rhizoma Anemarrhenae (*Sheng Zhi Mu*) and uncooked Radix Albus Paeoniae Lactiflorae (*Sheng Bai Shao Yao*) as in *Gui Zhi Shao Yao Zhi Mu Tang* (Cinnamon Twig, Peony & Anemarrhena Decoction [128])

Dosage: For flu, 2-6g; for rheumatic pain, 6-10g, and up to 30g for severe cases

—————————— Honey Mix-fried (*Mi Zhi*) ——————————

Names: *Zhi Gui Zhi, Mi Zhi Gui Zhi*

Flavors & nature: Sweet and slightly acrid; warm, slightly moistening

Functions: Warms the center, supplements vacuity

Indications: Epigastric and/or abdominal pain due to either 1) middle burner vacuity cold or 2) vacuity cold and qi vacuity of the middle burner

Typical combinations:

1) With Saccharum Granorum (*Yi Tang*) and wine[-processed] Radix Albus Paeoniae Lactiflorae (*Jiu Bai Shao Yao*) as in *Xiao Jian Zhong Tang* (Minor Fortify the Center Decoction [376])

2) With the above two ingredients plus honey mix-fried Radix Astragali Membranacei (*Mi Zhi Huang Qi*) as in *Huang Qi Jian Zhong Tang* (Astragalus Fortify the Center Decoction [157])

Dosage: 5-12g and up to 30g in severe cases

—————————— Stir-fried [till] Yellow (*Chao Huang*) ——————————

Names: *Chao Gui Zhi*

Flavors & nature: Sweet and slightly acrid; warm, slightly drying

Functions: Warms and quickens yang, scatters cold, stimulates the functions of the transformation of qi, disinhibits urination, warms the channels, quickens the blood

Indications:

1. Amenorrhea due to blood stasis with fixed pain in the lower abdomen

2. Infertility due to cold accumulated in the uterus with pain and a sensation of cold in the lower abdomen, menstrual irregularity, dysmenorrhea...

3. Cold, purplish extremities due to blood vacuity and cold in the channels

4. Cold phlegm due to an excess of dampness caused by spleen vacuity with chronic bronchitis, cough with expectoration of clear, liquid mucus, chest and epigastric distention, palpitations...

5. Edema due to accumulation of dampness caused by spleen and kidney yang vacuity with oliguria, edema, a feeling of heaviness...

6. Pain in the chest (*i.e.*, chest *bi*) due to either A) phlegm obstruction and deficient chest yang with thoracic pain and oppression, heart pain, shortness of breath, excessive mucus or B) heart yang vacuity with palpitations, heart pain which

Ramulus Cinnamomi continued. . .

radiates to the left arm, a pale complexion, a knotted (*jie*) and regularly interrupted (*dai*) pulse...

Typical combinations:

1. With wine[-processed] Cortex Radicis Moutan (*Jiu Mu Dan Pi*), uncooked Semen Pruni Persicae (*Sheng Tao Ren*), and wine[-processed] Radix Albus Paeoniae Lactiflorae (*Jiu Bai Shao Yao*) as in *Gui Zhi Fu Ling Wan* (Cinnamon Twig & Poria Pills [123])

2. With processed Fructus Evodiae Rutecarpae (*Zhi Wu Zhu Yu*), wine[-processed] Radix Ligustici Wallichii (*Jiu Chuan Xiong*), and wine[-processed] Radix Angelicae Sinensis (*Jiu Dang Gui*) as in *Wen Jing Tang* (Warm the Channels [or Menses] Decoction [341])

3. With uncooked Herba Cum Radice Asari (*Sheng Xi Xin*) and wine[-processed] Radix Angelicae Sinensis (*Jiu Dang Gui*) as in *Dang Gui Si Ni Tang* (Dang Gui Four Counterflows Decoction [79])

4. With uncooked Sclerotium Poriae Cocos (*Sheng Fu Ling*) and uncooked Rhizoma Atractylodis Macrocephalae (*Sheng Bai Zhu*) as in *Ling Gui Zhu Gan Tang* (Poria, Cinnamon, Atractylodes & Licorice Decoction [201])

5. With Sclerotium Polypori Umbellati (*Zhu Ling*), uncooked Rhizoma Alismatis (*Sheng Ze Xie*), and uncooked Sclerotium Poriae Cocos (*Sheng Fu Ling*) as in *Wu Ling San* (Five [Ingredients] *Ling* Powder [348])

6. A) With stir-fried Pericarpium Trichosanthis Kirlowii (*Chao Gua Lou Pi*), Bulbus Allii Macrostemi (*Xie Bai*), and uncooked Fructus Immaturus Citri Seu Ponciri (*Sheng Zhi Shi*) as in *Zhi Shi Xie Bai Gui Zhi Tang* (Immature Citrus, Allium & Cinnamon Twig Decoction [436])
B) With mix-fried Radix Glycyrrhizae (*Zhi Gan Cao*) as in *Gui Zhi Gan Cao Tang* (Cinnamon Twig & Licorice Decoction [125])

Dosage: 3-10g and up to 30g in severe cases

Herba Schizonepetae Tenuifoliae *(Jing Jie)*

Uncooked *(Sheng)*

Names: *Jing Jie*

Flavors & nature: Acrid; slightly warm

Functions: Dispels wind, resolves the exterior, induces perspiration

Indications:

1. Flu and common cold due to either A) wind cold with aversion to cold, fever, no sweating, and headache or B) wind heat with slight aversion to wind or cold, high fever, slight sweating, thirst, sore throat...

2. Measles (initial stage) due to wind heat accompanied by toxins with eruptions which come out poorly, fever, sore, swollen throat...

3. Cough due to external wind, which damages the lung with itchy throat, fever or no fever, aversion to cold, a floating (*fu*), relaxed/retarded (*huan*) pulse...

4. Sore throat due to wind heat or wind cold, which attacks the lungs with a swollen throat, aphonia...

Herba Schizonepetae Tenuifoliae continued . . .

Typical combinations:

1. A) With uncooked Radix Ledebouriellae Sesloidis (*Sheng Fang Feng*) and uncooked Radix Ligustici Wallichii (*Sheng Chuan Xiong*) as in *Jing Fang Bai Du San* (Schizonepeta & Ledebouriella Vanquish Toxins Powder [183])
B) With Herba Menthae Haplocalycis (*Bo He*), uncooked Flos Lonicerae Japonicae (*Sheng Jin Yin Hua*), and uncooked Fructus Forsythiae Suspensae (*Sheng Lian Qiao*) as in *Yin Qiao San* (Lonicera & Forsythia Powder [412])

2. With Periostracum Cicadae (*Chan Tui*) and uncooked Fructus Arctii Lappae (*Sheng Niu Bang Zi*) as in *Zhu Ye Liu Bang Tang* (Bamboo Leaf, Tamarisk, & Arctium Decoction [446])

3. With uncooked Radix Platycodi Grandiflori (*Sheng Jie Geng*), uncooked Radix Cynanchi Stautonii (*Sheng Bai Qian*), and uncooked Radix Stemonae (*Sheng Bai Bu*) as in *Zhi Sou San* (Stop Cough Powder [437])

4. With uncooked Radix Platycodi Grandiflori (*Sheng Jie Geng*) and uncooked Radix Glycyrrhizae (*Sheng Gan Cao*) as in *Jing Jie Tang* (Schizonepeta Decoction [184])

Dosage: 5-10g and up to 30g in severe cases

_____**Stir-fried [till] Carbonized** *(Chao Tan)* _____

Names: *Jing Jie Tan, Hei Jing Jie*

Flavors & nature: Slightly astringent; slightly warm

Functions: Stops bleeding, harmonizes the blood

Indications:

1. Hematemesis due to stomach vacuity cold with vomiting of purplish black blood, epigastric pain, melena...

2. Epistaxis due to heat in the liver and lungs with bleeding gums

3. Metrorrhagia due to *chong* and *ren* not securing

Typical combinations:

1. With Radix Pseudoginseng (*San Qi*), Terra Flava Usta (*Fu Long Gan*), and blast-fried Rhizoma Zingiberis (*Pao Jiang*)

2. With uncooked Cortex Radicis Moutan (*Sheng Mu Dan Pi*), uncooked Radix Scutellariae Baicalensis (*Sheng Huang Qin*), and carbonized Radix Rubiae Cordifoliae (*Qian Cao Gen Tan*)

3. With carbonized Radix Angelicae Sinensis (*Dang Gui Tan*), carbonized Folium Et Petiolus Trachycarpi (*Zong Lu Tan*), and uncooked Radix Sanguisorbae (*Sheng Di Yu*)

Dosage: 8-12g and up to 30g in severe cases

Herba Ephedrae *(Ma Huang)*

_____ **Uncooked** *(Sheng)* _____

Names: *Ma Huang, Jing Ma Huang, Xi Ma Huang*

Flavors & nature: Acrid and slightly bitter; warm

Functions: Resolves the exterior, induces perspiration, disinhibits urination, disperses swelling

Indications:

1. Flu and colds[1] due to wind cold repletion with

Herba Ephedrae continued . . .

fever, aversion to cold, no sweating, stiffness in the entire body, headache...

2. Edema due to external wind with sudden edema in the eyelids and face eventually extending to the entire body, oliguria, aversion to wind...

3. Jaundice due to external wind accompanied by damp heat with fever, aversion to cold, no sweating...

4. Rheumatic complaints due to wind dampness with evening fever, generalized pain, slight aversion to wind, a floating (*fu*), slippery (*hua*) pulse...

Typical combinations:

1. With uncooked Ramulus Cinnamomi (*Sheng Gui Zhi*) as in *Ma Huang Tang* (Ephedra Decoction [215])

2. With uncooked Gypsum Fibrosum (*Sheng Shi Gao*) and uncooked Rhizoma Zingiberis (*Sheng Jiang*) as in *Yue Bi Tang* (Maidservant from Yue Decoction [423])

3. With uncooked Gypsum Fibrosum (*Sheng Shi Gao*), Herba Artemisiae Capillaris (*Yin Chen Hao*), and uncooked Radix Puerariae (*Sheng Ge Gen*) or with uncooked Fructus Forsythiae Suspensae (*Sheng Lian Qiao*) and Semen Phaseoli Calcarati (*Chi Xiao Dou*) as in *Ma Huang Lian Qiao Chi Xiao Dou Tang* (Ephedra, Forsythia & Aduki Bean Decoction [214])

4. With uncooked Semen Coicis Lachryma-jobi (*Sheng Yi Yi Ren*) as in *Ma Xing Yi Gan Tang* (Ephedra, Armeniaca, Coix & Licorice Decoction [217])

Dosage: 2-6g and up to 15g in severe cases

Note: 1. Herba Ephedrae (*Ma Huang*) is sudorific, but Radix Ephedrae (*Ma Huang Gen*) and Nodus Ephedrae (*Ma Huang Jie*) are anti-sudorific. This is why the original text in which this formula was recorded, the *Shang Han Lun (Treatise on Cold Damage)* suggests that, in prescribing *Ma Huang Tang* for the purpose of promoting diaphoresis, one should use Herba Ephedrae without the nodes on the stems: "*Yong Ma Huang qu jie, i.e.* use Herba Ephedrae without the nodes."

Honey Mix-fried (*Mi Zhi*)

Names: *Zhi Ma Huang, Mi Zhi Ma Huang*

Flavors & nature: Acrid, sweet, and bitter; warm, slightly moistening

Functions: Diffuses and frees the flow of lung qi, calms dyspnea

Indications:

Cough and/or asthma due to: 1) wind cold with abundant phlegm, thoracic distention, headache, generalized pain, 2) accumulation of cold phlegm in the lungs with abundant, clear mucus, or 3) phlegm heat and/or heat in the lungs with thick, yellow mucus, fever, and a dry mouth

Typical combinations:

1. With uncooked Semen Pruni Armeniacae (*Xing Ren*) and uncooked Radix Glycyrrhizae (*Sheng Gan Cao*) as in *San Ao Tang* (Three [Ingredients] Unbinding Decoction [271])

2. With dry Rhizoma Zingiberis (*Gan Jiang*) and honey mix-fried Herba Cum Radice Asari (*Mi Zhi Xi Xin*) as in *Xiao Qing Long Tang* (Minor Blue Dragon Decoction [377])

3. With uncooked Gypsum Fibrosum (*Sheng Shi Gao*) and uncooked Semen Pruni Armeniacae (*Sheng Xing Ren*) as in *Ma Xing Shi Gan Tang* (Ephedra, Armeniaca, Gypsum & Licorice Decoction [216])

Dosage: 3-10g and up to 20g in severe cases

Uncooked Rhizoma Zingiberis *(Sheng Jiang)*

Fresh *(Xian)*[1]

Names: *Sheng Jiang, Xian Sheng Jiang*

Flavors & nature: Acrid; warm

Functions: Resolves the exterior, scatters cold, warms the stomach, stops vomiting, transforms phlegm, stops cough

Indications:

1. Flu and common colds due to wind cold of the vacuity type with disharmony of the constructive and defensive manifesting as fever, aversion to wind, slight sweating, headache...

2. Vomiting due to accumulation of dampness and cold in the middle burner with nausea, epigastric distention, absence of thirst...

3. Cough due to accumulation of phlegm with abundant mucus, epigastric and thoracic distention, possible slight aversion to wind and cold

4. Disharmony of the constructive and defensive with spontaneous perspiration

5. Food poisoning due to crab or fish

Typical combinations:

1. With uncooked Ramulus Cinnamomi (*Sheng Gui Zhi*) and Fructus Zizyphi Jujubae (*Da Zao*) as in *Gui Zhi Tang* (Cinnamon Twig Decoction [129])

2. Ginger[-processed] Rhizoma Pinelliae Ternatae (*Jiang Ban Xia*) as in *Xiao Ban Xia Tang* (Minor Pinellia Decoction [372])

3. With uncooked (*Sheng*) or stir-fried (*Chao*) Semen Pruni Armeniacae (*Xing Ren*), uncooked Sclerotium Poriae Cocos (*Sheng Fu Ling*), and uncooked Pericarpium Citri Reticulatae (*Sheng Chen Pi*)

4. With Fructus Zizyphi Jujubae (*Da Zao*) as in *Gui Zhi Tang* (Cinnamon Twig Decoction [129]) or *Xiao Jian Zhong Tang* (Minor Fortify the Center Decoction [376])

5. With Folium Perillae Frutescentis (*Zi Su Ye*) and Rhizoma Phragmitis Communis (*Lu Gen*)

Dosage: 3-10g or 2-6 slices and up to 20g in severe cases or in case of food poisoning

Note: 1. This refers to the fresh and crude form of this medicinal.

Roasted *(Wei)*[1]

Names: *Wei Jiang, Wei Sheng Jiang*

Flavors & nature: Moderately acrid; warm or slightly hot

Functions: Warms the middle burner, stops pain, stops bleeding

Indications:

1. Epigastric and abdominal pain due to middle burner vacuity cold with diarrhea

2. Vomiting of clear liquids, eructation, and nausea due to middle burner vacuity cold

3. Menstrual irregularity due to disharmony of the qi, blood, spleen, and liver with dysmenorrhea and premenstrual syndrome...

4. Abdominal distention due to cold dampness invading the spleen or to a disharmony of the liver and spleen with abdominal pain, loose stools...

Uncooked Rhizoma Zingiberis continued . . .

Typical combinations:

With earth stir-fried Rhizoma Alpiniae Officinari (*Tu Chao Gao Liang Jiang*), roasted Semen Myristicae Fragrantis (*Wei Rou Dou Kou*), and uncooked Radix Saussureae Seu Vladimiriae (*Sheng Mu Xiang*)

2. With ginger[-processed] Rhizoma Pinelliae Ternatae (*Jiang Ban Xia*) and processed Fructus Evodiae Rutecarpae (*Zhi Wu Zhu Yu*) as in *Wu Zhu Yu Tang* (Evodia Decoction)

3. With stir-fried Radix Bupleuri (*Chao Chai Hu*), wine[-processed] Radix Angelicae Sinensis (*Jiu Dang Gui*), and wine[-processed] Radix Albus Paeoniae Lactiflorae (*Jiu Bai Shao Yao*) as in *Xiao Yao San* (Rambling Powder [380])

4. With ginger[-processed] Cortex Magnoliae Officinalis (*Jiang Hou Po*) and Rhizoma Pinelliae Ternatae (*Fa Ban Xia*) as in *Hou Po Sheng Jiang Ban Xia Gan Cao Ren Shen Tang* (Magnolia, Fresh Ginger, Licorice & Ginseng Decoction [139])

Dosage: 5-10g or 3-6 slices and up to 30g in severe cases

Note: 1. This refers to the fresh and crude medicinal which is roasted under coals.

Juice (Zhi)[1]

Names: *Sheng Jiang Zhi, Jiang Zhi*

Flavors & nature: Acrid; warm

Functions: Disperses phlegm wind, stops vomiting

Indications:

1. Wind stroke due to phlegm wind with loss of consciousness and the sound of phlegm rattling in the throat

2. Vomiting of clear liquids due to accumulation of cold dampness and middle burner yang vacuity

Typical combinations:

1. With Succus Bambusae (*Zhu Li*)

2. With ginger[-processed] Rhizoma Pinelliae Ternatae (*Jiang Ban Xia*) as in *Sheng Jiang Ban Xia Tang* (Uncooked Ginger & Pinellia Decoction [296])

Dosage: 5-15 drops

Note: 1. This refers to the juice of fresh ginger.

Ginger Skin (Jiang Pi)[1]

Names: *Jiang Pi, Sheng Jiang Pi*

Flavors & nature: Slightly acrid; cool

Functions: Disinhibits urination, disperses swelling

Indications: Edema due to spleen vacuity with heavy limbs, oliguria, dysuria, abdominal and epigastric distention...

Typical combinations: With uncooked Cortex Radicis Mori Albi (*Sheng Sang Bai Pi*), Cortex Sclerotii Poriae Cocos (*Fu Ling Pi*), and Pericarpium Arecae Catechu (*Da Fu Pi*) as in *Wu Pi San* (Five Skins Powder [351]) or with Cortex Sclerotii Poriae Cocos (*Fu Ling Pi*), uncooked Rhizoma Atractylodis Macrocephalae (*Sheng Bai Zhu*), and Pericarpium Arecae Catechu (*Da Fu Pi*) as in *Bai Zhu San* (Atractylodes Powder [23])

Dosage: 3-10g

Note: 1. This refers to the skin of fresh ginger.

Herba Cum Radice Asari (Xi Xin)

—————————— Uncooked (Sheng) ——————————

Names: *Xi Xin, Sheng Xi Xin, Bei Xi Xin, Liao Xi Xin*

Flavors & nature: Acrid; warm

Functions: Resolves the exterior, scatters cold, dispels wind, stops pain, opens the portals of the nose

Indications:

1. Flu and common cold due to wind cold with aversion to cold, headache, nasal congestion...

2. Sinusitis and rhinitis due to wind cold with obstruction and congestion of the nose, abundant runny nose, diminished ability to smell, frontal headache...

3. Toothache due to A) wind heat or stomach heat with bad breath, red, swollen gums, thirst or B) wind cold with gums which are neither red nor swollen but rather pale...

4. Aphthae and glossitis due to a pattern of mixed cold and heat

5. Headache due to external wind

Typical combinations:

1. With uncooked Radix Ledebouriellae Sesloidis (*Sheng Fang Feng*), uncooked Herba Schizonepetae Tenuifoliae (*Sheng Jing Jie*), and uncooked Radix Ligustici Wallichii (*Sheng Chuan Xiong*) as in *Chuan Xiong Cha Tiao San* (Ligusticum Wallichium & Tea Regulating Powder [52])

2. With Radix Angelicae Dahuricae (*Bai Zhi*) and Flos Magnoliae Liliflorae (*Xin Yi Hua*) as in *Xin Yi San* (Flos Magnoliae Powder [380])

3. A) With uncooked Gypsum Fibrosum (*Sheng Shi Gao*) and uncooked Rhizoma Anemarrhenae (*Sheng Zhi Mu*) B) With Radix Lateralis Praeparatus Aconiti Carmichaeli (*Fu Zi*), Radix Angelicae Dahuricae (*Bai Zhi*), and Resina Olibani (*Ru Xiang*)

4. With wine mix-fried Rhizoma Coptidis Chinensis (*Jiu Zhi Huang Lian*), uncooked Radix Scutellariae Baicalensis (*Sheng Huang Qin*), and dry Rhizoma Zingiberis (*Gan Jiang*)

5. With uncooked Radix Ligustici Wallichii (*Sheng Chuan Xiong*) and Radix Angelicae Dahuricae (*Bai Zhi*) as in *Chuan Xiong Cha Tiao San* (Ligusticum Wallichium & Tea Powder [52])

Dosage: 1-3g[1] and up to 6g in severe cases

Note: 1. That one should never prescribe a large dose of *Sheng Xi Xin* is confirmed by the traditional saying, "[With] *Xi Xin* do not go beyond [1] *qian*." One *qian* equals approximately 3g.

—————————— Honey Mix-fried (Mi Zhi) ——————————

Names: *Mi Zhi Xi Xin, Mi Xi Xin, Zhi Xi Xin*

Flavors & nature: Acrid and slightly sweet; warm, slightly moistening

Functions: Warms the lungs, transforms phlegm and eliminates rheum, stops cough

Indications: Cough and asthma[1] due to accumulation of phlegm rheum and cold in the lung with abundant rheum and clear fluids

Typical combinations: With vinegar[-processed] Fructus Schizandrae Chinensis (*Cu Wu Wei Zi*),

Herba Cum Radice Asari continued . . .

dry Rhizoma Zingiberis (*Gan Jiang*), and honey mix-fried Herba Ephedrae (*Mi Zhi Ma Huang*) as in *Xiao Qing Long Tang* (Minor Blue Dragon Decoction [377]) or with vinegar[-processed] Fructus Schizandrae Chinensis (*Cu Wu Wei Zi*), dry Rhizoma Zingiberis (*Gan Jiang*), and uncooked Sclerotium Poriae Cocos (*Sheng Fu Ling*) as in *Ling Gan Wu Wei Jiang Xin Tang* (Poria, Licorice, Schizandra, Ginger & Asarum Decoction [200])

Note: 1. In case of a very pronounced external pattern, prescribe uncooked Herba Cum Radice Asari (*Sheng Xi Xin*).

2
Cool, Acrid Exterior-resolving Medicinals

Radix Bupleuri (Chai Hu)
_____ Uncooked (Sheng) _____

Names: *Chai Hu, Ruan Chai Hu, Ying Chai Hu, Nan Chai Hu, Bei Chai Hu*

Flavors & nature: Bitter and slightly acrid; slightly cold

Functions: Clears heat, harmonizes the *shao yang*

Indications:

1. Fever due to external damage (*i.e.*, wind cold which has transformed into heat, wind heat, warm diseases) associated with internal heat with headache, dry nose, irritability, a bitter taste in the mouth...

2. *Shao yang* pattern (half external/half internal) with either A) alternating fever and chills, chest and hypochondriac distention, dry throat, a bitter taste in the mouth, nausea, and agitation or B) accumulation of heat in the liver and gallbladder with alternating fever and chills, pain in the chest and hypochondrium, nausea, vomiting, constipation...

3. Malaria with alternating fever and chills...

Typical combinations:

1. With Radix Angelicae Dahuricae (*Bai Zhi*), Radix Et Rhizoma Notopterygii (*Qiang Huo*), and uncooked Gypsum Fibrosum (*Sheng Shi Gao*) as in *Chai Ge Jie Ji Tang* (Bupleurum & Pueraria Resolve the Muscles Decoction [43])

2. A) With uncooked Radix Scutellariae Baicalensis (*Sheng Huang Qin*) and clear Rhizoma Pinelliae Ternatae (*Qing Ban Xia*) as in *Xiao Chai Hu Tang* (Minor Bupleurum Decoction [374])
B) With uncooked Radix Scutellariae Baicalensis (*Sheng Huang Qin*), clear Rhizoma Pinelliae Ternatae (*Qing Ban Xia*), and uncooked Radix Et Rhizoma Rhei (*Sheng Da Huang*) as in *Da Chai Hu Tang* (Major Bupleurum Decoction [60])

3. With bran stir-fried Radix Dichroae Febrifugae (*Fu Chao Chang Shan*), stir-fried Fructus Amomi Tsao-ko (*Chao Cao Guo*), and uncooked Radix Scutellariae Baicalensis (*Sheng Huang Qing*)

Dosage: 5-15g and up to 60g in severe cases

_____ Stir-fried (Chao)[1] _____

Names: *Cu Chai Hu, Chao Chai Hu, Qing Chao Chai Hu*

Flavors & nature: Bitter and slightly sour (in the case of *Cu Chao* or vinegar stir-fried); neutral

Functions: Drains the liver,[2] eliminates stagnation,[2] and upbears (clear) yang[3]

Indications:

1. Lateral costal, epigastric, or abdominal pain and distention due to liver depression, qi stagnation[2]

2. Disharmony of the liver and spleen with simultaneous blood vacuity and lateral costal

Radix Bupleuri continued . . .

pain, dizziness, vertigo, menstrual irregularity, breast distention, premenstrual syndrome[2]. . .

3. Fall of spleen qi due to middle burner qi vacuity with ptosis of the internal organs, chronic diarrhea, frequent urination[3] . . .

Typical combinations:

1. With uncooked Fructus Immaturus Citri Seu Ponciri (*Sheng Zhi Shi*), uncooked Rhizoma Cyperi Rotundi (*Sheng Xiang Fu*), and wine[-processed] Radix Albus Paeoniae Lactiflorae (*Jiu Bai Shao Yao*) as in *Chai Hu Shu Gan San* (Bupleurum Soothe the Liver Powder [44])

2. With wine[-processed] Radix Albus Paeoniae Lactiflorae (*Jiu Bai Shao Yao*), wine[-processed] Radix Angelicae Sinensis (*Jiu Dang Gui*), and Herba Menthae Haplocalycis (*Bo He*) as in *Xiao Yao San* (Rambling Powder [380])

3. With honey mix-fried Radix Astragali Membranacei (*Mi Zhi Huang Qi*) and honey mix-fried Rhizoma Cimicifugae (*Mi Zhi Sheng Ma*) as in *Bu Zhong Yi Qi Tang* (Supplement the Center & Boost the Qi Decoction [38])

Dosage: 3-10g and up to 60g in severe cases

Notes: 1. Stir-frying Bupleurum weakens its sudorific function. 2. One uses vinegar stir-fried, or more exactly, vinegar mix-fried Bupleurum to drain the liver, eliminate stagnation, and for indications 1 & 2 above. 3. One uses stir-fried [till] scorched Bupleurum to raise yang qi as in indication 3 above.

Amyda Blood [Processed] (*Bei Xue*)[1]

Names: *Bei Xue Chai Hu, Bei Xue Ban Chai Hu*

Flavors & nature: Bitter and salty; slightly cold

Functions: Harmonizes the exterior and interior, clears vacuity heat

Indications:

1. Evening fever due to damage of yin following a warm disease with dry mouth, night sweats, a fine (*xi*), rapid (*shu*) pulse...

2. Malaria with alternating fever and chills and simultaneous signs of yin vacuity

Typical combinations:

1. With Herba Artemisiae Apiaceae·(*Qing Hao*), Cortex Radicis Lycii (*Di Gu Pi*), uncooked Radix Albus Paeoniae Lactiflorae (*Sheng Bai Shao Yao*), and salt[-processed] Rhizoma Anemarrhenae (*Zhi Mu*)

2. With stir-fried Fructus Amomi Tsao-ko (*Chao Cao Guo*), bran stir-fried Radix Dichroae Febrifugae (*Fu Chao Chang Shan*), salt[-processed] Rhizoma Anemarrhenae (*Yan Zhi Mu*), and Herba Artemisiae Apiaceae (*Qing Hao*)

Dosage: 6-10g and up to 60g in severe cases

Note: 1. This refers to the blood of a species of tortoise (*Amyda Sinensis*) which is added to the Bupleurum.

Addendum: There are also other ways of preparing Bupleurum. These are not used as often, however. They include: *Mi Zhi Chai Hu* or honey mix-fried Bupleurum to moisten the lungs and stop cough or to strengthen the middle burner and *Jiu Chai Hu*, wine[-processed] Bupleurum to quicken the blood and to quicken the channels and vessels.

Radix Puerariae (Ge Gen)

Uncooked (Sheng)

Names: *Sheng Ge Gen, Ge Gen, Gan (i.e., dry) Gen, Gan (i.e., sweet) Gen, Fen Ge Gen*

Flavors & nature: Sweet and acrid; neutral

Functions: Resolves the muscles, clears heat, engenders fluids, stops thirst, promotes the emission of skin eruptions

Indications:

1. Stiff neck and generalized stiffness due to wind cold with fever, chills, aversion to cold, no sweating, headache...

2. Thirst due to either A) a wind cold which has penetrated to the interior and transformed into heat with fever, headache, agitation, insomnia, eye pain, dry nose, aversion to cold, no sweating or B) stomach heat with dry mouth, a red tongue with no coating...

3. Measles (initial stage) either A) due an external pattern with fever, headache, chills, stiffness, and eruptions which emit poorly or B) with fever, eruptions which emit poorly, no sweating or sweating which emits poorly . . .

Typical combinations:

1. With uncooked Herba Ephedrae (*Sheng Ma Huang*) and uncooked Ramulus Cinnamomi (*Sheng Gui Zhi*) as in *Ge Gen Tang* (Pueraria Decoction [113])

2. A) With uncooked Radix Bupleuri (*Sheng Chai Hu*), Radix Et Rhizoma Notopterygii (*Qiang Huo*), and uncooked Radix Scutellariae Baicalensis (*Sheng Chai Hu*) as in *Chai Ge Jie Ji Tang* (Bupleurum & Pueraria Resolve the Muscles Decoction [43])
B) With Radix Trichosanthis Kirlowii (*Tian Hua Fen*), Rhizoma Phragmitis Communis (*Lu Gen*), and uncooked Gypsum Fibrosum (*Sheng Shi Gao*)

3. A) With uncooked Rhizoma Cimicifugae (*Sheng Ma*) as in *Sheng Ma Ge Gen Tang* (Cimicifuga & Pueraria Decoction [297])
B) With uncooked Herba Schizonepetae Tenuifoliae (*Sheng Jing Jie*) and uncooked Fructus Arctii Lappae (*Sheng Niu Bang Zi*) as in *Xuan Du Jie Biao Tang* (Diffuse Toxins & Resolve the Exterior Decoction [387])

Dosage: 6-30g and up to 60g in severe cases

Roasted (Wei)

Names: *Wei Ge Gen, Chao Ge Gen, Chao Gan Gen*

Flavors & nature: Sweet; neutral or slightly warm

Functions: Upbears (clear) yang, stops diarrhea, treats dysentery

Indications:

1. Dysentery due to replete heat with fever, slight aversion to wind and cold, agitation, thirst...

2. Diarrhea due to spleen vacuity causing middle burner qi fall and an accumulation of dampness with weakness, shortness of breath...

Typical combinations:

1. With stir-fried Radix Scutellariae Baicalensis (*Chao Huang Qin*) and uncooked Rhizoma Coptidis Chinensis (*Sheng Huang Lian*) as in *Ge Gen Qin Lian Tang* (Pueraria, Scutellaria & Coptis Decoction [112])

2. With earth stir-fried Rhizoma Atractylodis Macrocephalae (*Tu Chao Bai Zhu*) and Radix Panacis Ginseng (*Ren Shen*) as in *Qi Wei Bai Zhu San* (Seven Flavors Atractylodes Powder [237])

Dosage: 5-20g and up to 50g in severe cases

Flos Chrysanthemi Morifolii (*Ju Hua*)

_____ Uncooked *(Sheng)* _____

Names: *Ju Hua, Gan Ju Hua*

Flavors & nature: Sweet and bitter; slightly cold

Functions: Dispels wind, clears heat, resolves toxins, treats skin inflammations

Indications:

1. Colds and flu[1] due to either A) wind heat with high fever, slight aversion to cold and wind, thirst, and sore throat or B) wind heat with severe headache...

2. Skin inflammations[2] due to heat toxins with redness, swelling, and pain

3. Headache[1] due to external wind with fever, chills...

Typical combinations:

1. A) With uncooked Folium Mori Albi (*Sheng Sang Ye*) and Herba Menthae Haplocalycis (*Bo He*) as in *Sang Ju Yin* (Morus & Chrysanthemum Drink [276])

B) With uncooked Fructus Viticis (*Sheng Man Jing Zi*) and Radix Et Rhizoma Notopterygii (*Qiang Huo*) as in *Ju Hua San* (Chrysanthemum Powder [189])

2. With Herba Cum Radice Taraxaci Mongolici (*Pu Gong Ying*), Herba Violae Yedoensis (*Zi Hua Di Ding*), and uncooked Flos Lonicerae Japonicae (*Sheng Jin Yin Hua*)

3. With uncooked Radix Ligustici Wallichii (*Sheng Chuan Xiong*), Radix Angelicae Dahuricae (*Bai Zhi*), and Herba Menthae Haplocalycis (*Bo He*) as in *Ju Hua Cha Tiao San* (Chrysanthemum & Tea Regulating Powder [188])

Dosage: 5-12g and up to 100g in severe cases

Notes: 1. For external damage, it is recommended that one use the yellow type of Chrysanthemum (*Huang Ju Hua*), which dispels wind and clears heat better as opposed to the white Chrysanthemum (*Bai Ju Hua*). 2. For skin inflammations, it is better to use the wild Chrysanthemum, *i.e.*, Flos Chrysanthemi Indici (*Ye Ju Hua*), which resolves toxins and disperses swelling better.

_____ Stir-fried [till] Scorched *(Chao Jiao)* _____

Names: *Chao Ju Hua, Chao Gan Ju*

Flavors & nature: Sweet and bitter; slightly cold tending toward neutral

Functions: Clears heat, brightens the eyes, extinguishes wind, stops convulsions

Indications:

1. Headache[1] due to either A) liver fire or B) liver yang hyperactivity

2. Vertigo or convulsion and spasms[1] due to either A) liver fire or B) liver yang hyperactivity

3. Eye diseases[2] due to either A) liver/kidney yin vacuity, B) wind heat in the liver channel, or C) liver fire

Typical combinations:

1. A) With Spica Prunellae Vulgaris (*Xia Gu Cao*) and wine[-processed] Radix Gentianae Scabrae (*Jiu Long Dan Cao*)
B) With stir-fried Rhizoma Gastrodiae Elatae (*Chao Tian Ma*) and uncooked Concha Haliotidis (*Sheng Shi Jue Ming*)

2. A) Same as 1.A) above
B) Same as 1.B) above

Flos Chrysanthemi Morifolii continued . . .

3. A) with Fructus Lycii Chinensis (*Gou Qi Zi*), uncooked Semen Cuscutae (*Sheng Tu Si Zi*), wine-steamed Fructus Ligustri Lucidi (*Jiu Zheng Nu Zhen Zi*)
B) With uncooked Folium Mori Albi (*Sheng Sang Ye*), Periostracum Cicadae (*Chan Tui*), and uncooked Fructus Viticis (*Sheng Man Jing Zi*)
C) With Spica Prunellae Vulgaris (*Xia Gu Cao*),

wine[-processed] Radix Gentianae Scabrae (*Jiu Long Dan Cao*), and uncooked Semen Cassiae Torae (*Sheng Jue Ming Zi*)

Dosage: 5-12g and up to 100g in severe cases

Note: 1. In case of severe liver heat, one should prescribe uncooked Chrysanthemum (*Sheng Ju Hua*). 2. For this indication, it is advisable to use if possible the white Chrysanthemum (*Bai Ju Hua*) since it calms or levels the liver and brightens the eyes.

Fructus Viticis (*Man Jing Zi*)

———————— Uncooked (*Sheng*) ————————

Names: *Sheng Man Jing, Man Jing Zi*

Flavors & nature: Bitter and acrid; cold

Functions: Dispels wind, clears heat

Indications:

1. Colds and flu due to wind heat with fever, slight aversion to wind and cold, slight perspiration, severe headache...

2. Headache due to wind heat with fever, chills, vertigo...

3. Red, swollen, painful eyes due to wind heat in the liver channel with lacrimation, headache...

Typical combinations:

1. With uncooked Flos Chrysanthemi Morifolii

(*Sheng Ju Hua*), uncooked Radix Ledebouriellae Sesloidis (*Sheng Fang Feng*), and Herba Menthae Haplocalycis (*Bo He*)

2. With uncooked Bombyx Batryticatus (*Sheng Jiang Can*), uncooked Folium Mori Albi (*Sheng Sang Ye*), uncooked Flos Chrysanthemi Morifolii (*Sheng Ju Hua*), and Herba Menthae Haplocalycis (*Bo He*)

3. With stir-fried Flos Chrysanthemi Morifolii (*Chao Ju Hua*), uncooked Semen Cassiae Torae (*Sheng Jue Ming Zi*), Flos Buddleiae Officinalis (*Mi Meng Hua*), and Herba Equiseti Hiemalis (*Mu Zei*) as in *Chan Hua San* (Cicada & Chrysanthemum Powder [45])

Dosage: 5-10g and up to 30g in severe cases

———————— Stir-fried [till] Yellow (*Chao Huang*) ————————

Name: *Chao Man Jing*

Flavors & nature: Bitter and slightly acrid; slightly cold

Functions: Brightens the eyes, improves hearing, treats *bi*

Indications:

1. Diminished visual and auditory acuity due to central qi vacuity and non-upbearing of clear yang to nourish the upper (*i.e.*, the head) with deafness, tinnitus, and problems with vision and "floaters" in the eyes...

Fructus Viticis continued . . .

2. Rheumatic complaints due to wind dampness with pain of the joints, muscles, and channels . . .

Typical combinations:

1. With Radix Panacis Ginseng (*Ren Shen*), honey mix-fried Radix Astragali Membranacei (*Mi Zhi Huang Qi*), honey mix-fried Rhizoma Cimicifugae (*Mi Zhi Sheng Ma*), and roasted Radix Puerariae (*Wei Ge Gen*) as in *Yi Qi Cong Ming Tang* (Boost the Qi & Increase Acuity Decoction [403])

2. With Radix Et Rhizoma Notopterygii (*Qiang Huo*), wine[-processed] Radix Gentianae Macrophyllae (*Jiu Jin Qiao*), and wine[-processed] Radix Clematidis (*Jiu Wei Ling Xian*) or with Radix Et Rhizoma Notopterygii (*Qiang Huo*), stir-fried Radix Ledebouriellae Sesloidis (*Chao Fang Feng*), and uncooked Radix Ligustici Wallichii (*Sheng Chuan Xiong*)

Dosage: 5-10g and up to 30g in severe cases

Fructus Arctii Lappae *(Niu Bang Zi)*

Uncooked *(Sheng)*

Names: *Sheng Niu Bang, Niu Bang Zi, Da Li Zi*

Flavors & nature: Acrid and bitter; cold

Functions: Dispels wind, clears heat, promotes the emission of skin eruptions, moistens the intestines, frees the stool

Indications:

1. Colds and flu due to wind heat with fever, slight aversion to wind and cold, cough, headache, sore throat . . .

2. Measles (initial stage) due to accumulation of heat with eruptions which come to the surface poorly, chest oppression, agitation, a dry mouth, fever . . .

3. Scarlatina due to wind heat and toxins with a red, sore, swollen throat, fever, aversion to cold...

4. Mumps due to toxic heat with fever, aversion to cold . . .

5. Constipation due to heat . . .

Typical combinations:

1. With uncooked Fructus Forsythiae Suspensae (*Sheng Lian Qiao*), uncooked Flos Lonicerae Japonicae (*Sheng Jin Yin Hua*), and Herba Menthae Haplocalycis (*Bo He*) as in *Yin Qiao San* (Lonicera & Forsythia Powder [412])

2. With Periostracum Cicadae (*Chan Tui*) and Herba Lophatheri Gracilis (*Dan Zhu Ye*) as in *Zhu Ye Liu Bang Tang* (Bamboo Leaf, Tamarisk & Arctium Decoction [446])

3. With uncooked Radix Platycodi Grandiflori (*Sheng Jie Geng*) and uncooked Radix Glycyrrhizae (*Sheng Gan Cao*) as in *Qing Yan Tang* (Clear the Throat Decoction [258])

4. With Radix Isatidis Seu Baphicacanthi (*Ban Lan Gen*) and Fructificatio Lasiosphaerae (*Ma Bo*) as in *Pu Ji Xiao Du Yin* (Universal Benefit Disperse Toxins Drink [234])

5. With uncooked Radix Et Rhizoma Rhei (*Sheng Da Huang*) and Mirabilitum (*Mang Xiao*)

Dosage: 5-10g and up to 30g in severe cases

_____ Stir-fried [till] Yellow *(Chao Huang)* _____

Names: *Chao Niu Bang, Chao Da Li Zi*

Flavors & nature: Bitter and slightly acrid; slightly cold

Functions: Clears the lungs, disinhibits the throat, transforms phlegm, stops cough

Indications:

1. Cough due to either A) wind heat in the lungs associated with yin vacuity and phlegm which is difficult to expectorate and/or bloody, dry mouth and throat or B) wind heat which stagnates in the lungs with asthmatic cough, abundant rhinorrhea, abundant phlegm which is thick and pasty, thirst, agitation, fever, a sore throat . . .

2. Sore, swollen throat due to wind heat . . .

Typical combinations:

1. A) With honey mix-fried Fructus Aristolochiae (*Mi Zhi Ma Dou Ling*), uncooked Semen Pruni Armeniacae (*Sheng Xing Ren*), and Concha Cyclinae powder stir-fried Gelatinum Corii Asini (*Ge Fen Chao E Jiao*) as in *Bu Fei E Jiao Tang* (Supplement the Lungs Donkey Skin Glue Decoction [32])
B) With uncooked Folium Eriobotryae Japonicae (*Sheng Pi Pa Ye*), uncooked Pericarpium Trichosanthis Kirlowii (*Sheng Gua Lou Pi*), and Bulbus Fritillariae Thunbergii (*Zhe Bei Mu*) each. With Herba Menthae Haplocalycis (*Bo He*), Periostracum Cicadae (*Chan Tui*), and uncooked Folium Mori Albi (*Sheng Sang Ye*)

Dosage: 6-12g and up to 30g in severe cases

Folium Mori Albi *(Sang Ye)*

_____ Uncooked *(Sheng)* _____

Names: *Sang Ye, Dong Sang Ye, Shuang Sang Ye*

Flavors & nature: Bitter and sweet; cold

Functions: Resolves the exterior, clears heat

Indications:

1. Colds and flu due to wind heat with fever, slight aversion to wind and cold, headache, thirst, itchy throat, cough...

2. Red, swollen, painful eyes due to wind heat with lacrimation, headache, vertigo...

Typical combinations:

1. With uncooked Flos Chrysanthemi Morifolii (*Sheng Ju Hua*), uncooked Fructus Forsythiae Suspensae (*Sheng Lian Qiao*), uncooked Semen Pruni Armeniacae (*Sheng Xing Ren*), and Herba Menthae Haplocalycis (*Bo He*) as in *Sang Ju Yin* (Morus & Chrysanthemum Drink [276])

2. With Flos Chrysanthemi Indici (*Ye Ju Hua*), uncooked Semen Cassiae Torae (*Sheng Jue Ming Zi*), and stir-fried Fructus Gardeniae Jasminoidis (*Chao Zhi Zi*)

_____ Stir-fried [till] Scorched *(Chao Jiao)* _____

Name: *Chao Sang Ye*

Flavors & nature: Sweet and bitter; slightly cold

Functions: Nourishes the liver, brightens the eyes

Folium Mori Albi continued . . .

Indications: Vertigo and blurred vision due to liver/kidney yin vacuity with tinnitus, dry eyes, headache...

Typical combinations: With Semen Sesami Indici (*Hei Zhi Ma*) as in *Sang Ma Wan* (Morus & Sesame Pills [277])

Dosage: 5-10g and up to 50g in severe cases

_____ **Honey Mix-fried** *(Mi Zhi)*_____

Names: *Mi Zhi Sang Ye, Zhi Sang Ye*

Flavors & nature: Sweet and slightly bitter; slightly cold

Functions: Clears the lungs, moistens dryness, stops cough

Indications: Cough due to dryness of the lungs caused by an attack of dry heat with dry cough

without mucus, fever, dry mouth...

Typical combinations: With uncooked Semen Pruni Armeniacae (*Sheng Xing Ren*), Bulbus Fritillariae Thunbergii (*Zhe Bei Mu*), and Radix Adenophorae Strictae (*Nan Sha Shen*) as in *Sang Xing Tang* (Morus & Armeniaca Decoction [279])

Dosage: 8-15g and up to 50g in severe cases

Rhizoma Cimicifugae *(Sheng Ma)*

_____ **Uncooked** *(Sheng)* _____

Names: *Lu Sheng Ma, Guan Sheng Ma, Chuan Sheng Ma, Hua Sheng Ma, Ji Gu Sheng Ma, Xi Sheng Ma*

Flavors & nature: Acrid and sweet; slightly cold

Functions: Resolves the exterior, promotes the emission of skin eruptions, clears heat, resolves toxins

Indications:

1. Measles (initial stage)[1] with poor emission of eruptions...

2. Swollen, painful throat to due accumulation of heat toxins...

3. Headache due to wind heat...

4. Aphthae and glossitis due to accumulation of heat in the stomach with possible gingivitis, bad breath...

5. Toothache due to fire in the stomach with red,

swollen gums, abscess...

Typical combinations:

1. With uncooked Radix Puerariae (*Sheng Ge Gen*) as in *Sheng Ma Ge Gen Tang* (Cimicifuga & Pueraria Decoction [297])

2. With Rhizoma Belamcandae (*She Gan*), uncooked Radix Platycodi Grandiflori (*Sheng Jie Geng*), and Folium Isatidis (*Da Qing Ye*)

3. With uncooked Fructus Viticis (*Sheng Man Jing Zi*) as in *Qing Zhen Tang* (Clear Tremors Decoction [261])

4. With wine[-processed] Rhizoma Coptidis Chinensis (*Jiu Huang Lian*) and uncooked Radix Rehmanniae (*Sheng Di Huang*) as in *Qing Wei San* (Clear the Stomach Powder [256])

5. With uncooked Gypsum Fibrosum (*Sheng Shi Gao*) and uncooked Rhizoma Coptidis Chinensis

Rhizoma Cimicifugae continued . . .

(*Sheng Huang Lian*) as in *Qing Wei San* (Clear the Stomach Powder [256])

Dosage: For resolving the exterior, 3-5g; for

clearing heat and resolving toxins, 6-15g

Note: 1. Uncooked Rhizoma Cimifugae may be used for all types of eruptive maladies as long as there is poor emission of the eruptions.

Honey Mix-fried *(Mi Zhi)*

Names: *Mi Zhi Sheng Ma, Zhi Sheng Ma*

Flavors & nature: Sweet; slightly cold tending toward neutral

Functions: Upbears yang

Indications:

1. Fall of qi due to spleen qi vacuity with stomach or abdominal ptosis, chronic diarrhea, rectal or uterine prolapse, low-grade fever...

2. Constipation[1] due to either A) blood vacuity or dryness of the large intestine or B) kidney vacuity

Typical combinations:

1. With Radix Panacis Ginseng (*Ren Shen*), honey mix-fried Radix Astragali Membranacei (*Mi Zhi Huang Qi*), stir-fried Radix Bupleuri (*Chao Chai Hu*), and bran stir-fried Rhizoma Atractylodis Macrocephalae (*Fu Chao Bai Zhu*)

as in *Bu Zhong Yi Qi Tang* (Supplement the Center & Boost the Qi Decoction [38])

2. A) With uncooked Radix Angelicae Sinensis (*Sheng Dang Gui*) and stir-fried Semen Cannabis Sativae (*Chao Huo Ma Ren*) as in *Run Zao Tang* (Moisten Dryness Decoction [270])
B) With uncooked Herba Cistanchis (*Sheng Rou Cong Rong*) and salt[-processed] Radix Achyranthis Bidentatae (*Yan Huai Niu Xi*) as in *Ji Chuan Jian* (Benefit the River [Flow] Decoction [165])

Dosage: 3-5g

Note: 1. Cimicifuga does not have the particular function of treating constipation. For this complaint it is used as the messenger. In this case, Cimicifuga guides the action of the other medicinals to the bowels of the *yang ming* and, more precisely in this case, to the large intestine. Honey mix-frying makes this medicinal more moistening.

3
Heat-clearing Medicinals

Radix Cynanchi Atrati *(Bai Wei)*

Uncooked *(Sheng)*

Names: *Bai Wei, Xiang Bai Wei, Nen Bai Wei*

Flavors & nature: Bitter and slightly salty; cold

Functions: Cools the blood, frees strangury (*lin*)

Indications:

1. Strangury with hematuria (*xue lin*) due to heat in the blood. In this case, heat damages the network vessels or *luo* causing dysuria, pricking pain...

2. Heat strangury (*re lin*) due to heat accumulating in the bladder with urgent need to urinate, frequent urination, dysuria, a burning sensation in the urethra...

Typical combinations:

1. With uncooked Rhizoma Imperatae Cylindricae (*Sheng Bai Mao Gen*), carbonized Cortex Radicis Moutan (*Mu Dan Pi Tan*), carbonized Herba Cirsii Japonici (*Da Ji Tan*), and Folium Pyrossiae (*Shi Wei*)

2. With Talcum (*Hua Shi*), Caulis Akebiae Mutong (*Mu Tong*), uncooked Fructus Gardeniae Jasminoidis (*Sheng Shan Zhi Zi*), and Herba Dianthi (*Qu Mai*)

Dosage: 5-10g and up to 30g in severe cases

Honey Mix-fried *(Mi Zhi)*

Names: *Mi Zhi Bai Wei, Zhi Bai Wei*

Flavors & nature: Sweet, bitter, and slightly salty; cold

Functions: Enriches yin, clears vacuity heat

Indications:

1. Postpartum fever[1] due to blood vacuity with vertigo, fainting...

2. Evening fever due to either A) lung/kidney yin vacuity with red cheeks, cough, shortness of breath, difficult to expectorate mucus or bloody mucus or B) liver/kidney yin vacuity with dizziness, vertigo, tinnitus, soreness and weakness of the low back and knees, spermatorrhea...

3. Low-grade, persistent fever due to damage of yin fluids by heat. The signs appearing in the convalescent stage of a warm disease include thirst, red tongue, dry mouth...

Typical combinations:

1. With uncooked Radix Angelicae Sinensis (-*Sheng Dang Gui*) and Radix Panacis Ginseng (*Ren Shen*) as in *Bai Wei Tang* (Cynanchus Decoction [19])

Radix Cynanchi Atrati continued . . .

2. A) With Amyda tortoise blood processed Radix Stellariae (*Bie Xue Ban Yin Chai Hu*), Cortex Radicis Lycii (*Di Gu Pi*), uncooked Carapax Amydae Sinensis (*Sheng Bie Jia*), and uncooked Tuber Ophiopogonis Japonicae (*Sheng Mai Men Dong*)

B) With Fructus Lycii Chinensis (*Gou Qi Zi*), steamed Fructus Corni Officinalis (*Zheng Shan Zhu Yu*), prepared Radix Rehmanniae (*Shu Di Huang*), and uncooked Radix Albus Paeoniae Lactiflorae (*Sheng Bai Shao Yao*)

3. With Amyda tortoise blood processed Herba Artemisiae Apiaceae (*Bie Xue Ban Qing Hao*), stir-fried Rhizoma Anemarrhenae (*Chao Zhi Mu*), uncooked Radix Rehmanniae (*Sheng Di Huang*), and uncooked Cortex Radicis Moutan (*Sheng Mu Dan Pi*).

Dosage: 6-15g and up to 30g in severe cases

Note: 1. The use of stir-fried [till] yellow Radix Cynanchi Atrati (*Chao Huang Bai Wei*) for this indication can be advantageous.

Radix Rubrus Paeoniae Lactiflorae *(Chi Shao Yao)*

—————————— Uncooked *(Sheng)* ——————————

Names: *Sheng Chi Shao, Chi Shao Yao, Chi Shao*

Flavors & nature: Bitter; slightly cold

Functions: Clears heat, cools the blood, quickens the blood

Indications:

1. Fever due to heat in the blood level with macules, hematemesis, epistaxis...

2. Red, swollen, painful eyes due to wind heat, which attacks the top of the body, or liver fire, which rises upward with photophobia, lacrimation...

3. Inflammation of the skin (pyogenic) due to heat toxins in the blood with pain, redness, heat, swelling, production of pus, abscess...

Typical combinations:

1. With uncooked Cortex Radicis Moutan (*Sheng Mu Dan Pi*), Cornu Rhinocerotis (*Xi Jiao*)

[substitute Cornu Bubali (*Shui Niu Jiao*)], and uncooked Radix Rehmanniae (*Sheng Di Huang*) as in *Xi Jiao Di Huang Tang* (Rhinoceros Horn & Rehmannia Decoction [362])

2. With Herba Menthae Haplocalycis (*Bo He*), stir-fried Flos Chrysanthemi Morifolii (*Chao Ju Hua*), Spica Prunellae Vulgaris (*Xia Gu Cao*), and uncooked Semen Cassiae Torae (*Sheng Jue Ming Zi*)

3. With Spina Gleditschiae Chinensis (*Zao Jiao Ci*), uncooked Flos Lonicerae Japonicae (*Sheng Jin Yin Hua*), Radix Trichosanthis Kirlowii (*Tian Hua Fen*), and Radix Angelicae Dahuricae (*Bai Zhi*) as in *Xian Fang Huo Ming Yin* (Immortal Formula for Saving Life Drink [364])

Dosage: 5-10g and up to 30g in severe cases

Addendum: When a large dose of blood-cooling medicinals are used, Red Peony should be prescribed in order to quicken the blood and thus prevent stasis due to the cold nature of such medicinals.

Radix Rubrus Paeoniae Lactiflorae continued . . .

Wine Mix-fried (*Jiu Zhi*)

Names: *Jiu Zhi Chi Shao, Jiu Chi Shao*

Flavors & nature: Bitter; neutral

Functions: Quickens the blood, dispels stasis

Indications:

1. Dysmenorrhea, amenorrhea due to qi stagnation, blood stasis, which causes a disharmony of the *chong* and *ren* with pain in the lower abdomen, scanty menstruation, dark colored blood...

2. Pain in the chest and lateral costal regions due to heart blood stasis with severe pain, cold limbs...

3. Headache due to blood stasis with fixed pain, recalcitrant, chronic, worse in the evening...

4. Traumatic injury with blood stasis, pain, swelling...

5. Epigastric pain due to blood stasis in the stomach with fixed, severe pain, acid vomiting...

Typical combinations:

1. With wine[-processed] Radix Angelicae Sinensis (*Jiu Dang Gui*), uncooked Semen Pruni Persicae (*Sheng Tao Ren*), and Flos Carthami Tinctorii (*Hong Hua*)

2. With Flos Carthami Tinctorii (*Hong Hua*), Radix Pseudoginseng (*San Qi*), vinegar[-processed] Resina Olibani (*Cu Ru Xiang*), and wine[-processed] Radix Salviae Miltiorrhizae (*Jiu Dan Shen*)

3. With wine[-processed] Radix Ligustici Wallichii (*Jiu Chuan Xiong*), Radix Angelicae Dahuricae (*Bai Zhi*), and Flos Carthami Tinctorii (*Hong Hua*)

4. With vinegar[-processed] Resina Myrrha (*Cu Mo Yao*), vinegar[-processed] Resina Olibani (*Cu Ru Xiang*), and Lignum Sappanis (*Su Mu*)

5. With vinegar[-processed] Rhizoma Corydalis Yanhusuo (*Cu Yan Hu Suo*), stir-fried Resina Olibani (*Chao Ru Xiang*), and uncooked Os Sepiae Seu Sepiellae (*Sheng Hai Piao Xiao*)

Dosage: 5-10g and up to 30g in severe cases

Cortex Phellodendri (*Huang Bai*)

Uncooked (*Sheng*)

Names: *Sheng Huang Bai, Huang Bai, Chuan Huang Bai*

Flavors & nature: Bitter; cold, drying, and downbearing

Functions: Clears heat, eliminates dampness, resolves toxins

Indications:

1. Vexation due to heat toxins with anxiety, insomnia, disturbed sleep or hematemesis, epistaxis, skin eruptions...

2. Jaundice due to damp heat with fever, agitation, concentrated urine...

Cortex Phellodendri continued . . .

3. Abnormal vaginal discharge[1] due to damp heat with deficiency of the *dai mai*, low back pain...

4. Dysentery or diarrhea[1] due to heat toxins with pussy, bloody stools, abdominal pain, a burning sensation around the anus...

5. Skin inflammation due to damp heat with oozing dermatoses, pruritus...

Typical combinations:

1. With uncooked Rhizoma Coptidis Chinensis (*Sheng Huang Lian*), uncooked Radix Scutellariae Baicalensis (*Sheng Huang Qin*), and stir-fried Fructus Gardeniae Jasminoidis (*Chao Zhi Zi*) as in *Huang Lian Jie Du Tang* (Coptis Resolve Toxins Decoction [152])

2. With uncooked Fructus Gardeniae Jasminoidis (*Sheng Shan Zhi Zi*) as in *Zhi Zi Bai Pi Tang* (Gardenia & Phellodendron Decoction [440])

3. With stir-fried Semen Plantaginis (*Chao Che Qian Zi*), uncooked Semen Euryalis Ferocis (-*Sheng Qian Shi*), and stir-fried Semen Gingkonis Bilobae (*Chao Bai Guo*) as in *Yi Huang San* (-Change Yellow Powder [400])

4. With Radix Pulsatillae Chinensis (*Bai Tou Weng*), stir-fried Rhizoma Coptidis Chinensis (*Chao Huang Lian*), and Cortex Fraxini (*Qin Pi*) as in *Bai Tou Weng Tang* (Pulsatilla Decoction [18])

5. With Radix Sophorae Flavescentis (*Ku Shen*), Fructus Cnidii Monnieri (*She Chuang Zi*), and Cortex Radicis Dictamni (*Bai Xian Pi*)

Dosage: 6-5g and up to 30g in severe cases

Note: 1. Stir-fried [till] scorched Phellodendron (*Chao Jiao Huang Bai*) can be used to reinforce this medicinal's astringing function.

Salt Mix-fried (Yan Zhi)

Names: *Yan Huang Bai, Yan Zhi Huang Bai, Zhi Huang Bai*

Flavors & nature: Bitter and slightly salty; cold; drying

Functions: Drains heat, eliminates dampness

Indications:

1. Vacuity fire due to either A) kidney yin vacuity with steaming bone fever, evening fever, spermatorrhea or B) kidney yin vacuity with evening fever, night sweats, cough, hemoptysis...

2. Dysuria due to damp heat in the bladder and kidney vacuity with oliguria, dark colored urine...

3. Atony of the feet and knees due to damp heat in the lower burner, which damages the sinews with weakness of the lower extremities, paralysis or atony of the legs...

Typical combinations:

1. A) With salt[-processed] Rhizoma Anemarrhenae (*Yan Zhi Mu*) and prepared Radix Rehmanniae (*Shu Di Huang*) as in *Zhi Bai Di Huang Wan* (Anemarrhena & Phellodendron Rehmannia Pills [431])
B) With vinegar dip calcined Plastrum Testudinis (*Cu Cui Gui Ban*), salt[-processed] Rhizoma Anemarrhenae (*Yan Zhi Mu*), and prepared Radix Rehmanniae (*Shu Di Huang*) as in *Da Bu Yin Wan* (Great Supplement Yin Pills [59])

Cortex Phellodendri continued . . .

2. With salt[-processed] Rhizoma Anemarrhenae (*Yan Zhi Mu*) and Cortex Cinnamomi (*Rou Gui*) as in *Tong Guan Wan* (Open the Gate Pills [330])

3. With salt[-processed] Radix Achyranthis Bidentatae (*Yan Huai Niu Xi*) and uncooked Rhizoma Atractylodis (*Sheng Cang Zhu*) as in *San Miao Wan* (Three Marvels Pills [273])

Dosage: 6-15g and up to 30g in severe cases

_____ **Stir-fried [till] Carbonized** *(Chao Tan)* _____

Names: *Huang Bai Tan, Chuan Bai Tan*

Flavors & nature: Bitter and astringent; cold tending to neutral

Functions: Clears heat, eliminates dampness, stops bleeding

Indications:

1. Bloody stools due to damp heat in the large intestine with loss of bright red colored blood...

2. Metrorrhagia, menorrhagia due to heat in the blood, which disturbs the *chong* and *ren* with loss of bright red colored blood...

Typical combinations:

1. With uncooked Radix Sanguisorbae (*Sheng Di Yu*), carbonized Fructus Immaturus Sophorae Japonicae (*Huai Jiao Tan*), and uncooked Rhizoma Coptidis Chinensis (*Sheng Huang Lian*)

2. With carbonized Radix Scutellariae Baicalensis (*Huang Qin Tan*), uncooked Radix Albus Paeoniae Lactiflorae (*Sheng Bai Shao Yao*), and stir-fried Cortex Ailanthi Altissimi (*Chao Chun Gen Pi*)

Dosage: 6-15g and up to 30g in severe cases

Addenda: Wine mix-fried Phellodendron (*Jiu Zhi Huang Bai*) can also be used to treat diseases in the upper part of the body and is more effective for quickening the blood.

Honey mix-fried Phellodendron (*Mi Zhi Huang Bai*) can be used to treat diseases located in the middle burner.

Rhizoma Coptidis Chinensis *(Huang Lian)*

_____ **Uncooked** *(Sheng)* _____

Names: *Sheng Huang Lian, Huang Lian, Chuan Huang Lian, Ji Zhao Lian*

Flavors & nature: Very bitter; very cold

Functions: Drains fire, resolves toxins, clears heat, eliminates dampness

Indications:

1. Heat toxins with high fever, agitation, de-lirium, loss of consciousness...

2. Heat simultaneously in the qi and blood levels with high fever, agitation, thirst, skin eruptions, hematemesis, epistaxis...

3. Hemorrhage due to heat in the blood with hematemesis, epistaxis, hematuria, and/or bloody stools...

Rhizoma Coptidis Chinensis continued . . .

4. Diarrhea or dysentery[1] due to either A) heat toxins or damp heat with pussy, bloody stools, a burning sensation around the anus or B) damp heat and stagnation of qi in the large intestine with abdominal pain, tenesmus...

5. Toothache due to replete heat in the stomach with red, swollen gums, abscess...

Typical combinations:

1. With uncooked Radix Scutellariae Baicalensis (*Sheng Huang Qin*) and uncooked Cortex Phellodendri (*Sheng Huang Bai*) as in *Huang Lian Jie Du Tang* (Coptis Resolve Toxins Decoction [152])

2. With uncooked Gypsum Fibrosum (*Sheng Shi Gao*) and Cornu Rhinocerotis (*Xi Jiao*) [substitute Cornu Bubali (*Shui Niu Jiao*)] as in *Qing Wen Bai Du Yin* (Clear Warmth & Vanquish Toxins Drink [257])

3. With wine[-processed] Radix Et Rhizoma Rhei (*Jiu Da Huang*) and carbonized Radix Scutellariae Baicalensis (*Huang Qin Tan*) as in *Xie Xin Tang* (Drain the Heart Decoction [382])

4. A) With Radix Pulsatillae Chinensis (*Bai Tou Weng*) and Cortex Fraxini (*Qin Pi* as in *Bai Tou Weng Tang* (Pulsatilla Decoction [18])
B) With roasted Radix Saussureae Seu Vladimiriae (*Wei Mu Xiang*) as in *Xiang Lian Wan* (Saussurea & Coptis Pills [367])

5. With uncooked Gypsum Fibrosum (*Sheng Shi Gao*) and uncooked Rhizoma Cimicifugae (*Sheng Sheng Ma*) as in *Qing Wei San* (Clear the Stomach Powder [256])

Dosage: 3-10g and up to 15g in severe cases

Note: 1. In this case, one can equally use stir-fried [till] yellow Coptis (*Chao Huang Huang Lian*) in order to increase this medicinal's astringent effect.

─────────────── **Ginger Mix-fried (*Jiang Zhi*)** ───────────────

Names: *Jiang Zhi Huang Lian, Jiang Chuan Lian, Jiang Huang Lian*

Flavors & nature: Bitter and slightly acrid; cool tending to neutral

Functions: Clears heat, eliminates dampness, harmonizes the stomach, stops vomiting

Indications: Nausea and vomiting due to 1) damp heat in the middle burner with fullness and oppression of the chest and epigastrium, 2) stomach heat with regurgitation, thirst, 3) liver attacking the stomach with acid vomiting, or 4) vomiting during pregnancy

Typical combinations:

1. With ginger[-processed] Rhizoma Pinelliae Ternatae (*Jiang Ban Xia*) as in *Ban Xia Xie Xin Tang* (Pinellia Drain the Heart Decoction [28])

2. With ginger[-processed] Caulis In Taeniis Bambusae (*Jiang Zhu Ru*)

3. With processed Fructus Evodiae Rutecarpae (*Zhi Wu Zhu Yu*)

4. With Caulis Et Folium Perillae Frutescentis (*Zi Su*)

Dosage: 3-10g and up to 15g in severe cases

Rhizoma Coptidis Chinensis continued . .

_____ Wine Mix-fried *(Jiu Zhi)* _____

Names: *Jiu Zhi Huang Lian, Jiu Huang Lian*

Flavors & nature: Bitter and slightly acrid; cool tending to neutral

Functions: Clears the heart, resolves vexation, clears the head and eyes

Indications:

1. Heart palpitations and insomnia due to A) effulgent heart fire damaging yin and blood with vexation, B) non-communication of the heart and kidneys with vexation, cold limbs, C) non-communication of the heart and kidneys with anxiety, night sweats, heat in the five centers, tidal heat...

2. Red, swollen, painful eyes due to accumulation of heat or damp heat in the liver channel with lacrimation, photophobia, aphthae, glossitis...

Typical combinations:

1. A) With Cinnabar (*Zhu Sha*) and uncooked Radix Rehmanniae (*Sheng Di Huang*) as in *An Shen Wan* (Quiet the Spirit Pills [2])
B) With Cortex Cinnamomi (*Rou Gui*) as in *Jiao Tai Wan* (Supreme Communication Pills [174])
C) With uncooked Gelatinum Corii Asini (*Sheng E Jiao*) and Egg Yolk (*Ji Zi Huang*) as in *Huang Lian E Jiao Tang* (Coptis & Donkey Skin Glue Decoction [151])

2. With Fructus Gardeniae Jasminoidis (*Shan Zhi Zi*), Herba Equiseti Hiemalis (*Mu Zei*), and Flos Buddleiae Officinalis (*Mi Meng Hua*)

Dosage: 3-10g and up to 15g in severe cases

_____ Evodia Mix-fried *(Zhu Yu Zhi)*[1] _____

Names: *Zhu Yu Huang Lian, Zhu Yu Zhi Huang Lian*

Flavors & nature: Bitter; cool tending to neutral

Functions: Clears and resolves depressive heat in the liver, clears heat and eliminates dampness

Indications:

1. Acid vomiting due to depressive heat in the liver and disharmony between the liver and stomach with acid regurgitation, epigastric and lateral costal distention and pain...

2. Food stagnation with accumulation of dampness which has transformed into heat, epigastric distention, diarrhea (if dampness predominates), constipation (if heat predominates), abdominal pain with a sensation of heaviness...

Typical combinations:

1. With processed Fructus Evodiae Rutecarpae (*Zhi Wu Zhu Yu*) as in *Zuo Jin Wan* (Left Gold Pills [452])

2. With stir-fried Semen Arecae Catechu (*Chao Bing Lang*), uncooked Radix Saussureae Seu Vladimiriae (*Sheng Mu Xiang*), and uncooked Pericarpium Viridis Citri Reticulatae (*Sheng Qing Pi*) as in *Mu Xiang Bing Lang Wan* (Saussurea & Arecae Pills [225])

Dosage: 3-10g and up to 15g in severe cases

Note: 1. This refers to Coptis treated with Fructus Evodiae Rutecarpae (*Wu Zhu Yu*). This prepara-

Rhizoma Coptidis Chinensis continued . . .

tion lessens the cold nature of Coptis, which tends to damage the stomach, while it also helps to downbear counterflow qi of the stomach.

Addendum: Other methods of preparation of this medicinal are used. For instance, stir-fried [till]

yellow Coptis (*Chao Huang Huang Lian*) is used to lessen Coptis' bitter flavor and cold nature in order to protect the middle burner. This is most notably used in case of abdominal pain. Among others, carbonized Coptis (*Huang Lian Tan*) is sometimes used to clear heat and stop bleeding.

Radix Scutellariae Baicalensis *(Huang Qin)*

_____ Uncooked *(Sheng)* _____

Names: *Sheng Huang Qin, Huang Qin, Dan Qin, Ku Qin, Tiao Qin, Zi Qin*

Flavors & nature: Bitter; cold

Functions: Clears heat, drains fire, resolves toxins

Indications:

1. High fever due to either A) heat in the triple heater with delirium, irritability, agitation, dry mouth and throat, insomnia or B) heat in the level of the qi and blood with skin eruptions, epistaxis, hematemesis, headache, intense thirst, irritability, delirium...

2. Alternating fever and chills due to *shao yang* pattern with nausea, vomiting, a bitter taste in the mouth, lateral costal pain...

3. Jaundice due to accumulation of damp heat in the liver and gallbladder with yellow skin and eyes, darkish urine...

Typical combinations:

1. A) With uncooked Rhizoma Coptidis Chinensis (*Sheng Huang Lian*) and uncooked Cortex Phellodendri (*Sheng Huang Bai*) as in *Huang Lian Jie Du Tang* (Coptis Resolve Toxins Decoction [152]) B) With Cornu Rhinocerotis (*Xi Jiao*) [substitute Cornu Bubali (*Shui Niu Jiao*)] and uncooked Gypsum Fibrosum (*Sheng Shi Gao*) as in *Qing Wen Bai Du San* (Clear Warmth & Vanquish Toxins Powder [257])

2. With uncooked Fructus Amomi Tsao-ko (*Sheng Cao Guo*), uncooked Radix Bupleuri (*Sheng Chai Hu*), and ginger[-processed] Cortex Magnoliae Officinalis (*Jiang Hou Po*) as in *Qing Pi Tang* (Clear the Spleen Decoction [253])

3. With Herba Artemisiae Capillaris (*Yin Chen Hao*), uncooked Fructus Gardeniae Jasminoidis (*Sheng Shan Zhi Zi*), and Radix Gentianae Scabrae (*Long Dan Cao*) as in *Bi Xiao Wan* (Compelling Results Pills [30])

Dosage: 6-12g and up to 30g in severe cases

_____ Stir-fried [till] Scorched *(Chao Jiao)* _____

Names: *Chao Huang Qin, Chao Dan Qin*

Flavors & nature: Bitter; cool tending to neutral

Functions: Clears heat, eliminates dampness, harmonizes the stomach, quiets the fetus

Indications:

1. Dysentery due to accumulation of damp heat with abdominal pain, pussy, bloody diarrhea, tenesmus...

Radix Scutellariae Baicalensis continued . . .

2. Fever due to evil damp heat (*e.g.*, a *wen bing* or warm disease) with latent fever aggravated in the afternoon, to the touch the patient's skin feels only initially warm but becomes increasingly hot, chest and epigastric oppression and distention, no thirst...

3. Threatened spontaneous abortion or restless fetus caused by qi and blood vacuity accompanied by heat with loss of appetite, nausea, vomiting, a pale tongue, pale complexion...

Typical combinations:

1. With stir-fried Radix Albus Paeoniae Lacti-florae (*Chao Bai Shao Yao*) and uncooked Rhizoma Coptidis Chinensis (*Sheng Huang Lian*) as in *Shao Yao Tang* (Peony Decoction [285])

2. With Talcum (*Hua Shi*) and Medulla Tetrapanacis Papyriferi (*Tong Cao*) as in *Huang Qin Hua Shi Tang* (Scutellaria & Talcum Decoction [159])

3. With uncooked Radix Angelicae Sinensis (*Sheng Dang Gui*), wine[-processed] Radix Albus Paeoniae Lactiflorae (*Jiu Bai Shao Yao*), and bran stir-fried Rhizoma Atractylodis Macrocephalae (*Fu Chao Bai Zhu*) as in *Dang Gui San* (Dang Gui Powder [71])

Dosage: 6-12g and up to 30g in severe cases

Wine Mix-fried (Jiu Zhi)

Names: *Jiu Zhi Huang Qin, Jiu Huang Qin, Jiu Qin*

Flavors & nature: Bitter and slightly acrid; cool

Functions: Clears the upper burner, clears the lungs, clears the liver

Indications:

1. Cough due to lung heat and stagnation of phlegm heat with chest oppression, thick, yellow mucus, possible constipation...

2. Headache due to liver fire with vertigo, a bitter taste in the mouth, irritability...

3. Red, swollen, painful eyes due to heat in the liver channel with headache, a bitter taste in the mouth, irritability...

Typical combinations:

1. With uncooked Semen Pruni Armeniacae (*Sheng Xing Ren*), uncooked Radix Platycodi Grandiflori (*Sheng Jie Geng*), and uncooked Fructus Gardeniae Jasminoidis (*Sheng Shan Zhi Zi*) as in *Huang Qin Xie Fei Tang* (Scutellaria Drain the Lungs Decoction [161])

2. With wine[-processed] Radix Gentianae Scabrae (*Jiu Long Dan Cao*), uncooked Bombyx Batryticatus (*Sheng Jiang Can*), white Flos Chrysanthemi Morifolii (*Bai Ju Hua*), and Spica Prunellae Vulgaris (*Xia Ku Cao*)

3. With uncooked Semen Cassiae Torae (*Sheng Jue Ming Zi*), wine[-processed] Radix Gentianae Scabrae (*Jiu Long Dan Cao*), Spica Prunellae Vulgaris (*Xia Ku Cao*), and Herba Equiseti Hiemalis (*Mu Zei*)

Stir-fried [till] Carbonized (Chao Tan)

Names: *Huang Qin Tan, Qin Tan, Ku Qin Tan*

Flavors & nature: Bitter and slightly astringent; slightly cold

Functions: Clears heat, stops bleeding

Indications:

1. Hemorrhages due to heat stirring the blood and damaging the network vessels with hematemesis,

Radix Scutellariae Baicalensis continued . . .

epistaxis, hemoptysis, hematuria, bloody hemorrhoids...

2. Metrorrhagia and menorrhagia due to heat penetrating the *chong* and *ren* with bleeding of bright red blood

Typical combinations:

1. With carbonized Radix Rubiae Cordifoliae (*Qian Cao Gen Tan*), uncooked Cacumen Biotae Orientalis (*Sheng Ce Bai Ye*), uncooked Nodus Nelumbinis Nuciferae (*Sheng Ou Jie*), and uncooked Rhizoma Imperatae Cylindricae (*Sheng Bai Mao Gen*)

2. With carbonized Radix Angelicae Sinensis (*Dang Gui Tan*), uncooked Radix Rehmanniae (*Sheng Di Huang*), Pollen Typhae stir-fried Gelatinum Corii Asini (*Pu Huang Chao E Jiao*), and stir-fried Cortex Ailanthi Altissimi (*Chao Chun Gen Pi*)

Dosage: 3-13g and up to 30g in severe cases

Addenda: There are two types of Scutellaria. *Ku Qin* or withered Scutellaria is light and hollow. Its color is dark. Its propensity is centrifugal and its tropism is for the hand *tai yin* channel. It drains fire from the lungs, clears the upper burner, and resolves heat from the muscle layer and the exterior. This function is expressed in the formula *Jiu Wei Qiang Huo Tang* (Nine Flavors Notopterygium Decoction [185]).

Zi Qin or young Scutellaria and *Tiao Qin* or strip Scutellaria is dense, full, and hard. Its color is yellow and slightly green. Its propensity is centripetal and its tropism is for the hand *yang ming* channel. It drains fire from the large intestine, clears the lower burner, and treats heat type dysentery. This function is expressed, for example, in the formula *Huang Qin Tang* (Scutellaria Decoction [160]).

Bran stir-frying Scutellaria (*Fu Chao Huang Qin*) lessens its cooling nature if there is a stomach deficiency. Ginger mix-fried Scutellaria can be prescribed in case of vomiting due to stomach heat. In addition, Scutellaria prepared with bile (either pig or cow) is sometimes used to clear heat from the liver and gallbladder, most notably in the case of cholecystitis, hepatitis, etc.

Flos Lonicerae Japonicae (*Jin Yin Hua*)

—————————— Uncooked (*Sheng*) ——————————

Names: *Jin Yin Hua, Yin Hua, Er Hua, Shuang Hua, Er Zhi Hua, Ren Dong Hua*

Flavors & nature: Sweet and slightly bitter; cold

Functions: Clears heat, resolves toxins. Its tropism is for the upper burner and exterior.

Indications:

1. Warm diseases due to wind heat accompanied by toxins with fever, slight aversion to wind and cold, headache, thirst, sore throat...

2. Skin inflammation due to heat toxins with pain, redness, and swelling (furuncles, *yong*, skin lesions, purulent abscesses)...

3. High fever due to evil heat in the constructive qi and blood levels with thirst, skin eruptions, a dry, scarlet red tongue, mental confusion, insomnia...

4. Mastitis of the inflammatory and purulent stage...

Typical combinations:

1. With uncooked Fructus Forsythiae Suspensae

Flos Lonicerae Japonicae continued . . .

(*Sheng Lian Qiao*) and Herba Menthae Haplocalycis (*Bo He*) as in *Yin Qiao San* (Lonicera & Forsythia Powder [412])

2. With Herba Cum Radice Taraxaci Mongolici (*Pu Gong Ying*), Herba Violae Yedoensis (*Zi Hua Di Ding*), and Flos Chrysanthemi Indici (*Ye Ju Hua*) as in *Wu Wei Xiao Du Yin* (Five Flavors Disperse Toxins Drink [358])

3. With uncooked Gypsum Fibrosum (*Sheng Shi Gao*), uncooked Radix Rehmanniae (*Sheng Di Huang*), and uncooked Cortex Radicis Moutan (*Sheng Mu Dan Pi*)

4. With uncooked Fructus Forsythiae Suspensae (*Sheng Lian Qiao*), Herba Cum Radice Taraxaci Mongolici (*Pu Gong Ying*), and uncooked Fructus Trichosanthis Kirlowii (*Sheng Gua Lou*)

Dosage: 10-30g and up to 100g in severe cases

_____ Stir-fried [till] Yellow *(Chao Huang)* _____

Names: *Chao Yin Hua, Chao Shuang Hua, Chao Ren Dong Hua*

Flavors & nature: Sweet and slightly bitter; cool tending to neutral

Functions: Clears heat, resolves toxins. Its tropism is for the middle burner and qi level.

Indications: Warm diseases accompanied by stomach troubles with fever, vexation, chest and diaphragm oppression and distention, thirst,

regurgitation, nausea, a red tongue with dry coating, a rapid (*shu*), slippery (*hua*) pulse...

Typical combinations: With bran stir-fried Radix Scutellariae Baicalensis (*Fu Chao Huang Qin*), uncooked Fructus Gardeniae Jasminoidis (*Sheng Shan Zhi Zi*), uncooked Gypsum Fibrosum (*Sheng Shi Gao*), ginger[-processed] Caulis In Taeniis Bambusae (*Jiang Zhu Ru*), and Rhizoma Phragmitis Communis (*Lu Gen*)

Dosage: 10-20g and up to 60g in severe cases

_____ Stir-fried [till] Carbonized *(Chao Tan)* _____

Names: *Yin Hua Tan, Er Hua Tan*

Flavors & nature: Sweet, bitter, and astringent; slightly cold

Functions: Clears heat, resolves toxins, cools the blood, stops bleeding. Its tropism is for the lower burner and the blood level.

Indications:

1. Bloody dysentery due to damp heat in the large intestine with pussy, bloody diarrhea with more blood than pus, abdominal pain, tenesmus...

2. Epidemic dysentery due to heat toxins with

stools accompanied by fresh blood, purple and pussy, high fever, thirst, vexation, loss of consciousness or delirium if severe...

Typical combinations:

1. With uncooked Rhizoma Coptidis Chinensis (*Sheng Huang Lian*), Herba Portulacae Oleraceae (*Ma Chi Xian*), roasted Radix Saussureae Seu Vladimiriae (*Wei Mu Xiang*), and Radix Rubrus Paeoniae Lactiflorae (*Chi Shao Yao*)

2. With uncooked Rhizoma Coptidis Chinensis (*Sheng Huang Lian*), uncooked Radix Reh-

Flos Lonicerae Japonicae continued . . .

manniae (*Sheng Di Huang*), Radix Pulsatillae Chinensis (*Bai Tou Weng*), uncooked Cortex Phellodendri (*Sheng Huang Bai*), uncooked Cortex Radicis Moutan (*Sheng Mu Dan Pi*), and uncooked Radix Rubrus Paeoniae Lactiflorae (*Sheng Chi Shao Yao*)

Dosage: 10-15g and up to 60g in severe cases

Semen Cassiae Torae (*Jue Ming Zi*)

Uncooked (*Sheng*)

Names: *Jue Ming Zi, Sheng Jue Ming, Cao Jue Ming*

Flavors & nature: Sweet, bitter, and salty; slightly cold

Functions: Dispels wind, clears the liver, brightens the eyes, moistens the intestines, frees the stool

Indications:

1. Red, swollen, painful eyes due to either A) wind heat affecting the upper body with headache, vertigo or B) liver fire attacking the upper body with dry eyes, photophobia, lacrimation...

2. Constipation due to heat with dry stools

Typical combinations:

1. A) With stir-fried Flos Chrysanthemi Morifolii (*Chao Ju Hua*), uncooked Fructus Viticis (*Sheng Man Jing Zi*), Herba Equiseti Hiemalis (*Mu Zei*), and wine[-processed] Radix Scutellariae Baicalensis (*Jiu Huang Qin*) as in *Jue Ming Zi San* (Cassia Seed Powder [193])
B) With wine[-processed] Radix Gentianae Scabrae (*Jiu Long Dan Cao*), wine[-processed] Rhizoma Coptidis Chinensis (*Jiu Huang Lian*), uncooked Radix Bupleuri (*Sheng Chai Hu*), stir-fried Flos Chrysanthemi Morifolii (*Chao Ju Hua*), and Spica Prunellae Vulgaris (*Xia Ku Cao*)

2. With uncooked Semen Trichosanthis Kirlowii (*Sheng Gua Lou Ren*) and uncooked Semen Cannabis Sativae (*Sheng Huo Ma Ren*)

Dosage: 10-15g and up to 30g in severe cases

Stir-fried [till] Scorched (*Chao Jiao*)

Names: *Chao Jue Ming Zi, Chao Jue Ming, Chao Cao Jue Ming*

Flavors & nature: Sweet, bitter, and salty; neutral

Functions: Nourishes the kidneys, brightens the eyes

Indications: Optic atrophy due to liver/kidney vacuity

Typical combinations: With Fructus Lycii Chinensis (*Gou Qi Zi*), uncooked Semen Astragali (*Sheng Sha Yuan Zi*), uncooked Semen Cuscutae (*Sheng Tu Si Zi*), uncooked Fructus Ligustri Lucidi (*Sheng Nu Zhen Zi*), Fructus Mori Albi (*Sang Shen Zi*), and prepared Radix Rehmanniae (*Shu Di Huang*)

Dosage: 10-15g and up to 30g in severe cases

Fructus Forsythiae Suspensae (Lian Qiao)

_____ Uncooked (Sheng) _____

Names: _Lian Qiao, Qing Lian Qiao, Lian Ke_

Flavors & nature: Bitter; slightly cold

Functions: Clears heat, resolves toxins, disperses swelling, scatters nodulations

Indications:

1. Fever due to wind heat (heat in the defensive qi level) with slight aversion to wind and cold, slight perspiration, headache, slight thirst, sore throat...

2. Erysipelas due to heat toxins with skin inflammation, red, raised macules...

3. Goiter, scrofula, subcutaneous nodules with pain of the neck and nuchal region...

4. Mastitis of the inflammatory and purulent stage

5. _Yong_ due to heat toxins

Typical combinations:

1. With uncooked Flos Lonicerae Japonicae (_Sheng Jin Yin Hua_) and Herba Menthae Haplocalycis (_Bo He_) as in _Yin Qiao San_ (Lonicera & Forsythia Powder [412])

2. With Herba Cum Radice Taraxaci Mongolici (_Pu Gong Ying_), Herba Violae Yedoensis (_Zi Hua Di Ding_), uncooked Cortex Radicis Moutan (_Sheng Mu Dan Pi_), and uncooked Flos Lonicerae Japonicae (_Sheng Jin Yin Hua_)

3. With Radix Scrophulariae Ningpoensis (_Xuan Shen_), Thallus Algae (_Kun Bu_), and Bulbus Fritillariae Thunbergii (_Zhe Bei Mu_)

4. With uncooked Flos Lonicerae Japonicae (_Sheng Jin Yin Hua_), Flos Chrysanthemi Indici (_Ye Ju Hua_), and Herba Cum Radice Taraxaci Mongolici (_Pu Gong Ying_)

5. With Herba Cum Radice Taraxaci Mongolici (_Pu Gong Ying_), Herba Violae Yedoensis (_Zi Hua Di Ding_), and Spina Gleditschiae Chinensis (_Zao Jiao Ci_)

Dosage: 3-15g and up to 30g in severe cases

_____ Cinnabar [Processed] (Zhu Sha)[1] _____

Names: _Zhu Sha Ban Lian Qiao, Zhu Lian Qiao_

Flavors & nature: Bitter and slightly sweet; slightly cold

Functions: Clears heat, resolves toxins, calms the heart, quiets the spirit

Indications: Vexation due to evil heat penetrating the pericardium with high fever, thirst, irritability, insomnia, agitation...

Typical combinations: With uncooked Rhizoma Coptidis Chinensis (_Sheng Huang Lian_), stir-fried Fructus Gardeniae Jasminoidis (_Chao Zhi Zi_), and uncooked Radix Salviae Miltiorrhizae (_Sheng Dan Shen_) as in _Qing Ying Tang_ (Clear the Constructive Decoction [259])

Dosage: 10-15g and up to 20g in severe cases

Note: 1. _Zhu Sha_ refers to Cinnabar. In the preparation of this medicinal, the Forsythia is mixed in a solution of Cinnabar in order to reinforce its function of calming the spirit.

Addenda: 1. For the pattern of evil heat penetrating the pericardium with high fever, delirium, loss of consciousness, etc., one can prescribe either *Lian Qiao Xin* (*i.e.*, the heart or, in other words, the small seed found in the interior of the Fructus Forsythiae Suspensae) or *Zhu Sha Lian Qiao Xin* (the heart of the Forsythia fruit prepared with Cinnabar).

2. There exist two types of Forsythia: *Qing Lian Qiao* (green Forsythia) which is superior for clearing heat and resolving toxins and for treating fever and erysipelas, and *Huang Lian Qiao* (yellow Forsythia) which is better for dispersing swelling, scattering nodulations, and for treating goiter, scrofula, subcutaneous nodules, skin inflammations, *yong...*

Cortex Radicis Moutan *(Mu Dan Pi)*

Uncooked *(Sheng)*

Names: *Mu Dan Pi, Dan Pi, Sheng Dan Pi, Fen Dan Pi*

Flavors & nature: Acrid and bitter; slightly cold

Functions: Clears heat, cools the blood, quickens the blood, dispels stasis

Indications:

1. Fever due to either A) heat in the constructive and blood levels with fever aggravated at night, a dry mouth, delirium, loss of consciousness, skin eruptions, hemorrhages or B) vacuity heat caused by a warm disease which has damaged yin with a low-grade fever without perspiration...

2. Traumatic injury with blood stasis, pain, swelling, and hematoma...

3. Gingivitis due to stomach fire with red, swollen, painful gums, bleeding gums, thirst, fetid breath...

4. Acute appendicitis due to accumulation of heat and blood stasis in the intestines with swollen, painful abdomen, pain aggravated by pressure, constipation...

5. Abdominal mass due to qi stagnation and blood stasis with fixed, palpable mass...

Typical combinations:

1. A) With uncooked Radix Rehmanniae (*Sheng Di Huang*) and uncooked Radix Rubrus Paeoniae Lactiflorae (*Sheng Chi Shao Yao*) as in *Xi Jiao Di Huang Tang* (Rhinoceros Horn & Rehmannia Decoction [362])
B) With Amyda tortoise blood processed Herba Artemisiae Apiaceae (*Bie Xue Ban Qing Hao*) and uncooked Carapax Amydae Sinensis (*Sheng Bie Jia*) as in *Qing Hao Bie Jia Tang* (Artemisia Apiacea & Carapax Amydae Decoction [252])

2. With wine[-processed] Radix Angelicae Sinensis (*Jiu Dang Gui*) and vinegar[-processed] Resina Olibani (*Cu Ru Xiang*) as in *Mu Dan Pi San* (Moutan Powder [221])

3. With uncooked Rhizoma Cimicifugae (*Sheng Sheng Ma*) and uncooked Radix Rehmanniae (-*Sheng Di Huang*)

4. With uncooked Radix Et Rhizoma Rhei (*Sheng Da Huang*) and scalded Semen Pruni Persicae (*Dan Tao Ren*) as in *Da Huang Mu Dan Pi Tang* (Rhubarb & Moutan Decoction [64])

5. With Ramulus Cinnamomi (*Gui Zhi*) and uncooked Semen Pruni Persicae (*Sheng Tao Ren*) as in *Gui Zhi Fu Ling Wan* (Cinnamon Twig & Poria Pills [123])

Dosage: 6-12g and up to 30g in severe cases

_____ Stir-fried [till] Carbonized *(Chao Tan)* _____

Name: *Mu Dan Tan*

Flavors & nature: Bitter and slightly astringent; slightly cold tending to neutral

Functions: Cools the blood, stops bleeding

Indications:

1. Metrorrhagia, menorrhagia[1] due to blood vacuity and cold penetrating the blood with menstrual irregularity, pain in the lower abdomen, dysmenorrhea...

2. Hemorrhage due to heat stirring the blood and damaging the network vessels with hematemesis, epistaxis, hemoptysis, bloody stools, hematuria, metrorrhagia...

Typical combinations:

1. With uncooked Radix Sanguisorbae (*Sheng Di Yu*), carbonized Radix Angelicae Sinensis (*Dang Gui Tan*), and processed Fructus Evodiae Rutecarpae (*Zhi Wu Zhu Yu*) as in *Wen Jing Tang* (Warm the Channels [or Menses] Decoction [341])

2. With uncooked Cacumen Biotae Orientalis (*Sheng Ce Bai Ye*), carbonized Radix Rubiae Cordifoliae (*Qian Cao Gen Tan*, and carbonized Folium Et Petiolus Trachycarpi (*Zong Lu Tan*) as in *Shi Hui San* (Ten Ashes Powder [299])

Dosage: 5-10g and up to 20g in severe cases

Note: 1. Stir-fried [till] yellow Moutan harmonizes the blood and is prescribed for menstrual irregularity, as in *Wen Jing Tang* (Warm the Channels [or Menses] Decoction). It is, therefore, advantageous to prescribe stir-fried [till] yellow Moutan when irregularity of the menstrual cycle is more important in comparison to metrorrhagia. In addition, some practitioners use stir-fried [till] yellow Moutan to reinforce Moutan's action of quickening the blood and dispelling stasis.

Gypsum Fibrosum *(Shi Gao)*

_____ Uncooked *(Sheng)* _____

Names: *Shi Gao, Sheng Shi Gao*

Flavors & nature: Sweet and acrid; very cold

Functions: Clears heat, drains fire, resolves vexation, engenders fluids, stops thirst

Indications:

1. High fever due to either A) heat in the qi level with profuse perspiration, strong thirst, a flooding (*hong*) pulse or B) heat which has penetrated simultaneously the qi and blood levels with ruby red skin eruptions, mental confusion, loss of consciousness, thirst...

2. Cough, asthma due to replete heat in the lungs or wind heat stagnating in the lungs with fever, thirst...

3. Toothache due to stomach fire with agitation, a sensation of heat in the upper body, fetid breath, thirst...

4. Rheumatic complaints of the heat *bi* (*re bi*) type with severe pain, heat, swelling, and redness of the joints, possible fever...

Gypsum Fibrosum continued . . .

Typical combinations:

1. A) With uncooked Rhizoma Anemarrhenae (*Sheng Zhi Mu*) as in *Bai Hu Tang* (White Tiger Decoction [15])
B) With Cornu Rhinocerotis (*Xi Jiao*) [substitute Cornu Bubali (*Shui Niu Jiao*)], uncooked Radix Rehmanniae (*Sheng Di Huang*), and uncooked Rhizoma Anemarrhenae (*Sheng Zhi Mu*) as in *Hua Ban Tang* (Transform Macules Decoction [146])

2. With honey mix-fried Herba Ephedrae (*Mi Zhi Ma Huang*) and uncooked Semen Pruni Armeniacae (*Sheng Xing Ren*) as in *Ma Xing Shi Gan Tang* (Ephedra, Armeniaca, Gypsum & Licorice Decoction [216])

3. With uncooked Rhizoma Anemarrhenae (*Sheng Zhi Mu*), uncooked Tuber Ophiopogonis Japonicae (*Sheng Mai Men Dong*), and uncooked Radix Rehmanniae (*Sheng Di Huang*) as in *Yu Nu Jian* (Jade Maiden Decoction [416])

4. With Caulis Lonicerae Japonicae (*Ren Dong Teng*), Lumbricus (*Di Long*), and Caulis Sargentodoxae (*Hong Teng*)

Dosage: 30-60g and up to 250g in case of a severe heat affection in the qi level or in case of inflammatory rheumatic complaints

───────────── Honey Mix-fried *(Mi Zhi)* ─────────────

Names: *Mi Zhi Shi Gao, Mi Shi Gao*

Flavors & nature: Sweet; cold

Functions: Clears heat, precipitates fire, engenders fluids, moistens dryness

Indications:

1. Vacuity fire of the stomach due to stomach yin vacuity with low-grade fever, thirst, vexation, regurgitation, a scarlet red tongue with no coating, a fine (*xi*), rapid (*shu*) pulse...

2. Vacuity heat of the lungs due to yin vacuity of the lungs with evening fever, red cheeks, night sweats, cough with little mucus or mucus streaked with blood...

Typical combinations:

1. With uncooked Tuber Ophiopogonis Japonicae (*Sheng Mai Men Dong*), uncooked Radix Rehmanniae (*Sheng Di Huang*), Rhizoma Phragmitis Communis (*Lu Gen*), and uncooked Rhizoma Polygonati Odorati (*Sheng Yu Zhu*)

2. With Cortex Radicis Lycii (*Di Gu Pi*), honey mix-fried Radix Adenophorae Strictae (*Mi Zhi Nan Sha Shen*), uncooked Semen Pruni Armeniacae (*Sheng Xing Ren*), honey mix-fried Bulbus Lilii (*Mi Zhi Bai He*), and Concha Cyclinae powder stir-fried Gelatinum Corii Asini (*Ge Fen Chao E Jiao*)

Dosage: 15-30g and up to 100g in severe cases

───────────── Calcined *(Duan)*[1] ─────────────

Name: *Duan Shi Gao*

Flavors & nature: Sweet and slightly astringent; cool tending to neutral

Functions: Treats sores and dermatoses, engenders new tissue

Gypsum Fibrosum continued . . .

Indications:

1. Purulent skin infections for which Gypsum clears heat and eliminates necrotic tissue, evacuates pus and engenders new tissue

2. Purulent eczema for which Gypsum purifies sores, eliminates necrotic tissue, and engenders new tissue

Typical combinations:

1. With *Sheng Yao* (Divine Medicine)[2] as in *Jiu Yi Dan* (Nine [to] One Powder [187]) or used by itself

2. With calcined Smithsonitum (*Duan Lu Gan Shi*) and uncooked Hallyositum Rubrum (*Sheng Chi Shi Zhi*) as in *San Shi San* (Three Stones Powder [273a])

Dosage: Use externally as necessary. The quantity should be equal to the need. It is not possible to overdose when used topically.

Notes: 1. Calcined Gypsum is only used externally. 2. *Sheng Yao* (a.k.a. *Ling Yao* [Sacred Medicine] or *San Xian Dan* [Three Immortals Elixir]) is composed of several minerals: Alumen (*Ming Fan*), Mercury (*Shui Yin*), and Nitre (*Xiao Shi*). Toxic, this remedy is only used externally to resolve toxins, evacuate pus, eliminate necrotic tissue, and engender new tissue.

Rhizoma Anemarrhenae *(Zhi Mu)*
———————— Uncooked *(Sheng)* ————————

Names: *Zhi Mu, Zhi Mu Rou, Fei Zhi Mu*

Flavors & nature: Bitter; cold

Functions: Clears heat, drains fire, resolves toxins

Indications:

1. Cough, asthma due to replete heat in the lungs with chest oppression, vexation, fever, dry mouth, a slippery (*hua*), rapid (*shu*) pulse...

2. High fever due to heat in the qi level with no chills, profuse perspiration, strong thirst, a flooding (*hong*), rapid (*shu*) pulse...

3. Constipation due to warm disease which has damaged the fluids and dryness of the large intestine with dry mouth and throat, dry, hard stools...

Typical combinations:

1. With honey mix-fried Cortex Radicis Mori Albi (*Mi Zhi Sang Bai Pi*), wine[-processed] Radix Scutellariae Baicalensis (*Jiu Huang Qin*), and uncooked Radix Peucedani (*Sheng Qian Hu*) or honey mix-fried Cortex Radicis Mori Albi (*Mi Zhi Sang Bai Pi*), uncooked Flos Tussilaginis Farfarae (*Sheng Kuan Dong Hua*), and Bulbus Fritillariae Thunbergii (*Zhe Bei Mu*) as in *Zhi Mu San* (Anemarrhena Powder [433])

2. With uncooked Gypsum Fibrosum (*Sheng Shi Gao*) as in *Bai Hu Tang* (White Tiger Decoction [15])

3. With uncooked Radix Et Rhizoma Rhei (*Sheng Da Huang*), Radix Scrophulariae Ningpoensis (*Xuan Shen*), and uncooked Tuber Ophiopogonis Japonicae (*Sheng Mai Men Dong*) as in *Hu Wei Cheng Qi Tang* (Protect the Stomach & Seize the Qi Decoction [145])

Dosage: 10-15g and up to 30g in severe cases

Rhizoma Anemarrhenae continued . . .

_____ Stir-fried _(Chao)_ _____

Names: _Qing Chao Zhi Mu[1], Fu Chao Zhi Mu[2], Chao Zhi Mu_

Flavors & nature: Bitter; cool tending to neutral

Functions: Enriches yin, moistens dryness

Indications:

1. Cough[1] due to dryness of the lungs caused by heat which has damaged the fluids of the lungs with dry cough, dry mouth and throat, possible yellow phlegm which is difficult to expectorate...

2. Thirst[2] due to heat which has damaged the fluids of the stomach with dry mouth, a desire to drink cool liquids...

Typical combinations:

1. With Bulbus Fritillariae Cirrhosae (_Chuan Bei Mu_) as in _Er Mu San_ (Two _Mu_ Powder [99])

2. With Radix Trichosanthis Kirlowii (_Tian Hua Fen_) and uncooked Radix Dioscoreae Oppositae (_Sheng Shan Yao_) as in _Yu Ye Tang_ (Jade Humors Decoction [419])

Dosage: 10-15g and up to 30g in severe cases

Notes: 1. For cough, stir-fried [till] scorched Anemarrhena (_Chao Jiao Zhi Mu_) is prescribed. 2. For thirst, bran stir-fried Anemarrhena (_Fu Chao Zhi Mu_) is prescribed.

Addendum: Stir-frying Anemarrhena lessens the cooling nature of uncooked Anemarrhena.

_____ Salt Mix-fried _(Yan Zhi)_ _____

Names: _Yan Shui Zhi Mu, Yan Zhi Zhi Mu, Yan Zhi Mu, Xian Zhi Mu_

Flavors & nature: Bitter and slightly salty; cold

Functions: Nourishes the kidneys, downbears fire, moistens dryness

Indications:

1. Evening fever due to vacuity heat caused by yin vacuity of the kidneys with steaming bone fever, night sweats, spermatorrhea, tidal heat, heat in the five centers...

2. Oliguria, anuria due to kidney yin vacuity

accompanied by damp heat in the bladder

Typical combinations:

1. With salt[-processed] Cortex Phellodendri and prepared Radix Rehmanniae (_Shu Di Huang_) as in _Zhi Bai Di Huang Wan_ (Anemarrhena & Phellodendron Rehmannia Pills [431])

2. With Cortex Cinnamomi (_Rou Gui_) and salt[-processed] Cortex Phellodendri (_Yan Huang Bai_) as in _Zi Shen Wan_ (Enrich the Kidneys Pills [447])

Dosage: 10-15g and up to 30g in severe cases

Fructus Gardeniae Jasminoidis (Shan Zhi Zi)

———————— Uncooked (Sheng) ————————

Names: *Zhi Zi, Shan Zhi Zi, Shan Zhi*

Flavors & nature: Bitter; cold

Functions: Drains fire, resolve toxins, disinhibits the bladder, treats jaundice

Indications:

1. High fever[1] due to accumulation of heat in the triple heater with vexation, mental confusion, fever, regurgitation, insomnia, a dry mouth and throat...

2. Jaundice due to damp heat with yellow complexion and eyes, yellow colored, concentrated urine...

3. Dysuria due to damp heat in the bladder or heat strangury (*re lin*) with oliguria, abdominal distention, agitation...

Typical combinations:

1. With uncooked Rhizoma Coptidis Chinensis (*Sheng Huang Lian*), uncooked Cortex Phellodendri (*Sheng Huang Bai*), and uncooked Radix Scutellariae Baicalensis (*Sheng Huang Qin*) as in *Huang Lian Jie Du Tang* (Coptis Resolve Toxins Decoction [152])

2. With Herba Artemisiae Capillaris (*Yin Chen Hao*) and uncooked Radix Et Rhizoma Rhei (*Sheng Da Huang*) as in *Yin Chen Hao Tang* (Artemisia Capillaris Decoction [409])

3. With uncooked Rhizoma Imperatae Cylindricae (*Sheng Bai Mao Gen*) and uncooked Semen Benincasae Hispidae (*Sheng Dong Gua Zi*) as in *Zhi Zi Ren San* (Gardenia Powder [442])

Dosage: 5-10g and up to 20g in severe cases

Note: 1. In case of vacuity heat due to kidney yin vacuity, salt-fried Gardenia (*Yan Zhi Zhi Zi*) is prescribed.

Addenda: 1. In case of heart fire, it is necessary to remove the epicarpium of the fruit.
2. In case of lung fire, it is necessary to keep the epicarpium of the fruit.

———————— Stir-fried [till] Scorched (Chao Jiao) ————————

Names: *Chao Jiao Zhi Zi, Chao Zhi Zi, Jiao Zhi Zi*

Flavors & nature: Less bitter; slightly cold

Functions: Clears heat, resolves vexation, clears the liver

Indications:

1. Red, swollen, painful eyes due to liver heat with photophobia, tearing...

2. Vexation due to warm disease with insomnia, chest and epigastric oppression, a sensation of malaise and of heat in the stomach, acid regurgitation, loss of appetite...

Typical combinations:

1. With Periostracum Cicadae (*Chan Tui*), Fructus Tribuli Terrestris (*Bai Ji Li*), uncooked Semen Cassiae Torae (*Sheng Jue Ming Zi*), and Scapus Et Inflorescentia Eriocaulonis Buergeriani (*Gu Jing Cao*) as in *Zhi Zi Sheng Ji Tang* (Gardenia Overcome Accumulation Decoction [443])

Fructus Gardeniae Jasminoidis continued . . .

2. With clear Semen Praeparatum Sojae (*Qing Dan Dou Chi*) as in *Zhi Zi Chi Tang* (Gardenia & Prepared Soy Beans Decoction [441])

Dosage: 5-10g and up to 20g in severe cases

Addendum: In case of stomach weakness and vomiting, one can prescribe ginger mix-fried Gardenia (*Jiang Zhi Zhi Zi*).

_____ Stir-fried [till] Carbonized *(Chao Tan)* _____

Names: *Zhi Zi Tan, Hei Zhi Zi*

Flavors & nature: Bitter and slightly astringent; slightly cold

Functions: Cools the blood, stops bleeding

Indications:

1. Hemorrhage due to heat which stirs the blood and damages the network vessels with hemoptysis, epistaxis, hematuria, hematemesis...

2. Metrorrhagia, menorrhagia due to heat in the blood

Typical combinations:

1. With uncooked Cacumen Biotae Orientalis (*Sheng Ce Bai Ye*), uncooked Rhizoma Imperatae Cylindricae (*Sheng Bai Mao Gen*), and uncooked Rhizoma Anemarrhenae (*Sheng Zhi Mu*) as in *Liang Xue Tang* (Cool the Blood Decoction [198])

2. With carbonized Radix Et Rhizoma Rhei (*Da Huang Tan*), carbonized Cortex Radicis Moutan (*Mu Dan Pi Tan*), and uncooked Cacumen Biotae Orientalis (*Sheng Ce Bai Ye*) as in *Shi Hui San* (Ten Ashes Powder [299])

4
Precipitating (*i.e.*, Purging) Medicinals

Radix Et Rhizoma Rhei *(Da Huang)*

_____ Uncooked *(Sheng)* _____

Names: *Sheng Da Huang, Da Huang, Sheng Chuan Jun, Sheng Jin Wen*

Flavors & nature: Bitter; cold

Functions: Drains fire, resolves toxins, precipitates accumulations

Indications:

1. Constipation due to: A) replete heat in the stomach and large intestine with dry stool, abdominal distention and pain aggravated by pressure, evening fever, B) accumulation of cold with aversion to cold, cold extremities, or C) food stagnation with epigastric and abdominal distention, indigestion...

2. Acute appendicitis[1] due to heat toxins and blood stasis with pain, distention, and swelling of the abdomen, which is aggravated by pressure...

3. Skin infection, burns[2] due to heat toxins

Typical combinations:

1. A) With Mirabilitum (*Mang Xiao*) and uncooked Fructus Immaturus Citri Seu Ponciri (*Sheng Zhi Shi*) as in *Da Cheng Qi Tang* (Major Seize the Qi Decoction [61])
B) With processed Radix Lateralis Praeparatus

Aconiti Carmichaeli (*Zhi Fu Zi*) as in *Da Huang Fu Zi Tang* (Rhubarb & Aconite Decoction [63])
C) With uncooked Radix Saussureae Seu Vladimiriae (*Sheng Mu Xiang*) and uncooked Pericarpium Viridis Citri Reticulatae (*Sheng Qing Pi*) as in *Mu Xiang Bing Lang Wan* (Saussurea & Areca Pills [225])

2. With uncooked Cortex Radicis Moutan (*Sheng Mu Dan Pi*), scalded Semen Pruni Persicae (*Dan Tao Ren*), and uncooked Semen Benincasae Hispidae (*Sheng Dong Gua Ren*) as in *Da Huang Mu Dan Pi Tang* (Rhubarb & Moutan Decoction [64])

3. For skin infections, use a powder of this ingredient with uncooked Cortex Phellodendri (*Sheng Huang Bai*), uncooked Radix Glycyrrhizae (*Sheng Gan Cao*), and Radix Trichosanthis Kirlowii (*Tian Hua Fen*) mixed in an oil base. For burns, soak Rhubarb in vinegar for 1-3 days and then apply this to the burn. This preparation is contraindicated in case of open sores.

Dosage: 3-30g depending on the degree of severity; 0.5-2g as a powder taken orally

Notes: 1. If heat is less important and blood stasis is more severe, one should prescribe wine mix-fried Rhubarb (*Jiu Zhi Da Huang*). 2. Used externally

Radix Et Rhizoma Rhei continued . . .

_____ Prepared *(Shu)*[1] _____

Names: *Zhi Da Huang, Shu Da Huang, Zhi* or *Shu Chuan Jun, Zhi* or *Shu Jin Wen*

Flavors & nature: Bitter; cool tending to neutral

Functions: Clears heat, eliminates dampness

Indications:

1. Jaundice[2] due to damp heat with yellowish orange complexion and eyes, thirst, abdominal distention, oliguria, constipation...

2. Strangury, dysuria due to damp heat in the bladder with acute pain and distention of the lower abdomen, dark, turbid, or reddish urine, urgent, frequent micturition, oliguria...

3. Abdominal and epigastric distention and fullness due to accumulation of damp heat in the stomach and large intestine followed by food stagnation with diarrhea or constipation, dark, scanty urine...

4. Dysentery, diarrhea due to damp heat in the large intestine with a burning sensation around the anus, abdominal pain, tenesmus, pussy, bloody stools...

Typical combinations:

1. With Herba Artemisiae Capillaris (*Yin Chen Hao*) and uncooked Fructus Gardeniae Jasminoidis (*Sheng Shan Zhi Zi*) as in *Yin Chen Hao Tang* (Artemisia Capillaris Decoction [409])

2 With salt[-processed] Semen Plantaginis (*Yan Che Qian Zi*) and Herba Dianthi (*Qu Mai*) in *Ba Zheng San* (Eight Righteous [Medicinals] Powder [5])

3. With bran stir-fried Fructus Immaturus Citri Seu Ponciri (*Fu Chao Zhi Shi*) and stir-fried Massa Medica Fermentata (*Chao Shen Qu*) as in *Zhi Shi Dao Zhi Wan* (Immature Citrus Abduct Stagnation Pills [434])

4. With roasted Radix Saussureae Seu Vladimiriae (*Wei Mu Xiang*), stir-fried Radix Albus Paeoniae Lactiflorae (*Chao Bai Shao Yao*), and uncooked Rhizoma Coptidis Chinensis (*Sheng Huang Lian*) as in *Shao Yao Tang* (Peony Decoction [285])

Dosage: 5-15g

Notes: 1. This refers to Rhubarb which has been steamed or stewed in rice wine. 2. If heat predominates and jaundice is accompanied by severe constipation, one should prescribe uncooked Rhubarb (*Sheng Da Huang*).

_____ Wine Mix-fried *(Jiu Zhi)* _____

Names: *Jiu Da Huang, Jiu Zhi Da huang, Jiu Chuan Jun*

Flavors & nature: Bitter and slightly acrid; cool tending to neutral

Functions: Quickens the blood, dispels stasis, clears the upper burner

Indications:

1. Mental troubles due to an accumulation of blood with delirium, mental confusion, madness

aggravated at night, fullness and masses in the lower abdomen, oliguria, blackish stools...

2. Abdominal pain postpartum due to blood stasis with pain aggravated by pressure, retention of lochia...

3. Amenorrhea due to blood stasis with dry skin, desquamation, emaciation, a darkish color surrounding the eyes...

4. Traumatic injury with blood stasis

Radix Et Rhizoma Rhei continued . . .

5. Epistaxis, hematemesis[1] due to fire toxins which rise up and damage the network vessels with constipation, vexation...

6. Red, swollen eyes, aphthae, *yong*[1] due to accumulation of heat in the three burners

Typical combinations:

1. With stone-baked Hirudo (*Bei Shui Zhi*), stone-baked Tabanus (*Bei Meng Chong*), and uncooked Semen Pruni Persicae (*Sheng Tao Ren*) as in *Di Dang Tang* (Resistance Decoction [82])

2. With uncooked Semen Pruni Persicae (*Sheng Tao Ren*) and stone-baked Eupolyphaga Seu Opisthoplatia (*Bei Zhe Chong*) as in *Xia Yu Xue Tang* (Precipitate Static Blood Decoction [363])

3. With uncooked Semen Pruni Persicae (*Sheng Tao Ren*) and stone-baked Tabanus (*Bei Meng Chong*) as in *Da Huang Zhe Chong Wan* (Rhubarb & Eupolyphaga Pills [65])

4. With Flos Carthami Tinctorii (*Hong Hua*) and wine[-processed] Radix Angelicae Sinensis (*Jiu Dang Gui*) as in *Fu Yuan Huo Xue Tang* (Restore the Source & Quicken the Blood Decoction [106])

5. With wine[-processed] Rhizoma Coptidis Chinensis (*Jiu Huang Lian*) and wine[-processed] Radix Scutellariae Baicalensis (*Jiu Huang Qin*) as in *Xie Xin Tang* (Drain the Heart Decoction [382])

6. With the same ingredients as in #5 above

Dosage: 5-15g

Note: 1. For this indication, uncooked Rhubarb (*Sheng Da Huang*) is certainly more powerful for clearing heat but its tropism is mainly for the lower burner. Thus the use of wine mix-fried Rhubarb allows this ingredient's actions to be focused on the upper burner.

Stir-fried [till] Carbonized (Chao Tan)

Names: *Da Huang Tan, Chuan Jun Tan*

Flavors & nature: Bitter and slightly astringent; cool tending to neutral

Functions: Harmonizes the blood, stops bleeding

Indications:

1. Hematemesis, hemoptysis due to heat stirring the blood and damaging the network vessels

2. Bloody diarrhea due to food stagnation with epigastric fullness and distention, abdominal pain...

Typical combinations:

1. With uncooked Cacumen Biotae Orientalis (*Sheng Ce Bai Ye*), carbonized Radix Rubiae Cordifoliae (*Qian Cao Gen Tan*), and carbonized Folium Et Petiolus Trachycarpi (*Zong Lu Tan*) as in *Shi Hui San* (Ten Ashes Powder [299])

2. With stir-fried Fructus Crataegi (*Chao Shan Zha*), bran stir-fried Fructus Citri Seu Ponciri (*Fu Chao Zhi Ke*), stir-fried Massa Medica Fermentata (*Chao Shen Qu*), and stir-fried Fructus Germinatus Hordei Vulgaris (*Chao Mai Ya*)

Dosage: 5-15g

Radix Euphorbiae Kansui (*Gan Sui*)

_____ Uncooked *(Sheng)*[1] _____

Names: *Gan Sui, Sheng Gan Sui*

Flavors & nature: Bitter; cold; toxic

Functions: Disperses swelling, scatters nodulations

Indications: Pyogenic infection due to accumulation of damp heat and toxins with redness, swelling, and pain

Typical combinations:

Apply locally a paste made from powdered

Gan Sui and water.

Dosage: Use topically as much as necessary. There is no toxicity or overdosage when this medicinal is used topically.

Note: 1. Uncooked *Gan Sui* is only prescribed topically. Taking the uncooked form orally is strongly counselled against because of the toxicity of *Gan Sui*. One can use other medicinals taken orally in order to treat pyogenic infection.

_____ Prepared *(Shu)*[1] _____

Names: *Shu Gan Sui, Zhi Gan Sui*

Flavors & nature: Bitter; cold; slightly toxic

Functions: Precipitates water, expels phlegm

Indications:

1. Severe chest pain due to either A) depression of phlegm rheum in the chest and lateral costal regions with cough, shortness of breath, pain in the chest and lateral costal regions radiating to the back, constipation, dysuria, or B) accumulation of phlegm in one part or another of the diaphragm with hypersalivation, stertorous breathing

2. Mental troubles due to phlegm misting the portals of the heart with mental confusion, psychosis, schizophrenia, agitation...

Typical combinations:

1. A) with vinegar[-processed] Radix Euphorbiae Pekinensis (*Cu Jing Da Ji*), vinegar[-processed]

Flos Genkwae (*Cu Yuan Hua*), and Fructus Zizyphi Jujubae (*Da Zao*) as in *Shi Zao Tang* (Ten Dates Decoction [302])
B) With vinegar[-processed] Radix Euphorbiae Pekinensis (*Cu Jing Da Ji*) and stir-fried Semen Sinapis Albae (*Chao Bai Jie Zi0* as in *Kong Xian Dan* (Control Drool Elixir [195])

2. With Cinnabar (*Zhu Sha*) as in *Sui Xin Dan* (Follow [Your] Heart Elixir [318])

Dosage: 0.5-1.5g in powder; 1.5-3g in decoction and up to 8g in decoction in severe cases with strict surveillance for side effects

Note: 1. Prepared *Gan Sui* is soaked for several days in clear water and then boiled with tofu until the center of the root is no longer white. Then the *Gan Sui* is allowed to dry slowly over a very mild fire. This method of drying is the same as that called *hong*.

Radix Euphorbiae Kansui continued . . .

_____ **Vinegar Mix-fried (*Cu Zhi*)** _____

Names: *Cu Zhi Gan Sui, Cu Gan Sui*

Flavors & nature: Bitter and slightly sour; cool tending to neutral; slightly toxic

Functions: Precipitates accumulations, drains liquids, scatters nodulations

Indications:

1. Ascites due to accumulation of dampness in the stomach involving stagnation of qi with abdominal distention, thirst, constipation, dysuria...

2. Constipation due to accumulation of damp heat which has built up from the refuse of food following a stagnation of qi in the stomach and intestines with severe abdominal distention, foul-smelling vomitus...

3. Inguinal hernia due to damp heat in the liver channel with pain in the lower abdomen, hernia which tends to be permanent and sinking downward...

Typical combinations:

1. With uncooked Semen Pharbitidis (*Sheng Qian Nu Zi*), prepared Radix Et Rhizoma Rhei (*Shu Da Huang*), and uncooked Pericarpium Viridis Citri Reticulatae (*Sheng Qing Pi*) as in *Zhou Che Wan* (Vessel & Vehicle Pills [444])

2. With uncooked Radix Et Rhizoma Rhei (*Sheng Da Huang*), ginger[-processed] Cortex Magnoliae Officinalis (*Jiang Hou Po*), and uncooked Radix Saussureae Seu Vladimiriae (*Sheng Mu Xiang*) as in *Gan Sui Tong Jie Tang* (Euphorbia Kansui Free the Bound Decoction [111])

3. With salt[-processed] Fructus Foeniculi Vulgaris (*Yan Xiao Hui Xiang*), salt[-processed] Radix Linderae Strychnifoliae (*Yan Wu Yao*), salt[-processed] Semen Litchi Chinensis (*Yan Li Zhi He*), and salt[-processed] Semen Citri Reticulatae (*Yan Ju He*)

Dosage: 0.5-1.5g in powder; 1.5-3g in decoction and up to 8g in decoction in severe cases with strict surveillance for side effects

Mirabilitum *(Mang Xiao)*

_____ *Mang Xiao*[1] _____

Name: *Mang Xiao*

Flavors & nature: Salty and bitter; cold

Functions: Moistens dryness, scatters nodulations, drains heat, frees the stool

Indications:

1. Constipation due to accumulation of heat in the intestines with dry, hard stools

2. Pain and fullness in the chest due to accumulation of heat and fluids or of phlegm in the chest

with chest oppression, shortness of breath, dyspnea, pain, fullness and masses in the epigastrium and abdomen, a dry mouth, thirst, constipation...

3. Eczema[2] of the damp heat type with pruritus, pain, and seeping...

Typical combinations:

1. With uncooked Radix Et Rhizoma Rhei (*Sheng Da Huang*) and bran stir-fried Fructus Immaturus Citri Seu Ponciri (*Fu Chao Zhi Shi*) as in *Da Cheng Qi Tang* (Major Support the Qi Decoction

Mirabilitum continued . . .

[61]) or *Tao Wei Cheng Qi Tang* (Regulate the Stomach & Support the Qi Decoction [327])

2. With uncooked Radix Et Rhizoma Rhei (*Sheng Da Huang*) and vinegar[-processed] Radix Euphorbiae Kansui (*Yan Gan Sui*) as in *Da Xian Xiong Tang* (Great Fell [*i.e.*, Drain] the Chest Decoction [68])

3. With calcined Alumen (*Duan Ming Fan*). The combination of these two substances may be applied locally as a powder.

Dosage: For internal use, 5-10g and up to 30g in severe cases; for external application, use whatever quantity is needed. It is not possible to overdose when this medicinal is used topically.

Notes: 1. This refers to the pure crystals of this medicinal used either internally or externally.
2. Used externally

Pi Xiao[1]

Names: *Pi Xiao, Pu Xiao*

Flavors & nature: Salty, acrid, and bitter; cold

Functions: Disperses food stagnation, eliminates abscess

Indications:

1. Food stagnation with epigastric and abdominal pain

2. Mastitis with swollen, hard, painful breasts (*i.e.*, the inflammatory phase of mastitis)

Typical combinations:

1. Apply locally a paste made from a powder of *Pi Xiao* mixed with water.

2. Same as above

Dosage: For external application, use whatever quantity is needed. Overdosage is not possible when this medicinal is used externally. Use 30-60g for food stagnation and apply topically.

Note: 1. This refers to the impure crystals which are only used externally.

Xuan Ming Fen[1]

Names: *Xuan Ming Fen, Yuan Ming Fen, Feng Hua Xiao*

Flavors & nature: Salty and bitter; cold

Functions: Clears heat, resolves toxins

Indications:

1. Aphthae, glossitis due to heat toxins

2. Sore throat due to heat toxins

3. Toothache due to heat toxins

Typical combinations:

1. With Cinnabar (*Zhu Sha*), Borneol (*Bing Pian*), and Borax (*Peng Sha*) as in *Bing Peng San* (Borneol & Borax Powder [31])

2. Same as above

3. Same as above

Note: 1. This refers to the pure, dehydrated crystals used externally in ophthalmology and stomatology.

Semen Pharbitidis (Qian Niu Zi)

Uncooked (Sheng)

Names: *Qian Niu Zi, Sheng Qian Niu, Er Chou, Hei Bai Chou*

Flavors & nature: Bitter; cold

Functions: Drains water, disperses swelling

Indications:

1. Edema due to accumulation of dampness with edematous limbs and body, constipation, oliguria, dyspnea...

2. Ascites due to accumulation of dampness with abdominal distention like a drum, thirst, raspy sounding breathing, constipation, oliguria...

Typical combinations:

1. With Caulis Akebiae Mutong (*Mu Tong*), uncooked Rhizoma Atractylodis Macrocephalae (*Sheng Bai Zhu*), uncooked Cortex Radicis Mori Albi (*Sheng Sang Bai Pi*), and Cortex Cinnamomi (*Rou Gui*) as in *Qian Niu Zi San* (Morning Glory Seed Powder [245])

2. With vinegar[-processed] Radix Euphorbiae Kansui (*Cu Gan Sui*), vinegar[-processed] Flos Daphnis Genkwae (*Cu Yuan Hua*), and prepared Radix Et Rhizoma Rhei (*Shu Da Huang*) as in *Zhou Che Wan* (Vessel & Vehicle Pills [444])

Dosage: 3-10g in decoction and up to 15g in severe cases; 1.5-3g in powder

Stir-fried (Chao)

Names: *Chao Qian Niu, Chao Er Chou, Chao Bai Chou, Chao Hei Chou*

Flavors & nature: Bitter; cold tending to neutral

Functions: Transforms phlegm, disperses food stagnation, expels parasites

Indications:

1. Cough, asthma due to accumulation of phlegm in the lungs with chest and abdominal distention, constipation, dyspnea...

2. Food stagnation with stagnation of qi, engenderment of damp heat, constipation, abdominal distention...

3. Intestinal parasites[1] with abdominal pain, constipation...

Typical combinations:

1. With stir-fried Semen Lepidii (*Chao Ting Li Zi*), uncooked Semen Pruni Armeniacae (*Sheng Xing Ren*), and uncooked Pericarpium Citri Reticulatae (*Sheng Chen Pi*)

2. With stir-fried Semen Arecae Catechu (*Chao Bing Lang*), uncooked Radix Saussureae Seu Vladimiriae (*Sheng Mu Xiang*), stir-fried Massa Medica Fermentata (*Chao Shen Qu*), stir-fried Fructus Crataegi (*Chao Shan Zha*), and stir-fried Fructus Germinatus Hordei Vulgaris (*Chao Mai Ya*)

3. With uncooked Semen Arecae Catechu (*Sheng Bing Lang*), uncooked Radix Et Rhizoma Rhei (*Sheng Da Huang*), and Realgar (*Xiong Huang*) as in *Qian Niu San* (Morning Glory Powder [244])

Dosage: 3-8g in decoction and up to 15g in severe cases; 1-3g in powder

Note: 1. For this indication, one can prescribe uncooked Pharbitidis (*Sheng Qian Niu*).

5
Center-warming Medicinals

Fructus Amomi Tsao-ko *(Cao Guo)*

Stir-fried [till] Yellow *(Chao Huang)*

Names: *Chao Cao Guo, Cao Guo, Cao Guo Ren*

Flavors & nature: Acrid; warm

Functions: Scatters cold, eliminates dampness, transforms phlegm

Indications:

1. Malaria[1] A) of the heat type with more fever than chills, a wiry (*xian*), rapid (*shu*) pulse, B) of the phlegm cold type, or C) which is incessant and will not heal with more fever than chills, loss of appetite, diarrhea, abundant urination...

2. Phlegm accumulation with headache, back pain, nausea or vomiting after meals...

Typical combinations:

1. A) With uncooked Radix Scutellariae Baicalensis (*Sheng Huang Qin*), uncooked Radix Bupleuri (*Sheng Chai Hu*), and clear Rhizoma Pinelliae Ternatae (*Qing Ban Xia*) as in *Qing Pi Tang* (Clear the Spleen Decoction [253])
B) With bran stir-fried Radix Dichroae Febrifugae (*Fu Chao Chang Shan*) and uncooked Semen Arecae Catechu (*Sheng Bing Lang*) as in *Cao Guo Yin* (Amomum Tsao-ko Drink [40])
C) With bran stir-fried Radix Dichroae Febrifugae (*Fu Chao Chang Shan*) and processed Radix Lateralis Praeparatus Aconiti Carmichaeli (*Zhi Fu Zi*)

2. With processed Rhizoma Arisaematis (*Zhi Tian Nan Xing*), clear Rhizoma Pinelliae Ternatae (*Qing Ban Xia*), uncooked Sclerotium Poriae Cocos (*Sheng Fu Ling*), and stir-fried Pericarpium Citri Reticulatae (*Chao Chen Pi*) as in *Qu Tan Yin Zi* (Dispel Phlegm Rheum Drink [265])

Dosage: 3-6g and up to 10g in severe cases

Note: 1. For indications 1.B) and 1.C), one can prescribe ginger mix-fried *Cao Guo* (*Jiang Zhi Cao Guo*) instead of stir-fried [till] yellow *Cao Guo*.

Ginger Mix-fried *(Jiang Zhi)*

Names: *Jiang Zhi Cao Guo, Jiang Cao Guo, Jiang Cao Guo Ren*

Flavors & nature: Acrid; warm

Functions: Warms the center, scatters cold, stops pain, disperses stagnant food

Indications:

1. Epigastric pain due to accumulation of cold dampness in the middle burner with cold extremities and a sensation of cold in the stomach or to the touch, epigastric distention...

2. Food stagnation due to food stagnation and cold with epigastric pain and distention, nausea, vomiting, acid vomiting or with a putrid odor...

3. Vomiting due to accumulation of phlegm in the middle burner with eructation, vomiting clear fluids...

Fructus Amomi Tsao-ko continued . . .

4. Diarrhea[1] due to cold dampness

Typical combinations:

1. With Flos Caryophylli (*Ding Xiang*), Rhizoma Alpiniae Officinari (*Gao Liang Jiang*), and ginger[-processed] Cortex Magnoliae Officinalis (*Jiang Hou Po*)

2. With ginger[-processed] Cortex Magnoliae Officinalis (*Jiang Hou Po*), uncooked Endothelium Corneum Gigeriae Galli (*Sheng Ji Nei Jin*), and stir-fried Pericarpium Citri Reticulatae (*Chao Chen Pi*)

3. With stir-fried Pericarpium Citri Reticulatae (*Chao Chen Pi*), bran stir-fried Rhizoma Atractylodis (*Fu Chao Cang Zhu*), and ginger[-processed] Cortex Magnoliae Officinalis (*Jiang Hou Po*)

4. With bran stir-fried Rhizoma Atractylodis (*Fu Chao Cang Zhu*), roasted Semen Alpiniae Katsumadai (*Wei Cao Dou Kou*), Fructus Amomi (*Sha Ren*)

Dosage: 3-6g and up to 10g in severe cases

Note: 1. For this indication, roasted *Cao Guo* (*Wei Cao Guo*) can also be prescribed advantageously.

Radix Aconiti Kusnezofii *(Cao Wu Tou)*[1]

─────── Uncooked *(Sheng)*[2] ───────

Names: *Sheng Cao Wu, Sheng Cao Wu Tou*

Flavors & nature: Acrid; hot; very toxic

Functions: Scatters cold, disperses swelling, stops pain

Indications:

1. Trismus due to attack by wind toxins which cause tetany

2. Scrofula, subcutaneous nodules due to stagnation of phlegm in the channels

3. *Yong* due to heat toxins

4. Rheumatic complaints due to wind cold dampness

Typical combinations:

1. With Fructus Gleditschiae Chinensis (*Zao Jiao*) and a small amount of Secretio Moschi Moschiferi (*She Xiang*). These three ingredients should be pulverized into a fine powder which is then daubed on the teeth and insufflated into the nostrils.

2. With Semen Momordicae Cochinensis (*Mu Bie Zi*) and a small amount of uncooked Concha Ostreae (*Sheng Mu Li*). These three substances should be pulverized and mixed with a small amount of water in order to make a plaster.

3. Powder *Cao Wu Tou* and mix with a small amount of water to make a plaster.

4. With wine[-processed] Radix Clematidis Chinensis (*Jiu Wei Ling Xian*), steamed Fructus Chaenomelis Lagenariae (*Zheng Mu Gua*) and Caulis Lonicerae Japonicae (*Ren Dong Teng*). Chop these four ingredients into small pieces. Then soak in rice wine at 50-60 (degrees) for 15 days. Leave the medicinals in the tincture. Only apply externally over the joints.

Dosage: Use externally only as much as is needed. There is no toxicity when used topically.

Notes: 1. See the following pages for the distinction between *Fu Zi, Wu Tou, Chuan Wu Tou,* and *Cao Wu Tou.* 2. Uncooked *Cao Wu Tou* is very toxic. This medicinal must be used strictly externally.

Processed (Zhi)[1]

Names: *Zhi Cao Wu, Zhi Cao Wu Tou*

Flavors & nature: Acrid and slightly sweet; warm; toxic

Functions: Scatters cold, disperses swelling, stops pain

Indications:

1. Rheumatic complaints due to either A) wind cold dampness with severe joint pain aggravated by cold, loss of mobility, or B) stagnation of cold dampness in the network vessels with sinew pain, loss of mobility...

2. Paralysis due to wind stroke (*zhong feng*)

3. Headache due to accumulation of internal cold with severe pain in the nuchal region and head

4. Vacuity cold of the spleen and stomach with loss of appetite, a tasteless mouth, loss of taste, borborygmus, loose stools, aversion to cold...

Typical combinations:

1. A) With uncooked Ramulus Cinnamomi (*Sheng Gui Zhi*) and uncooked Herba Cum Radice Asari (*Sheng Xi Xin*)

B) With Radix Praeparatus Aconiti Carmichaeli (*Zhi Chuan Wu Tou*) as in *Xiao Huo Luo Dan* (Minor Quicken the Network Vessels Elixir [375])

2. With uncooked Rhizoma Arisaematis (*Sheng Tian Nan Xing*), Lumbricus (*Di Long*), Radix Praeparatus Aconiti Carmichaeli (*Zhi Chuan Wu Tuo*) as in *Xiao Huo Luo Dan* (Minor Quicken the Network Vessels Elixir [375])

3. With uncooked Herba Cum Radice Asari (*Sheng Xi Xin*) and Secretio Moschi Moschiferi (*She Xiang*) as in *Wu Xiang San* (Five Fragrances Powder [359])

4. With bran stir-fried Rhizoma Atractylodis Macroce phalae (*Fu Chao Bai Zhu*), mix-fried Radix Glycyrrhizae (*Zhi Gan Cao*), honey mix-fried Radix Codonopsis Pilosulae (*Mi Zhi Dang Shen*), and Semen Glycinis Hispidae (*Hei Dou*)

Dosage: 2-6g and up to 10g in severe cases

Note: 1. *Cao Wu Tou* is made by soaking in clear water for 1 day. Then the small rootlets are taken off leaving only the large central root. This is boiled with Radix Glycyrrhizae (*Gan Cao*) and Semen Glycinis Hispidae (*Hei Dou*) until the heart of the root is cooked (approximately 4-6 hours).

Radix Aconiti Carmichaeli (*Chuan Wu Tou*)[1]

Uncooked (Sheng)[2]

Names: *Sheng Chuan Wu, Sheng Chuan Wu Tou*

Flavors & nature: Acrid; very hot; very toxic

Functions: Scatters cold, stops pain

Indications:

1. Pain in the low back and feet with loss of mobility, a sensation of cold in the low back and feet...

Radix Aconiti Carmichaeli continued . . .

2. Severe, persistent headache due to invasion of cold in the *tai yang*

3. Toothache due to wind cold with severe pain, pale red gums...

4. Mycoses, scabies with pruritus

5. *Yong*

Typical combinations:

1. Applied externally as a plaster made from finely powdered *Chuan Wu* and vinegar.

2. Applied externally on acupuncture points on the bladder channel in the form of a plaster made from *Chuan Wu* and Rhizoma Arisaematis (*Tian Nan Xing*) mixed with the juice of Chinese scallions

3. Applied externally as a plaster made from finely powdered Radix Lateralis Praeparatus Aconiti Carmichaeli (*Fu Zi*), *Chuan Wu*, and wheat flour

4. Applied externally as a plaster made from *Chuan Wu*

5. Applied externally as an alcohol tincture of *Chuan Wu*

Dosage: Use externally only. The amount should be equivalent to the need. There is no toxicity when applied topically.

Notes: 1. See the following pages for the distinction between *Fu Zi, Wu Tou, Chuan Wu Tou*, and *Cao Wu Tou*. 2. The uncooked form of this medicinal is extremely toxic and is strictly reserved for topical application.

_____ **Processed *(Zhi)***[1] _____

Names: *Zhi Chuan Wu, Zhi Chuan Wu Tou*

Flavors & nature: Acrid and slightly sweet; hot; toxic

Functions: Scatters cold, stops pain

Indications:

1. Rheumatic complaints due to wind cold dampness with cold predominating, severe joint pain aggravated by cold and at night, loss of mobility...

2. Deviated mouth and eyes due to wind stroke (*zhong feng*) with aphasia, difficulty moving the hands and feet, disorientation, uneven gait...

3. Heart pain radiating to the back due to accumulation of cold

4. Inguinal hernia, maladies of the testicles and scrotum due to cold stagnation in the liver channel with pain in the lower abdomen, cold hands and feet...

Typical combinations:

1. With uncooked Herba Ephedrae (*Sheng Ma Huang*) and uncooked Radix Astragali Membranacei (*Sheng Huang Qi*) as in *Wu Tou Tang* (Aconite Decoction [356]) or uncooked Rhizoma Atractylodis (*Sheng Cang Zhu*) and vinegar dip calcined Pyritum (*Cu Cui Zi Ran Tong*) as in *Wu Zhu Wan* (Aconite & Atractylodes Pills [360])

2. With Secretio Moschi Moschiferi (*She Xiang*) and Borneol (*Bing Pian*) as in *Wu Long Dan* (Aconite & Borneol Elixir [349])

3. With dry Rhizoma Zingiberis (*Gan Jiang*) and stir-fried Pericarpium Zanthoxyli Bungeani (*Chao Hua Jiao*) as in *Wu Tou Chi Shi Zhi Wan* (Aconite & Hallyositum Rubrum Pills [354])

4. With stir-fried Ramulus Cinnamomi (*Chao Gui Zhi*) and wine[-processed] Radix Albus Paeoniae Lactiflorae (*Jiu Bai Shao Yao*) as in *Wu Tou Gui Zhi Tang* (Aconite & Cinnamon Twig Decoction [355])

Dosage: 2-8g and up to 12g in severe cases

Note: 1. The method of preparing processed *Chuan Wu Tou* is approximately the same as for processed *Cao Wu Tou*.

Radix Lateralis Praeparatus Aconiti Carmichaeli *(Fu Zi)*[1]

_____ Scalded *(Dan)*[2] _____

Names: *Dan Fu Zi*[3], *Dan Fu Pian*[3]

Flavors & nature: Sweet and acrid; hot; toxic

Functions: Returns yang, scatters cold, stops pain

Indications:

1. Yang desertion due to accumulation of internal cold with abdominal pain, cold limbs, profuse, cold sweating, aversion to cold, a faint *(wei)* pulse...

2. Rheumatic complaints due to cold dampness with severe joint pain aggravated by cold, loss of mobility, aversion to cold, cold limbs and body...

3. Edema due to either A) spleen/kidney yang vacuity with oliguria, generalized edema, aversion to cold, loose stools or B) kidney yang vacuity with edema predominantly in the lower body, aversion to cold, impotence, pain in the low back and knees...

4. Epigastric pain due to cold strike *(zhong han)* to the stomach accompanied by stagnation of qi with borborygmus, diarrhea, cold limbs...

5. Infertility due to cold accumulated in the uterus with dysmenorrhea, oligomenorrhea, or amenorrhea, lower abdominal pain aggravated by cold...

6. Colds and flu due to wind cold accompanied by chronic yang vacuity with fever, severe aversion to cold and strong chills, cold limbs, a pale complexion, a deep *(chen)* pulse despite the exterior pattern...

Typical combinations:

1. With dry Rhizoma Zingiberis *(Gan Jiang)* and mix-fried Radix Glycyrrhizae *(Zhi Gan Cao)* as in

Si Ni Tang (Four Counterflows Decoction [312])

2. With uncooked Ramulus Cinnamomi *(Sheng Gui Zhi)* and uncooked Rhizoma Zingiberis *(Sheng Jiang)* as in *Gui Zhi Fu Zi Tang* (Cinnamon Twig & Aconite Decoction [124]) or uncooked Ramulus Cinnamomi *(Sheng Gui Zhi)*, uncooked Rhizoma Atractylodis Macrocephalae *(Sheng Bai Zhu)*, and mix-fried Radix Glycyrrhizae *(Zhi Gan Cao)* as in *Gan Cao Fu Zi Tang* (Licorice & Aconite Decoction [108])

3. A) With uncooked Rhizoma Atractylodis Macrocephalae *(Sheng Bai Zhu)* and uncooked Sclerotium Poriae Cocos *(Sheng Fu Ling)* as in *Zhen Wu Tang* (True Warrior Decoction [429]) B) With prepared Radix Rehmanniae *(Shu Di Huang)*, stir-fried Ramulus Cinnamomi *(Chao Gui Zhi)*, and steamed Fructus Corni Officinalis *(Zheng Shan Zhu Yu)* as in *Shen Qi Wan* (Kidney Qi Pills [291])

4. With roasted Radix Saussureae Seu Vladimiriae *(Wei Mu Xiang)* and vinegar[-processed] Rhizoma Corydalis Yanhusuo *(Cu Yan Hu Suo)* as in *Xuan Fu Tang* (Corydalis & Aconite Decoction [390])

5. With wine[-processed] Radix Angelicae Sinensis *(Jiu Dang Gui)*, processed Fructus Evodiae Rutecarpae *(Zhi Wu Zhu Yu)*, and vinegar[-processed] Folium Artemisiae Argyii *(Cu Ai Ye)*

6. With uncooked Herba Ephedrae *(Sheng Ma Huang)* and uncooked Herba Cum Radice Asari *(Sheng Xi Xin)* as in *Ma Huang Fu Zi Xi Xin Tang* (Ephedra, Aconite & Asarum Decoction [213])

Dosage: 5-10g to stimulate the lifegate fire; 10-15g to return yang; and up to 30g in severe cases and in a patient sufficiently strong to support such a dose

Radix Lateralis Praeparatus Aconiti Carmichaeli continued . . .

Notes: 1. See the following pages for the distinction between *Fu Zi, Wu Tou,* and *Tian Xiong.* 2. The roots first undergo treatment in salt (*Yan Fu Zi*) and are then boiled with Radix Glycyrrhizae (*Gan Cao*) and Semen Glycinis Hispidae (*Hei Dou*) in a very precise process. 3. Attention: The term *Fu Zi* in a prescription means uncooked *Fu Zi* (*Sheng Fu Zi*), which is very toxic and should only be used externally. The indications of *Sheng Fu Zi* are identical to those of *Sheng Cao Wu Tou* or *Sheng Chuan Wu Tou.*

Blast-fried (Pao)[1]

Names: *Pao Fu Zi, Pao Fu Pian*

Flavors & nature: Sweet, acrid, and slightly astringent; hot; a little toxic

Functions: Warms the kidneys and spleen

Indications:

1. Diarrhea due to spleen/kidney yang vacuity with aversion to cold, vomiting, intermittent diarrhea aggravated by eating uncooked or cold foods, fatigue, cold limbs...

2. Dysentery or constipation due to spleen yang vacuity accompanied by qi stagnation and cold in the intestines with abdominal pain and distention...

Typical combinations:

1. With dry Rhizoma Zingiberis (*Gan Jiang*), Radix Panacis Ginseng (*Ren Shen*), and earth stir-fried Rhizoma Atractylodis Macrocephalae (*Tu Chao Bai Zhu*) as in *Fu Zi Li Zhong Wan* (Aconite Rectify the Center Pills [107])

2. With dry Rhizoma Zingiberis (*Gan Jiang*) and uncooked Radix Et Rhizoma Rhei (*Sheng Da Huang*) as in *Wen Pi Tang* (Warm the Spleen Decoction [342])

Dosage: 2-10g and up to 20g in severe cases and if the patient is strong enough to support such a dose

Note: 1. First the roots are subjected to a treatment with salt (*Yan Fu Zi*) and then the bark is taken off. The roots are then cut into slices. Next the Aconite is subjected to several other treatments. They are soaked in water; then macerated in a Ginger decoction; next they are steamed; later they are dried over a slow fire; etc.

A Comparative Analysis Between *Fu Zi, Tian Xiong, Wu Tou, Cao Wu Tou & Chuan Wu Tou*

The existing Western literature is quite confused concerning the differences which exist between *Fu Zi, Tian Xiong, Wu Tou, Chuan Wu Tou,* and *Cao Wu Tou.* In fact, *Fu Zi, Tian Xiong,* and *Wu Tou* all come from the same plant. *Wu Tou* or Radix Praeparatus Aconiti Carmichaeli is the principle root. *Fu Zi* or Radix Lateralis Praeparatus Aconiti Carmichaeli, on the other hand, is made from the lateral or secondary roots of *Wu Tou.* Literally, *fu* means annex and *zi* means child. When there is only a single lateral root, this medicinal is then called *Tian Xiong.* Literally, this means heavenly male and is so named because it is reputed to be very powerful. It has the same actions and indications as *Fu Zi.*

In addition, *Wu Tou* is a generic term for a very numerous group of varieties of Aconite (approximately 15), the two best known being: 1) *Cao Wu Tou* or *Cao Wu* (Radix Aconiti Carmichaeli or Radix Aconiti Kusnezofii). These come from northeastern provinces [of China], such as Shanxi, Hebei, and Liaoning. They are wild aconites and the most toxic. 2) *Chuan Wu Tou* or *Chuan Wu* (Radix Aconiti Carmichaeli). This is cultivated aconite principally grown in the province of Sichuan. It is proportionately less toxic than *Cao Wu Tou.*

Dry Rhizoma Zingiberis (Gan Jiang)

Dry (Gan)[1]

Names: *Gan Jiang, Dan Gan Jiang, Jun Jiang, Chuan Gan Jiang*

Flavors & nature: Acrid; hot

Functions: Warms the center, scatters cold, returns yang, warms the lungs, transforms phlegm rheum

Indications:

1. Diarrhea and/or vomiting due to spleen yang vacuity with aversion to cold, cold limbs, abdominal pain, loss of appetite...

2. Yang desertion with cold limbs, watery diarrhea, lethargy, a faint (*wei*) pulse, and possible loss of consciousness...

3. Epigastric and abdominal pain due to vacuity cold of the spleen and stomach with severe pain of the chest and heart, vomiting, a cold sensation in the abdomen...

4. Cough, asthma due to lung yang vacuity and accumulation of phlegm rheum in the lungs with excessive, clear, thin mucus. Sometimes this pattern is accompanied by attack of wind cold.

Typical combinations:

1. With earth stir-fried Rhizoma Atractylodis Macrocephalae (*Tu Chao Bai Zhu*) and Radix Panacis Ginseng (*Ren Shen*) as in *Li Zhong Wan* (Rectify the Center Pills [196])

2. With processed Radix Lateralis Praeparatus Aconiti Carmichaeli (*Zhi Fu Zi*) as in *Si Ni Tang* (Four Counterflows Decoction [312])

3. With stir-fried Pericarpium Zanthoxyli Bungeani (*Chao Hua Jiao*) and Radix Panacis Ginseng (*Ren Shen*) as in *Da Jian Zhong Tang* (Major Fortify the Center Decoction [66])

4. With clear Rhizoma Pinelliae Ternatae (*Qing Ban Xia*), honey mix-fried Herba Ephedrae (*Mi Zhi Ma Huang*), wine-steamed Fructus Schizandrae Chinensis (*Jiu Zheng Wu Wei Zi*), and honey mix-fried Herba Cum Radice Asari (*Mi Zhi Xi Xin*) as in *Xiao Qing Long Tang* (Minor Blue Dragon Decoction [377])

Dosage: 3-10g and up to 20g in severe cases or for returning yang

Note: 1. This refers to the mature, dried rhizome of ginger, while *Sheng Jiang* refers to the young, fresh rhizome.

Blast-fried (Pao)[1]

Names: *Pao Jiang, Pao Jiang Tan, Hei Jiang*

Flavors & nature: Slightly acrid, bitter; warm

Functions: Warms the channels, stops bleeding, warms the center, stops diarrhea

Indications:

1. Metrorrhagia, menorrhagia due to *chong* and *ren* not securing with scanty, continuous bleeding

2. Hematemesis with vomiting of blackish blood, epigastric oppression...

3. Postpartum abdominal pain due to blood stasis caused by cold with retention of the lochia, pain in the lower abdomen aggravated by pressure and cold...

4. Diarrhea due to vacuity cold of the spleen and stomach with abdominal pain...

Dry Rhizoma Zingiberis continued . . .

Typical combinations:

1. With carbonized Folium Artemisiae Argyii (*Ai Ye Tan*), carbonized Radix Angelicae Sinensis (*Dang Gui Tan*), Pollen Typhae stir-fried Gelatinum Corii Asini (*Pu Huang Chao E Jiao*), and Terra Flava Usta (*Fu Long Gan*)

2. With Radix Pseudoginseng (*San Qi*), carbonized Folium Et Petiolus Trachycarpi (*Zong Lu Tan*), and Terra Flava Usta (*Fu Long Gan*)

3. With wine[-processed] Radix Angelicae Sinensis (*Jiu Dang Gui*), wine[-processed] Radix Ligus-tici Wallichii (*Jiu Chuan Xiong*), and uncooked Semen Pruni Persicae (*Sheng Tao Ren*) as in *Sheng Hua Tang* (Engender & Transform Decoction [294])

4. With earth stir-fried Rhizoma Atractylodis Macrocephalae (*Tu Chao Bai Zhu*), roasted Radix Saussureae Seu Vladimiriae (*Wei Mu Xiang*), Fructus Amomi (*Sha Ren*), and Rhizoma Alpiniae Officinari (*Gao Liang Jiang*)

Dosage: 3-12g and up to 20g in severe cases

Note: 1. This refers to dry ginger (*Gan Jiang*) which has been charred.

Fructus Evodiae Rutecarpae (*Wu Zhu Yu*)

Uncooked (*Sheng*)[1]

Names: *Sheng Wu Zhu Yu, Sheng Wu Yu*

Flavors & nature: Acrid and bitter; warm; toxic

Functions: Scatters cold, stops pain

Indications:

1. Aphthae due to heat in the heart and spleen

2. Pruritus due to eczema

3. Toothache due to wind cold with pale gums which are not swollen...

Typical combinations:

1. Applied locally as a plaster made from finely powdered Evodia and vinegar

2. With uncooked Os Sepiae Seu Sepiellae (*Sheng Hai Piao Xiao*) and uncooked Sulfur (*Sheng Liu Huang*). Reduce these three substances to a powder. If the eczema is purulent, place the powder directly on the affected area. If the eczema is dry, mix this powder in sesame oil and apply this unguent locally.

3. Applied locally as an alcoholic tincture of Evodia

Dosage: For external use only, in which case use whatever amount necessary. There is no overdosage when used topically.

Note: 1. For external use only

Processed (*Zhi*)[1]

Names: *Pao Wu Yu, Wu Zhu Yu, Chao Wu Yu, Zhi Wu Yu, Dan Wu Yu*

Flavors & nature: Acrid, bitter, and slightly sweet; warm; slightly toxic

Functions: Scatters cold, stops pain, warms the center, stops diarrhea, drains the liver, downbears counterflow qi

Fructus Evodiae Rutecarpae continued . . .

Indications:

1. Vomiting[2] due to either A) stomach cold with epigastric fullness and pain, regurgitation, nausea, vomiting clear liquids or B) accumulation of heat in the liver channel with acid vomiting, eructation, lateral costal pain...

2. Headache due to external cold attacking the upper body with pain in the nuchal region, incessant headache...

3. Inguinal hernia, maladies of the scrotum or of the testicles[3] due to stagnation of cold in the liver channel with swollen, cold scrotum, pain in the lower abdomen...

4. Dysmenorrhea[4] due to qi stagnation, blood stasis, and vacuity cold of the *chong* and *ren*

5. Diarrhea due to invasion of cold dampness of the spleen with abdominal pain, diarrhea with undigested food...

Typical combinations:

1. A) With uncooked Rhizoma Zingiberis (*Sheng Jiang*) and Radix Panacis Ginseng (*Ren Shen*) as in *Wu Zhu Yu Tang* (Evodia Decoction [361])
B) With ginger[-processed] Rhizoma Coptidis Chinensis (*Jiang Huang Lian*) as in *Zuo Jin Wan* (Left Gold Pills [452])

2. With uncooked Herba Cum Radice Asari (*Sheng Xi Xin*), uncooked Radix Ligustici Wallichii (*Sheng Chuan Xiong*), and Radix Et Rhizoma Ligustici Chinensis (*Gao Ben*)

3. With salt[-processed] Fructus Foeniculi Vulgaris (*Yan Xiao Hui Xiang*) and salt[-processed] Fructus Meliae Toosendan (*Yan Chuan Lian Zi*) as in *Dao Qi Tang* (Abduct the Qi Decoction [80])

4. With stir-fried Ramulus Cinnamomi (*Chao Gui Zhi*), wine[-processed] Radix Angelicae Sinensis (*Jiu Dang Gui*), and wine[-processed] Radix Ligustici Wallichii (*Jiu Chuan Xiong*) as in *Wen Jing Tang* (Warm the Channels Decoction [341])

5. With uncooked Rhizoma Coptidis Chinensis (*Sheng Huang Lian*) and stir-fried Radix Albus Paeoniae Lactiflorae (*Chao Bai Shao Yao*) as in *Wu Ji Wan* (Five Accumulations Pills [345])

Dosage: 2-6g and up to 9-15g in severe cases

Notes: 1. Evodia is processed by several methods. The most important one is boiling in a Licorice decoction and then drying it slowly (*hong*). 2. For this indication, processed Evodia refers to that treated with ginger juice. 3. For this indication, processed Evodia refers to that treated by salt. 4. For this indication, processed Evodia refers to that treated by rice wine.

Fructus Foeniculi Vulgaris *(Xiao Hui Xiang)*

Uncooked *(Sheng)*

Names: *Xiao Hui Xiang, Sheng Hui Xiang, Gu Hui Xiang, Hui Xiang*

Flavors & nature: Acrid; warm

Functions: Rectifies the qi, harmonizes the center, stimulates the appetite

Indications:

1. Loss of appetite due to vacuity cold of the spleen and stomach with chest and diaphragm oppression, periumbilical pain...

2. Vomiting due to either A) disharmony of the stomach qi with nausea, eructation, loss of appe-

Fructus Foeniculi Vulgaris continued . . .

tite or B) vacuity cold of the spleen and stomach with vomiting clear liquids, pain and a sensation of cold in the epigastrium and abdomen...

Typical combinations:

1. With ginger[-processed] Cortex Magnoliae Officinalis (*Jiang Hou Po*), dry Rhizoma Zingiberis (*Gan Jiang*), and processed Radix Lateralis Praeparatus Aconiti Carmichaeli (*Zhi Fu Zi*)

2. A) With Fructus Cardamomi (*Bai Dou Kou*), ginger[-processed] Rhizoma Pinelliae Ternatae (*Jiang Ban Xia*), and stir-fried Pericarpium Citri Reticulatae (*Chao Chen Pi*)
B) With processed Radix Lateralis Praeparatus Aconiti Carmichaeli (*Zhi Fu Zi*), processed Fructus Evodiae Rutecarpae (*Zhi Wu Zhu Yu*), uncooked Rhizoma Zingiberis (*Sheng Jiang*), and honey mix-fried Radix Codonopsis Pilosulae (*Mi Zhi Dang Shen*)

Dosage: 3-5g and up to 5-10g in severe cases

Salt Mix-fried (Yan Zhi)

Names: *Yan Zhi Hui Xiang, Yan Xiao Hui Xiang*

Flavors & nature: Acrid and slightly salty; warm

Functions: Scatters cold, stops pain, warms the kidneys, soothes the liver

Indications:

1. Inguinal hernia, maladies of the scrotum or the testicles due to stagnation of cold and qi in the liver channel with lower abdominal pain, inflation, distention, and pain of the scrotum...

2. Low back pain due to kidney yang vacuity with a cold sensation in the lumbar region...

Typical combinations:

1. With processed Fructus Evodiae Rutecarpae

(*Zhi Wu Zhu Yu*), uncooked Radix Saussureae Seu Vladimiriae (*Sheng Mu Xiang*), and salt[-processed] Fructus Meliae Toosendan (*Yan Chuan Lian Zi*) as in *Dao Qi Tang* (Abduct the Qi Decoction [80] or salt[-processed] Semen Citri Reticulatae (*Yan Ju He*), salt[-processed] Semen Litchi Sinensis (*Yan Li Zhi He*), and salt[-processed] Radix Linderae Strychnifoliae (*Yan Wu Yao*)

2. With processed Radix Lateralis Praeparatus Aconiti Carmichaeli (*Zhi Fu Zi*), salt[-processed] Cortex Eucommiae Ulmoidis (*Yan Du Zhong*), salt[-processed] Radix Dipsaci (*Yan Xu Duan*), and wine[-processed] Cortex Radicis Acanthopanacis (*Yan Wu Jia Pi*)

Dosage: 3-5g and up to 5-10g in severe cases

6
Wind Dampness Dispelling Medicinals

Agkistrodon Seu Bungarus (Bai Hua She)

Uncooked (Sheng)[1]

Names: *Sheng Bai Hua She, Sheng Jin Qian Bai Hua She*

Flavors & nature: Sweet and salty; warm; toxic

Functions: Dispels wind, stops itching

Indications: Scabies, mycoses, leprosy[2] with severe pruritus

Typical combinations: With Buthus Martensi (*Quan Xie*), uncooked Rhizoma Gastrodiae Elatae (*Sheng Tian Ma*), and uncooked Radix Angelicae Sinensis (*Sheng Dang Gui*) applied topically as an alcohol tincture or with Radix Sophorae Flavescentis (*Ku Shen*), Zaocys Dhumnades (*Wu Shao She*), and Elaphe (*Jin Qian Bai Hua She*) as in *Yu Feng Dan* (Heal Wind Elixir [414]). These pills are placed in rice wine in order to make an alcohol tincture for external use.

Dosage: For external use. Use whatever quantity necessary. There is no overdosage when used topically.

Notes: 1. Uncooked Agkistrodon is toxic. It is strictly reserved for external use. 2. Agkistrodon treats both internal and external wind based on the adage:

> Internally, (Agkistrodon) is directed
> at the viscera and bowels;
> Externally, (Agkistrodon) is directed
> toward the skin.

Wine Mix-fried (Jiu Zhi)

Names: *Jiu Zhi Bai Hua She, Jiu Bai Hua She, Bai Hua She, Jin Qian Bai Hua She*

Flavors & nature: Sweet, salty, and slightly acrid; warm; toxic

Functions: Dispels wind, eliminates dampness, opens the network vessels, stops pain

Indications:

1. Tremors

2. Rheumatic complaints due to wind dampness with joint pain aggravated by a damp climate, sinew contractions...

3. Hemiplegia due to wind stroke (*zhong feng*) with deviated mouth and eyes...

4. Leprosy, scabies, scrofula, mycoses, syphilis, urticaria, vitiligo due to wind and toxins

Typical combinations:

1. With uncooked Zaocys Dhummades (*Wu Shao She*) and stone-baked Scolopendra Subspinipes (*Bei Wu Gong*) as in *Ding Ming San* (Determine Destiny Powder [86])

2. With Radix Et Rhizoma Notopterygii (*Qiang Huo*), Radix Angelicae Pubescentis (*Du Huo*), steamed Fructus Chaenomelis Lagenariae (*Zheng Mu Gua*), uncooked Rhizoma Atractylodis (*Sheng*

Agkistrodon Seu Bungarus continued . . .

Cang Zhu), and wine[-processed] Radix Clematidis Chinensis (*Jiu Wei Ling Xian*)

3. With Buthus Martensi (*Quan Xie*), uncooked Rhizoma Gastrodiae Elatae (*Sheng Tian Ma*), and uncooked Radix Ledebouriellae Sesloidis (*Sheng Fang Feng*) as in *Bai Hua She Jiu* (Agkistrodon Wine [16a])

4. With Herba Menthae Haplocalycis (*Bo He*), uncooked Herba Schizonepetae Tenuifoliae (*Sheng Jing Jie*), uncooked Rhizoma Gastrodiae Elatae (*Sheng Tian Ma*), and uncooked Radix Ledebouriellae Sesloidis (*Sheng Fang Feng*) as in *Qu Feng Gao* (Expel Wind Paste [262])

Dosage: 3-9g in decoction; 0.5-1g in powder

Fructus Xanthii *(Cang Er Zi)*

_____ Uncooked *(Sheng)* _____

Names: *Sheng Cang Er Zi, Sheng Cang Zi*

Flavors & nature: Acrid, sweet, and slightly bitter; slightly warm; slightly toxic

Functions: Dispels wind, stops itching

Indications: Urticaria, mycoses, scrofula due to wind with itching

Typical combinations: With Fructus Kochiae Scopariae (*Di Fu Zi*), Radix Ledebouriellae Sesloidis (*Fang Feng*), Cortex Radicis Dictamni (*Bai Xian Pi*), and Fructus Tribuli Terrestris (*Bai Ji Li*)

Dosage: 5-10g

_____ Stir-fried [till] Scorched *(Chao Jiao)* _____

Names: *Chao Cang Er Zi, Chao Cang Zi, Cang Er Zi*

Flavors & nature: Sweet, slightly acrid, and bitter; warm

Functions: Opens the portals of the nose, eliminates dampness, stops pain

Indications:

1. Sinusitis, rhinitis[1] due to wind cold which stagnates in the portals of the nose with nasal congestion, incessant rhinorrhea, frontal headache...

2. Rheumatic complaints due to A) wind dampness lodging in the muscles, the channels and network vessels, or the joints with generalized pain, painful limbs, loss of mobility, B) cold dampness with severe pain aggravated by cold or

at night, or C) damp heat with pain, redness, swelling, and hot joints...

Typical combinations:

1. With Flos Magnoliae Liliflorae (*Xin Yi Hua*), Radix Angelicae Dahuricae (*Bai Zhi*), and Herba Menthae Haplocalycis (*Bo He*) as in *Cang Er San* (Xanthium Powder [39])

2. A) With Radix Et Rhizoma Notopterygii (*Qiang Huo*), Radix Angelicae Pubescentis (*Du Huo*), and Radix Clematidis Chinensis (*Wei Ling Xian*)
B) With uncooked Ramulus Cinnamomi (*Sheng Gui Zhi*), processed Radix Aconiti (*Zhi Chuan Wu Tou*), and uncooked Herba Cum Radice Asari (*Sheng Xi Xin*)
C) With Caulis Sargentodoxae (*Hong Teng*), Caulis Lonicerae Japonicae (*Ren Dong Teng*), and Lumbricus (*Di Long*)

Fructus Xanthii continued . . .

Dosage: 5-10g and up to 30g in severe cases

Note: 1. Uncooked Xanthium (*Sheng Cang Er Zi*) can also be prescribed for sinusitis or rhinitis. However, stir-fried Xanthium (*Chao Cang Er Zi*) is preferable because there is no toxicity.

Rhizoma Atractylodis (Cang Zhu)

————— Uncooked (Sheng) —————

Names: *Sheng Cang Zhu, Sheng Mao Zhu*

Flavors & nature: Acrid, sweet, and slightly bitter; warm; drying

Functions: Dispels wind, induces perspiration, eliminates dampness

Indications:

1. Rheumatic complaints due to wind dampness stagnating in the channels and network vessels with joint pain and a sensation of heaviness, numbness of the limbs, loss of mobility...

2. Colds, flu due to wind cold blocking the exterior with headache radiating to the nuchal region, fever, chills, aching...

3. Fever due to damp heat with joint pain and the sensation of a heavy body...

4. Pain in the feet and knees[1] due to damp heat in the lower burner with feebleness of the extremities, painful, red, swollen, and engorged feet and knees...

Typical combinations:

1. With uncooked Semen Coicis Lachryma-jobi (*Sheng Yi Yi Ren*), Radix Angelicae Pubescentis (*Du Huo*), and Radix Et Rhizoma Notopterygii (*Qiang Huo*) as in *Yi Yi Ren Tang* (Coix Decoction [406])

2. With Radix Angelicae Dahuricae (*Bai Zhi*), uncooked Radix Ligustici Wallichii (*Sheng Chuan Xiong*), and uncooked Herba Cum Radice Asari (*Sheng Xi Xin*) as in *Shen Zhu San* (Magic Atractylodes Powder [293])

3. With uncooked Gypsum Fibrosum (*Sheng Shi Gao*) and uncooked Rhizoma Anemarrhenae (*Sheng Zhi Mu*) as in *Bai Hu Jia Cang Zhu Tang* (White Tiger Plus Atractylodes Decoction [14])

4. With salt[-processed] Cortex Phellodendri (*Yan Huang Bai*) and salt[-processed] Radix Achyranthis Bidentatae (*Yan Huai Niu Xi*) as in *San Miao Wan* (Three Marvels Pills [273])

Dosage: 5-10g and up to 30g in severe cases

Note: 1. For this indication, bran stir-fried Atractylodis (*Fu Chao Cang Zhu*) can also be prescribed.

————— Bran Stir-fried (Fu Chao) —————

Names: *Fu Chao Cang Zhu, Chao Cang Zhu*

Flavors & nature: Sweet, slightly acrid, and slightly bitter; warm

Functions: Fortifies the spleen, dries dampness, brightens the eyes

Indications:

1. Disharmony of the spleen and stomach due to either A) stagnation of damp turbidity in the middle burner with loss of appetite, epigastric and abdominal distention, nausea, vomiting, diarrhea, a thick, white tongue coating or B) summerheat

Rhizoma Atractylodis continued . . .

and dampness with fever, chills, vomiting, diarrhea, cough, and a thick, white tongue coating...

2. Optic atrophy, night blindness due to liver/-kidney vacuity

Typical combinations:

1. A) With ginger[-processed] Cortex Magnoliae Officinalis (*Jiang Hou Po*) and stir-fried Pericarpium Citri Reticulatae (*Chao Chen Pi*) as in *Ping Wei San* (Level the Stomach Powder [231]) B) With Herba Agastachis Seu Pogostemi (*Huo*

Xiang), ginger[-processed] Rhizoma Pinelliae Ternatae (*Jiang Ban Xia*), and ginger[-processed] Cortex Magnoliae Officinalis (*Jiang Hou Po*) as in *Bu Huan Jing Zheng Qi San* (More Valuable than Gold Righteous Qi Powder [35])

2. Feces Vespertilionis Murini (*Ye Ming Sha*), Pork Liver (*Zhu Gan*), Sheep Liver (*Yang Gan*), Fructus Lycii Chinensis (*Gou Qi Zi*), and prepared Radix Rehmanniae (*Shu Di Huang*)

Dosage: 5-10g and up to 30g in severe cases

Addendum: Bran stir-frying allows one to lessen the very drying quality of *Cang Zhu*.

_____ **Stir-fried [till] Scorched** *(Chao Jiao)* _____

Names: *Jiao Chao Cang Zhu, Jiao Cang Zhu*

Flavors & nature: Sweet, acrid, and bitter; drying; warm

Functions: Dries dampness, stops diarrhea, stops abnormal vaginal discharge

Indications:

1. Diarrhea due to spleen vacuity and stagnation of dampness in the middle burner

2. Abnormal vaginal discharge due to accumulation of dampness in the lower burner with white, clear, copious discharge

Typical combinations:

1. With stir-fried Pericarpium Zanthoxyli Bungeani (*Chao Hua Jiao*) as in *Jiao Zhu Wan* (Zanthoxylum & Atractylodes Pills [175]) or Fructus Amomi (*Sha Ren*), roasted Semen Apliniae Katsumadai (*Wei Cao Dou Kou*), and ginger[-processed] Cortex Magnoliae Officinalis (*Jiang Hou Po*)

2. With stir-fried Radix Angelicae Dahuricae (*Chao Bai Zhi*), bran stir-fried Rhizoma Atractylodis Macrocephalae (*Fu Chao Bai Zhu*), bran stir-fried Radix Dioscoreae Oppositae (*Fu Chao Shan Yao*), and uncooked Semen Euryalis Ferocis (*Sheng Qian Shi*)

Dosage: 5-10g and up to 30g in severe cases

Fructus Chaenomelis Lagenariae (*Mu Gua*)

_____ **Steamed** *(Zheng)*[1] _____

Names: *Xuang Mu Gua, Chuan Mu-Gua, Chen Mu Gua, Mu Gua, Zhi Mu Gua, Zheng Mu Gua*

Flavors & nature: Sour and astringent; warm

Functions: Soothes the network vessels, eliminates *bi*

Indications:

1. Rheumatic complaints due to wind dampness in the muscles, channels and network vessels, and joints with loss of mobility, sinew spasms...

Fructus Chaenomelis Lagenariae continued . . .

2. Beriberi due to wind dampness in the lower burner with painful, heavy feet and legs, lack of strength in the lower extemities, difficulty walking...

Typical combinations:

1. With wine[-processed] Radix Clematidis Chinensis (*Jiu Wei Ling Xian*), Radix Angelicae Pubescentis (*Du Huo*), Radix Et Rhizoma Notopterygii (*Qiang Huo*), and uncooked Cortex Radicis Acanthopanacis (*Sheng Wu Jia Pi*)

2. With uncooked Semen Arecae Catechu (*Sheng Bing Lang*), processed Fructus Evodiae Rutecarpae (*Zhi Wu Zhu Yu*), and Folium Perillae Frutescentis (*Zi Su Ye*) as in *Ji Ming San* (Cock Crow Powder [167])

Dosage: 5-12g and up to 20g in severe cases

Note: 1. Chaenomeles is first soaked for 1 hour in clear water and then steamed in vapor. Afterward, it is cut into slices and again heated and finally baked (*hong*) till dry.

_____ **Stir-fried [till] Yellow (*Chao Huang*)** _____

Names: *Qing Chao Mu Gua, Chao Mu Gua*

Flavors & nature: Sour; warm

Functions: Harmonizes the stomach, transforms dampness

Indications:

1. Vomiting, diarrhea due to either A) stagnation of evil dampness in the middle burner with chest oppression or B) stagnation of dampness in the middle burner with spasmodic pain in the abdomen...

2. Dysentery due to accumulation of dampness in the stomach and intestines with incessant dysentery...

Typical combinations:

1. A) With Herba Agastachis Seu Pogostemi (*Huo Xiang*) and ginger[-processed] Rhizoma Pinelliae Ternatae (*Jiang Ban Xia*)
B) With processed Fructus Evodiae Rutecarpae (*Zhi Wu Zhu Yu*), Fructus Foeniculi Vulgaris (*Xiao Hui Xiang*), Caulis Perillae Frutescentis (*Zi Su Geng*), and uncooked Rhizoma Zingiberis (*Sheng Jiang*) as in *Mu Gua Tang* (Chaenomeles Decoction [223])

2. With uncooked Pericarpium Papaveris Somniferi (*Sheng Ying Su Ke*) and stir-fried Semen Plantaginis (*Chao Che Qian Zi*) as in *Mu Gua San* (Chaenomeles Powder [222])

Dosage: 5-12g and up to 20g in severe cases

Ramulus Mori Albi (*Sang Zhi*)

_____ **Uncooked (*Sheng*)** _____

Names: *Sheng Sang Zhi, Ye Sang Zhi, Nen Sang Zhi*

Flavors & nature: Bitter; neutral

Functions: Clears heat, dispels wind, disinhibits urination

Indications:

1. Rheumatic complaints of the heat type with painful, red, swollen, hot joints...

2. Vertigo due to liver wind or liver fire with headache...

Ramulus Mori Albi continued . . .

3. Beriberi due to wind toxins and evil dampness with edema of the feet and ankles, weakness and feebleness of the limbs...

4. Vitiligo, tinea flava, pityriasis versicolor due to external wind attacking the skin accompanied by heat in the blood

Typical combinations:

1. With Caulis Lonicerae Japonicae (*Ren Dong Teng*), Lumbricus (*Di Long*), and Caulis Sargentodoxae (*Hong Teng*)

2. With stir-fried Folium Mori Albi (*Chao Sang Ye*) and stir-fried Semen Leonuri Heterophylli (*Chao Chong Wei Zi*) as in *Shuang Sang Tang* (Two Moruses Decoction [307])

3. With salt[-processed] Cortex Phellodendri (*Yan Huang Bai*), uncooked Rhizoma Atractylodis (*Sheng Cang Zhu*), and uncooked Cortex Rhizomatis Zingiberis (*Sheng Jiang Pi*)

4. Applied as a 40% alcoholic tincture of Ramulus Mori and Fructus Psoraleae Corylifoliae (*Bu Gu Zhi*)

Dosage: 10-30g and up to 250g in severe cases

Wine Mix-fried (*Jiu Zhi*)

Names: *Jiu Zhi Sang Zhi, Jiu Sang Zhi*

Flavors & nature: Bitter and slightly acrid; slightly warm

Functions: Opens the network vessels, disinhibits the joints, eliminates dampness, stops pain

Indications:

1. Rheumatic complaints due to either A) wind dampness with joint pain, loss of mobility, spasm and numbness of the limbs or B) blood stasis with severe, fixed, piercing pain...

2. Traumatic injury with qi stagnation, blood stasis

Typical combinations:

1. A) With wine[-processed] Radix Aristolochiae Fangchi (*Jiu Fang Ji*), uncooked Radix Achyranthis Bidentatae (*Sheng Huai Niu Xi*), and streamed Fructus Chaenomelis Lagenariae (*Zheng Mu Gua*)
B) With wine[-processed] Radix Angelicae Sinensis (*Jiu Dang Gui*) and wine[-processed] Caulis Millettiae Seu Spatholobi (*Jiu Ji Xue Teng*)

2. With Flos Carthami Tinctorii (*Hong Hua*), vinegar[-processed] Resina Olibani (*Cu Ru Xiang*), vinegar[-processed] Resina Myrrhae (*Cu Mo Yao*), wine[-processed] Radix Ligustici Wallichii (*Jiu Chuan Xiong*), and Radix Pseudoginseng (*San Qi*)

Dosage: 10-30g and up to 250g in severe cases

Radix Clematidis Chinensis (Wei Ling Xian)

Uncooked (Sheng)

Names: *Sheng Wei Ling Xian, Sheng Ling Xian, Wei Ling Xian*

Flavors & nature: Bitter and slightly acrid; warm

Functions: Eliminates dampness, treats jaundice, transforms phlegm, dissolves fishbones

Indications:

1. Jaundice due to damp heat with yellowish orange skin and eyes, dark yellow urine...

2. Accumulation of phlegm in the chest and diaphragm with nausea, vomiting, cough, asthma, anorexia...

3. Fishbone caught in the throat when it is small, soft, and located in the base of the throat or larynx

4. Dysphagia due to qi stagnation and phlegm with a sensation of obstruction when the patient swallows, diaphragmatic and epigastric oppression...

Typical combinations:

1. With Herba Artemisiae Capillaris (*Yin Chen Hao*), Radix Et Rhizoma Polygoni Cuspidati (*Hu Zhang*), uncooked Fructus Gardeniae Jasminoidis (*Sheng Shan Zhi Zi*), and Radix Gentianae Scabrae (*Long Dan Cao*)

2. With stir-fried Semen Lepidii (*Chao Ting Li Zi*), clear Rhizoma Pinelliae Ternatae (*Qing Ban Xia*), and Fructus Gleditschiae Chinensis (*Zao Jiao*)

3. With Fructus Pruni Mume (*Wu Mei*). Make a decoction of Clematis and Mume and add vinegar and sugar. Drink slowly in small swallows.

4. With clear Rhizoma Pinelliae Ternatae (*Qing Ban Xia*), ginger[-processed] Cortex Magnoliae Officinalis (*Jiang Hou Po*), and uncooked Rhizoma Zingiberis (*Sheng Jiang*)

Dosage: 5-15g and up to 30g in severe cases

Wine Mix-fried (Jiu Zhi)

Names: *Jiu Zhi Wei Ling Xian, Jiu Wei Ling Xian, Jiu Ling Xian*

Flavors & nature: Acrid and bitter; warm

Functions: Dispels wind, eliminates *bi*, opens the channels, stops pain

Indications:

1. Rheumatic complaints due to wind dampness in the muscles, channels and network vessels, and joints with joint pain, loss of mobility, spasms of the limbs...

2. Dysmenorrhea or amenorrhea due to disharmony of the *chong* and *ren* and blood stasis with a long cycle, loss of scanty menstruation but accompanied by clots...

3. Abdominal masses due to qi stagnation, blood stasis

Typical combinations:

1. With Radix Angelicae Pubescentis (*Du Huo*), Radix Et Rhizoma Notopterygii (*Qiang Huo*), uncooked Ramulus Cinnamomi (*Sheng Gui Zhi*), and steamed Fructus Chaenomelis Lagenariae (*Zheng Mu Gua*)

2. With wine[-processed] Radix Angelicae

Radix Clematidis Chinensis continued . . .

Sinensis (*Jiu Dang Gui*), wine[-processed] Radix Ligustici Wallichii (*Jiu Chuan Xiong*), and Flos Carthami Tinctorii (*Hong Hua*)

3. With wine[-processed] Radix Angelicae Sinensis (*Jiu Dang Gui*), vinegar[-processed] Resina Myrrha (*Cu Mo Yao*), vinegar[-processed] Resina Olibani (*Cu Ru Xiang*), and vinegar[-processed] Rhizoma Sparganii (*Cu San Leng*)

Dosage: 8-15g and up to 30g in severe cases

Cortex Radicis Acanthopanacis *(Wu Jia Pi)*

Uncooked *(Sheng)*

Names: *Sheng Wu Jia Pi, Sheng Nan Wu Jia Pi, Sheng Bei Wu Jia Pi*

Flavors & nature: Acrid and bitter; warm

Functions: Dispels wind, eliminates dampness, disinhibits urination

Indications:

1. Rheumatic complaints due to wind dampness with swollen, painful joints, loss of mobility, low back pain...

2. Arthrosis of the knee, *i.e.*, crane's knee wind (*he xi feng*), due to cold dampness stagnating in the joints with both knees very swollen and painful...

3. Edema[1] due to spleen vacuity with edema of the four limbs or genralized edema, anuria...

Typical combinations:

1. Steamed Fructus Chaenomelis Lagenariae (*Zheng Mu Gua*) and Nodus Ligni Pini (*Song Jie*)

as in *Wu Jia Pi San* (Acanthopanax Powder [346])

2. With salt[-processed] Radix Achyranthis Bidentatae (*Yan Huai Niu Xi*), Radix Angelicae Pubescentis (*Du Huo*), Nodus Ligni Pini (*Song Jie*), and wine[-processed] Radix Clematidis Chinensis (*jiu Wei Ling Xian*)

3. With uncooked Cortex Rhizomatis Zingiberis (*Sheng Jiang Pi*), Cortex Sclerotii Poriae Cocos (*Fu Ling Pi*), Pericarpium Citri Reticulatae (*Chen Pi*), and Pericarpium Arecae Catechu (*Da Fu Pi*) as in *Wu Pi San* (Five Peels Powder [351])

Dosage: 5-15g and up to 30g in severe cases

Note: 1. There are two types of *Wu Jia Pi*: Southern Acanthopanax (*Nan Wu Jia Pi*), which is superior for dispelling wind dampness, supplementing the liver and kidneys, and strengthening the sinews and bones; and Northern Acanthopanax (*Bei Wu Jia Pi*), which is better for disinhibiting the urination, eliminating dampness, and treating edema. In any case, Northern Acanthopanax is toxic and should always be used in a moderate dose.

Wine Mix-fried *(Jiu Zhi)*

Names: *Jiu Zhi Wu Jia Pi, Jiu Nan Wu Jia Pi, Jiu Wu Jia Pi*

Flavors & nature: Acrid and slightly bitter; warm

Functions: Supplements the liver and kidneys, strengthens the sinews and bones

Indications:

1. Weakness and pain of the knees and low back due to liver/kidney vacuity

Cortex Radicis Acanthopanacis continued . . .

2. Retarded growth in infants due to kidney vacuity with atonic lower limbs, retardation in learning to walk...

3. Chronic rheumatic complaints due to liver/-kidney vacuity with joint pain, which is not so severe but incessant, located in the low back, hips, knees, ankles...

4. Bone fractures

Typical combinations:

1. With salt[-processed] Cortex Eucommiae Ulmoidis (*Yan Du Zhong*), salt[-processed] Radix Dipsaci (*Yan Xu Duan*), and salt[-processed] Rhizoma Cibotii Barometz (*Yan Gou Ji*) as in *Wu Jia Pi San* (Acanthopanax Powder [346])

2. With salt[-processed] Radix Achyranthis Bidentatae (*Yan Huai Niu Xi*), vinegar[-processed] Plastrum Testudinis (*Cu Gui Ban*), salt[-processed] Cortex Eucommiae Ulmoidis (*Yan Du Zhong*), sand stir-fried Rhizoma Drynariae(*Gu Sui Bu*), and Cornu Parvum Cervi (*Lu Rong*)

3. With salt[-processed] Radix Achyranthis Bidentatae (*Yan Huai Niu Xi*), wine[-processed] Ramus Loranthi Seu Visci (*Jiu Sang Ji Sheng*), salt[-processed] Radix Dipsaci (*Jiu Xu Duan*), and wine[-processed] Radix Clematidis Chinensis (*Jiu Wei Ling Xian*)

4. With stone-baked Eupolyphaga Seu Opisthoplatia (*Bei Zhe Chong*), vinegar[-processed] Pyritum (*Cu Zi Ran Tong*), and sand stir-fried Rhizoma Drynariae (*Sha Chao Gu Sui Bu*)

Dosage: 9-15g and up to 30g in severe cases

Zaocys Dhumnades *(Wu Shao She)*

———————————— Uncooked *(Sheng)* ————————————

Names: *Sheng Wu Shao She, Wu Shao She*

Flavors & nature: Sweet; neutral

Functions: Dispels wind, stops itching, soothes tremors

Indications:

1. Urticaria due to wind dampness with severe itching and somewhat permanent...

2. Convulsions, spasms with muscular spasms, infantile convulsions, trismus, tetany, aphasia, epilepsy...

3. Leprosy, mycoses, scabies

4. Tinea flava, Pityriasis versicolor

Typical combinations:

1. With uncooked Herba Cum Radice Asari (*Sheng Xi Xin*), Buthus Martensi (*Quan Xie*), Radix Angelicae Dahuricae (*Bai Zhi*), and Cortex Radicis Dictamni (*Bai Xian Pi*)

2. With Buthus Martensi (*Quan Xie*), uncooked Bombyx Batryticatus (*Sheng Jiang Can*), uncooked Rhizoma Arisaematis (*Sheng Tian Nan Xing*), and stone-baked Scolopendra Subspinipes (*Bei Wu Gong*)

3. With wine[-processed] Agkistrodon Seu Bungarus (*Jiu Bai Hua She*) and wine[-processed] Elaphe (*Jiu Jin Qian Bai Hua She*) as in *Yu Feng Dan* (Heal Wind Elixir [414])

Zaocys Dhumnades continued . . .

4. Applied locally as a 40% alcohol tincture with Agkistrodon Seu Bungarus (*Bai Hua She*), Radix Clematidis Chinensis (*Wei Ling Xian*), and Fructus Psoraleae Corylifoliae (*Bu Gu Zhi*)

Dosage: 5-15g in decoction; 1-2g in powder

_____ **Wine Mix-fried** (*Jiu Zhi*) _____

Names: *Jiu Zhi Wu Shao She, Jiu Wu Shao She*

Flavors & nature: Sweet and slightly acrid; slightly warm

Functions: Dispels wind, frees the network vessels, stops pain

Indications: Rheumatic complaints due to wind dampness with joint pain, weakness of the hands and feet, loss of mobility...

Typical combinations: With Radix Et Rhizoma Notpterygii (*Qiang Huo*), uncooked Radix Ledebouriellae Sesloidis (*Sheng Fang Feng*), wine[-processed] Radix Clematidis Chinensis (*Jiu Wei Ling Xian*), Radix Angelicae Pubescentis (*Du Huo*), and processed Radix Aconiti Carmichaeli (*Zhi Chuan Wu Tou*)

Dosage: 5-15g in decoction and up to 30g in severe cases; 1-2g in powder

Herba Siegesbeckiae (*Xi Xian Cao*)

_____ Uncooked (*Sheng*) _____

Names: *Sheng Xi Xian Cao, Xi Xian Cao*

Flavors & nature: Bitter; cold

Functions: Clears liver heat, resolves toxins

Indications:

1. Vertigo due to liver yang rising with headache, irritability, insomnia...

2. Headache due to wind heat in the liver channel or liver yang rising

3. Jaundice due to damp heat in the liver and gallbladder

4. *Yong* due to hot toxins

Typical combinations:

1. With Fructus Tribuli Terrestris (*Bai Ji Li*), stir-fried Rhizoma Gastrodiae Elatae (*Chao Tian Ma*), Ramulus Uncariae Cum Uncis (*Gou Teng*), uncooked Haematitum (*Sheng Dai Zhe Shi*)

2. With uncooked Fructus Viticis (*Sheng Man Jing Zi*), uncooked Flos Chrysanthemi Morifolii (*Sheng Ju Hua*), Ramulus Uncariae Cum Uncis (*Gou Teng*), stir-fried Rhizoma Gastrodiae Elatae (*Chao Tian Ma*)

3. With Herba Artemisiae Capillaris (*Yin Chen Hao*), Herba Desmodii Seu Lysimachiae (*Jin Qian Cao*), Radix Et Rhizoma Polygoni Cuspidati (*Hu Zhang*), and uncooked Fructus Gardeniae Jasminoidis (*Sheng Shan Zhi Zi*)

Herba Siegesbeckiae continued . . .

4. With Herba Cum Radice Taraxaci Mongolici (*Pu Gong Ying*), Herba Violae Yedoensis (*Zi Hua Di Ding*), stir-fried Resina Olibani (*Chao Ru Xiang*), and uncooked Fructus Forsythiae Suspensae (*Sheng Lian Qiao*)

Dosage: 10-20g and up to 30-60g in severe cases

Wine Mix-fried (*Jiu Zhi*)

Names: *Jiu Zhi Xi Xian Cao, Jiu Xi Xian Cao, Zhi Xi Xian Cao*

Flavors & nature: Bitter and slightly acrid; neutral

Functions: Dispels wind, eliminates dampness, strengthens the sinews and bones

Indications:

1. Rheumatic complaints due to A) wind dampness in the muscles, sinews, or joints with joint pain, loss of mobility, B) heat with redness, pain, swelling, and heat of the joints, or C) cold and blood stasis with severe, fixed joint pain aggravated by cold...

2. Hemiplegia due to wind stroke (*zhong feng*) with deviated mouth and eyes, aphasia...

Typical combinations:

1. A) With uncooked Rhizoma Atractylodis (*Sheng Cang Zhu*), uncooked Semen Coicis Lachryma-jobi (*Sheng Yi Yi Ren*), and wine[-processed] Radix Clematidis Chinensis (*Jiu Wei Ling Xian*)
B) With Caulis Lonicerae Japonicae (*Ren Dong Teng*), uncooked Ramulus Mori Albi (*Sheng Sang Zhi*), stone-baked Lumbricus (*Bei Di Long*), and Caulis Sargentodoxae (*Hong Teng*)
C) With wine[-processed] Radix Angelicae Sinensis (*Jiu Dang Gui*), wine[-processed] Radix Ligustici Wallichii (*Jiu Chuan Xiong*), and processed Radix Aconiti Carmichaeli (*Jiu Chuan Wu Tou*)

2. With uncooked Radix Astragali Membranacei (*Sheng Huang Qi*), wine[-processed] Radix Angelicae Sinensis (*Jiu Dang Gui*), and wine[-processed] Agkistrodon Seu Bungarus (*Jiu Bai Hua She*)

Dosage: 10-20g and up to 30-60g in severe cases

7
Dampness-eliminating, Urination-disinhibiting Medicinals

Semen Plantaginis (Che Qian Zi)

————————Stir-fried (Chao)————————

Names: *Chao Che Qian Zi, Che Qian Zi*

Flavors & nature: Sweet; cold tending to neutral

Functions: Eliminates dampness, stops diarrhea, transforms phlegm, stops cough

Indications:

1. Diarrhea due to accumulation of dampness with watery diarrhea, oliguria...

2. Cough due to lung heat and stagnant phlegm in the lungs with abundant expectoration...

Typical combinations:

1. With earth stir-fried Rhizoma Atractylodis Macrocephalae (*Tu Chao Bai Zhu*), uncooked Sclerotium Poriae Cocos (*Sheng Fu Ling*), Fructus Amomi (*Sha Ren*), and bran stir-fried Rhizoma Atractylodis (*Fu Chao Cang Zhu*)

2. With uncooked Semen Pruni Armeniacae (*Sheng Xing Ren*), uncooked Radix Peucedani (*Sheng Qian Hu*), and uncooked Radix Platycodi Grandiflori (*Sheng Jie Geng*)

Dosage: 5-15g and up to 30g in severe cases

————————Salt Mix-fried (Yan Zhi)————————

Names: *Yan Zhi Che Qian Zi, Yan Che Qian Zi*

Flavors & nature: Sweet and slightly salty; cold tending to neutral

Functions: Disinhibits urination, frees strangury, supplements the kidneys, brightens the eyes

Indications:

1. Strangury[1] due to damp heat in the bladder with urgent need to urinate, frequent urination, dysuria, urinating drop by drop, possible sensation of burning in the urethra...

2. Edema due to accumulation of dampness with oliguria...

3. Red, swollen, painful eyes due to liver heat with leucoma, albugo or white spots, photophobia...

4. Diminishment of visual acuity due to liver/-kidney vacuity with photophobia, blurred vision, tearing in the wind, leucoma...

5. Spermatorrhea, premature ejaculation, impotence due to kidney vacuity

Typical combinations:

1. With Herba Dianthi (*Qu Mai*), Herba Polygoni Avicularis (*Bian Xu*), and Talcum (*Hua Shi*) as in *Ba Zheng San* (Eight Righteous [Medicinals] Powder [5])

Semen Plantaginis continued . . .

2. With uncooked Sclerotium Poriae Cocos (*Sheng Fu Ling*), uncooked Rhizoma Alismatis (*Sheng Ze Xie*), Pericarpium Benincasae (*Dong Gua Pi*), and uncooked Rhizoma Atractylodis Macrocephalae (*Sheng Bai Zhu*)

3. Flos Buddleiae Officinalis (*Mi Meng Hua*), uncooked Semen Cassiae Torae (*Sheng Jue Ming Zi*), and stir-fried Flos Chrysanthemi Morifolii (*Chao Ju Hua*) as in *Che Qian San* (Plantago Powder [46])

4. With prepared Radix Rehmanniae (*Shu Di Huang*) and uncooked Semen Cuscutae (*Sheng Tu Si Zi*) as in *Zhu Jing Wan* (Preserve Vistas Pills [445])

5. With salt[-processed] Semen Cuscutae (*Yan Tu Si Zi*), Fructus Rubi (*Fu Pen Zi*), and wine[-processed] Herba Cistanchis (*Jiu Rou Cong Rong*)

Dosage: 5-15g and up to 30g in severe cases

Note: 1. Uncooked Plantago (*Sheng Che Qian Zi*) may also be prescribed equally for this indication.

Medulla Junci Effusi *(Deng Xin Cao)*

———————————— Uncooked *(Sheng)* ————————————

Names: *Sheng Deng Xin, Deng Xin Cao, Deng Cao*

Flavors & nature: Sweet and bland; slightly cold

Functions: Disinhibits urination, frees strangury, clears heat

Indications:

1. Anuria due to damp heat in the bladder

2. Strangury due to damp heat in the bladder with urgent need to urinate, frequent urination, oliguria, dysuria, urinating drop by drop, possible sensation of burning in the urethra...

3. Jaundice due to damp heat with scanty, dark urination...

4. Vomiting due to heat in the stomach with thirst, nausea...

Typical combinations:

1. With Caulis Akebiae Mutong (*Mu Tong*), uncooked Semen Benincasae Hispidae (*Sheng Dong Gua Zi*), and Talcum (*Hua Shi*) as in *Xuan Qi San* (Diffuse the Qi Powder [392])

2. With Sclerotium Polypori Umbellati (*Zhu Ling*), Herba Lophatheri Gracilis (*Dan Zhu Ye*), Herba Dianthi (*Qu Mai*), and salt[-processed] Semen Plantaginis (*Yan Che Qian Zi*)

3. With Herba Artemisiae Capillaris (*Yin Chen Hao*), Radix Et Rhizoma Polygoni Cuspidati (*Hu Zhang*), and Herba Desmodii Seu Lysimachiae (*Jin Qian Cao*)

4. With ginger[-processed] Caulis In Taeniis Bambusae (*Jiang Zhu Ru*) and ginger[-processed] Rhizoma Coptidis Chinensis (*Jiang Huang Lian*)

Dosage: 2-5g

———————————— Indigo [Processed] *(Qing Dai)*[1] ————————————

Name: *Qing Dai Ban Deng Xin Cao*

Flavors & nature: Sweet and slightly salty; cold

Functions: Clears heat, cools the blood

Indications:

1. Hemoptysis due to lung heat with scanty, concentrated urine...

Medulla Junci Effusi continued . . .

2. Hematuria due to damp heat damaging the net work vessels with clots in the urine, agitation, dry mouth...

Typical combinations:

1. With honey mix-fried Fructus Aristolochiae (*Mi Zhi Ma Dou Ling*), uncooked Concha Cyclinae (*Sheng Hai Ge Ke*), uncooked Rhizoma Imperatae Cylindricae (*Sheng Bai Mao Gen*), Cortex Radicis Moutan (*Sheng Mu Dan Pi*), and carbonized Fructus Gardeniae Jasminoidis (*Zhi Zi Tan*)

2. With carbonized Herba Cephalanoploris Segeti (*Xiao Ji Tan*), carbonized Herba Cirsii Japonici (*Da Ji Tan*), uncooked Nodus Nelumbinis Nuciferae (*Ou Jie*), and uncooked Rhizoma Imperatae Cylindricae (*Sheng Bai Mao Gen*)

Dosage: 2-5g

Note: 1. Juncus is first moistened in either alcohol or water. Then it is mixed with powdered Indigo (*Qing Dai*), 1 part Indigo to 2 parts Juncus.

Cinnabar [Processed] (*Zhu Sha*)

Names: *Zhu Sha Ban Deng Xin Cao, Zhu Deng Xin Cao, Zhu Deng Xin*

Flavors & nature: Sweet; cold

Functions: Downbears fire, clears the heart, quiets the spirit

Indications:

1. Insomnia due to either A) heart fire which agitates the spirit with vexation, a dry mouth, aphthae on the tip of the tongue or B) disharmony of the heart and kidneys

2. Night-crying in infants due to heart heat with agitated sleep and irritability...

Typical combinations:

1. A) With uncooked Rhizoma Coptidis Chinensis (*Sheng Huang Lian*) and stir-fried Fructus Gardeniae Jasminoidis (*Chao Shan Zhi Zi*)
B) With processed Radix Polygalae Tenuifoliae (*Zhi Yuan Zhi*), uncooked Rhizoma Coptidis Chinensis (*Sheng Huang Lian*), prepared Radix Rehmanniae (*Shu Di Huang*), and Egg Yolk (*Ji Zi Huang*)

2. With Cinnabar[-processed] Tuber Ophiopogonis Japonicae (*Zhu Sha Ban Mai Men Dong*) and Radix Scrophulariae Ningpoensis (*Xuan Shen*)

Dosage: 2-5g

Stir-fried [till] Carbonized (*Chao Tan*)

Names: *Deng Xin Cao Tan, Deng Xin Tan*

Flavors & nature: Sweet and slightly astringent; neutral

Functions: Clears heat, disinhibits the throat, promotes the healing of sores

Indications:

1. Sore throat[1] due to wind heat

2. Open sores with bleeding, hematoma, abscess

Typical combinations:

1. With Borneol (*Bing Pian*)

2. With uncooked Flos Lonicerae Japonicae (*Sheng Jin Yin Hua*), Calculus Bovis (*Niu Huang*), and Borneol (*Bing Pian*)

Dosage: 1-2g

Note: 1. For external use only

Addendum: Uncooked Juncus is white colored. Indigo[-processed] Juncus is blue colored. Cinnabar[-processed] Juncus is red colored, and carbonized Juncus is black colored.

Sclerotium Poriae Cocos (Fu Ling)

Uncooked (Sheng)

Names: *Fu Ling, Bai Fu Ling, Yun Ling*

Flavors & nature: Sweet and bland; neutral

Functions: Disinhibits urination, eliminates dampness, supplements the spleen, harmonizes the stomach

Indications:

1. Edema due to accumulation of dampness with oliguria...

2. Phlegm due to spleen vacuity with chest and lateral costal distention, dizziness, shortness of breath...

3. Vomiting due to stagnation of dampness in the middle burner involving disharmony of the stomach with nausea, vomiting of clear liquids, epigastric distention...

4. Diarrhea due to spleen and stomach vacuity with loss of appetite, nausea, a pale complexion...

Typical combinations:

1. With Sclerotium Polypori Umbellati (*Zhu Ling*), uncooked Rhizoma Atractylodis Macrocephalae (*Sheng Bai Zhu*), and uncooked Rhizoma Alismatis (*Sheng Ze Xie*) as in *Wu Ling San* (Five [Ingredients] *Ling* Powder [348])

2. With stir-fried Ramulus Cinnamomi (*Chao Gui Zhi*), uncooked Rhizoma Atractylodis Macrocephalae (*Sheng Bai Zhu*), and mix-fried Radix Glycyrrhizae (*Zhi Gan Cao*) as in *Ling Gui Zhu Gan Tang* (Poria, Cinnamon, Atractylodes & Licorice Decoction [201])

3. With ginger[-processed] Rhizoma Pinelliae Ternatae (*Jiang Ban Xia*) and uncooked Rhizoma Zingiberis (*Sheng Jiang*) as in *Xiao Ban Xia Jia Fu Ling Tang* (Minor Pinellia & Poria Decoction [371])

4. With earth stir-fried Rhizoma Atractylodis Macrocephalae (*Tu Chao Bai Zhu*), Radix Panacis Ginseng (*Ren Shen*), stir-fried Radix Dioscoreae Oppositae (*Chao Shan Yao*), and Fructus Amomi (*Sha Ren*) as in *Shen Ling Bai Zhu San* (Ginseng, Poria & Atractylodes Powder [288])

Dosage: 5-15g and up to 30-60g in severe edema or oliguria

Cinnabar [Processed] (Zhu Sha)[1]

Names: *Zhu Sha Ban Fu Ling, Zhu Fu Ling, Chen Fu Ling*

Flavors & nature: Sweet; neutral tending to cool

Functions: Calms the heart, quiets the spirit

Indications:

1. Insomnia due to agitation of the spirit

2. Heart palpitations due to agitation of the spirit

3. Poor memory due to heart vacuity with diminished concentration and intellectual capacity

Typical combinations:

1. With uncooked Semen Zizyphi Spinosae (*Sheng Suan Zao Ren*) as in *Suan Zao Ren Tang* (Zizyphus Spinosa Decoction [317])

2. With uncooked Semen Zizyphi Spinosae (*Sheng Suan Zao Ren*), Cinnabar[-processed] Sclerotium Pararadicis Poriae Cocos (*Zhu Sha Ban Fu Shen*), calcined Os Draconis (*Duan Long Gu*), and processed Radix Polygalae Tenuifoliae (*Zhi Yuan Zhi*) as in *Ping Bu Zhen Xin Dan* (Level & Supplement the True Heart Elixir [230])

Sclerotium Poriae Cocos continued . . .

3. With vinegar dip calcined Plastrum Testudinis (*Cu Cui Gui Ban*), processed Radix Polygalae Tenuifoliae (*Zhi Yuan Zhi*), and honey mix-fried

Radix Codonopsis Pilosulae (*Mi Zhi Dang Shen*)

Dosage: 10-15g

Note: 1. This refers to Poria prepared with Cinnabar (*Zhu Sha*).

Sclerotium Poriae Cocos (Fu Ling)

Fu Ling is a generic term for a fungus which parasitizes the roots of the pine trees, Pinus Densiflora and Pinus Massoniana. It covers several different medicinals:

1. Cortex Sclerotii Poriae Cocos (Fu Ling Pi): This refers to the blackish outer cortex of the fungus. It disinhibits urination without altering the qi and it disperses swelling. It treats edema and oliguria due to accumulation of severe dampness caused by spleen vacuity. Its action is draining and slightly supplementing. Its dosage is between 15-30g.

2. Sclerotium Rubrum Poriae Cocos (Chi Fu Ling or Chi Ling): This refers to the rosy meat located somewhat externally and just under the blackish cortex. It drains heat and disinhibits urination. It treats strangury (*lin*), oliguria, and reddish or darkish urine due to damp heat. Its action is draining. Its dosage is between 5-15g.

3. Sclerotium Album Poriae Cocos (Fu Ling or Bai Fu Ling or Yun Ling): This refers to the whit-

ish meat which constitutes the major portion of this fungus. It disinhibits urination, supplements the spleen, and quiets the spirit. For its indications and dosage, see *Sheng Fu Ling* and *Zhu Sha Ban Fu Ling* previously. Its action is supplementing and moderately draining without altering the qi.

4. Sclerotium Pararadicis Poriae Cocos (Fu Shen): This refers to the meat encircling the root. It calms the heart and quiets the spirit. It treats insomnia, agitated sleep, palpitations, poor memory, etc. Its action for quieting the spirit is superior to *Bai Fu Ling*. *Fu Shen* is often prepared with Cinnabar (*Zhu Sha*) to reinforce its action. Its dosage is between 5-15g.

5. Mother of Fu Shen (Fu Shen Mu) or Heart of Fu Shen (Fu Shen Xin): This refers to the parasitized root of the pine, which is at the heart of the fungus. It calms the liver and quiets the heart spirit. It treats poor memory, insomnia, heart pain, sinew spasms, etc. Its action for quieting the spirit is superior to *Bai Fu Ling* and *Fu Shen*. Its dosage is between 5-10g.

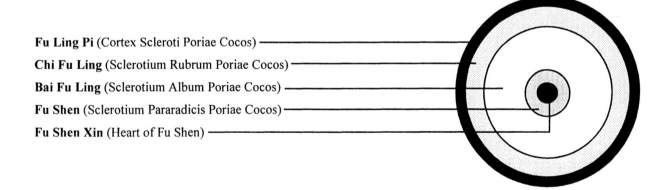

Fu Ling Pi (Cortex Scleroti Poriae Cocos) ————————————

Chi Fu Ling (Sclerotium Rubrum Poriae Cocos) ————————

Bai Fu Ling (Sclerotium Album Poriae Cocos) ————————

Fu Shen (Sclerotium Pararadicis Poriae Cocos) ————————

Fu Shen Xin (Heart of Fu Shen) ————————

Semen Coicis Lachryma-jobi *(Yi Yi Ren)*

Uncooked *(Sheng)*

Names: *Sheng Yi Yi Ren, Sheng Yi Ren, Sheng Mi Ren, Yi Yi Ren, Yi Ren, Mi Ren*

Flavors & nature: Sweet and bland; slightly cold

Functions: Disinhibits urination, eliminates dampness (and heat), evacuates pus, dissipates abscesses

Indications:

1. Edema due to either A) spleen vacuity involving accumulation of dampness with edematous limbs or B) kidney yang vacuity

2. Rheumatic complaints due to evil dampness with joint pain and a sensation of heaviness and numbness, loss of mobility...

3. Lung abscess due to stagnation of heat in the lungs with chest pain, cough with expectoration of pus and blood...

4. Appendicitis (*i.e.*, intestinal abscess) due to stagnation of qi and blood stasis in the intestines with severe pain in right side of the lower abdomen aggravated by pressure, stretched [tight] skin of the lower abdomen...

Typical combinations:

1. A) With uncooked Rhizoma Atractylodis Macrocephalae (*Sheng Bai Zhu*), uncooked Sclerotium Poriae Cocos (*Sheng Fu Ling*), and Semen Phaseoli Calcarati (*Chi Xiao Dou*)
B) With uncooked Cortex Eucommiae Ulmoidis (*Sheng Du Zhong*) and uncooked Radix Astragali Membranacei (*Sheng Huang Qi*) as in *Yi Yi Du Zhong Tang* (Coix & Eucommia Decoction [405])

2. With uncooked Rhizoma Atractylodis (*Sheng Cang Zhu*), Radix Et Rhizoma Notopterygii (*Qiang Huo*), and Radix Angelicae Pubescentis (*Du Huo*) as in *Yi Yi Ren Tang* (Coix Decoction [406])3. With Rhizoma Phragmitis Communis (*Lu Gen*) and uncooked Semen Benincasae Hispidae (*Sheng Dong Gua Ren*) as in *Wei Jing Tang* (Phragmites Decoction [338])

4. With uncooked Cortex Radicis Moutan (*Mu Dan Pi*), scalded Semen Pruni Persicae (*Dan Tao Ren*), and uncooked Pericarpium Trichosanthis Kirlowii (*Sheng Gua Lou Pi*) as in *Jin Jian Yi Yi Ren Tang* (Gold Mirror Coix Decoction [180])

Dosage: 10-30g and up to 50-100g in severe cases

Stir-fried [till] Yellow *(Chao Huang)*

Names: *Chao Yi Yi Ren[1], Chao Yi Ren, Chao Mi Ren*

Flavors & nature: Sweet and bland; neutral

Functions: Supplements the spleen, stops diarrhea

Indications: Diarrhea due to spleen vacuity involving an accumulation of dampness with fatigue, loss of appetite, borborygmus...

Typical combinations: With Radix Panacis Ginseng (*Ren Shen*), uncooked Sclerotium Poriae Cocos (*Sheng Fu Ling*), earth stir-fried Rhizoma Atractylodis Macrocephalae (*Tu Chao Bai Zhu*), and Fructus Amomi (*Sha Ren*) as in *Shen Ling Bai Zhu San* (Ginseng, Poria & Atractylodes Powder [288])

Dosage: 10-30g and up to 50-100g in severe cases

Note: 1. One can equally use bran stir-fried Coix (*Fu Chao Yi Yi Ren*) or earth stir-fried Coix (*Tu Chao Yi Yi Ren*).

Rhizoma Alismatis (Ze Xie)

Uncooked (Sheng)

Names: *Sheng Ze Xie, Ze Xie, Jian Ze Xie, Fu Ze Xie*

Flavors & nature: Sweet; cold

Functions: Eliminates dampness, disinhibits urination

Indications:

1. Strangury[1] due to damp heat in the bladder with urgent need to urinate, frequent urination, oliguria, dysuria, urinating drop by drop, possible sensation of burning in the urethra...

2. Edema due to accumulation of damp heat with edema in the lower body, dysuria, oliguria, lower abdominal distention...

3. Jaundice due to damp heat with yellow skin and eyes, oliguria, concentrated urine...

4. Abnormal vaginal discharge due to damp heat in the lower burner with thick, sticky, abundant, foul-smelling, yellow vaginal discharge...

Typical combinations:

1. With Herba Dianthi (*Qu Mai*), Folium Pyrrosiae (*Shi Wei*), salt[-processed] Semen Plantaginis (*Yan Che Qian Zi*), and Sclerotium Polypori Umbellati (*Zhu Ling*)

2. With uncooked Sclerotium Poriae Cocos (*Sheng Fu Ling*), Sclerotium Polypori Umbellati (*Zhu Ling*), Radix Stephaniae Tetrandrae (*Han Fang Ji*), and salt[-processed] Semen Plantaginis (*Yan Che Qian Zi*)

3. With Herba Artemisiae Capillaris (*Yin Chen Hao*) and Talcum (*Hua Shi*) as in an old version of *Yin Chen Wu Ling San* (Artemisia Capillaris Five [Ingredients] *Ling* Powder [410]) when dampness is more severe than heat

4. With Rhizoma Smilacis Glabrae (*Tu Fu Ling*), Radix Gentianae Scabrae (*Long Dan Cao*), and Radix Sophorae Flavescentis (*Ku Shen*)

Dosage: 5-15g and up to 30g in severe cases

Note: 1. For this indication, salt mix-fried Alisma (*Yan Zhi Ze Xie*) can also equally be prescribed.

Bran Stir-fried (Fu Chao)

Names: *Fu Chao Ze Xie, Chao Ze Xie, Chao Jian Ze Xie*

Flavors & nature: Sweet; cold tending to neutral

Functions: Eliminates dampness, harmonizes the spleen

Indications:

1. Diarrhea due to A) deficiency in the function of transportation and transformation of the spleen involving an accumulation of dampness with watery diarrhea, oliguria, loss of appetite, B) cold, C) heat, D) summerheat, or E) food stagnation

2. Vertigo due to accumulation of dampness in the middle burner and clear yang which cannot raise itself in order to nourish the upper part of the body

Typical combinations:

1. A) With earth stir-fried Rhizoma Atractylodis Macrocephalae (*Tu Chao Bai Zhu*), uncooked Sclerotium Poriae Cocos (*Sheng Fu Ling*), and stir-fried Semen Plantaginis (*Chao Che Qian Zi*)

Rhizoma Alismatis continued . . .

B) With dry Rhizoma Zingiberis (*Gan Jiang*), stir-fried Pericarpium Zanthoxyli Bungeani (*Chao Hua Jiao*), and roasted Radix Saussureae Seu Vladimiriae (*Wei Mu Xiang*)

C) With stir-fried Semen Plantaginis (*Chao Che Qian Zi*), uncooked Rhizoma Coptidis Chinensis (*Sheng Huang Lian*), and Cortex Fraxini (*Qin Pi*)

D) With Herba Elsholtziae (*Xiang Ru*), Herba Agastachis Seu Pogostemi (*Huo Xiang*), ginger[-processed] Cortex Magnoliae Officinalis (*Jiang Hou Po*), and stir-fried Semen Plantaginis (*Chao Che Qian Zi*)

E) With stir-fried Massa Medica Fermentata (*Chao Shen Qu*), stir-fried Fructus Crataegi (*Chao Shan Zha*), and uncooked Radix Et Rhizoma Rhei (*Sheng Da Huang*)

2. With bran stir-fried Rhizoma Atractylodis Macrocephalae (*Fu Chao Bai Zhu*) as in *Ze Xie Tang* (Alisma Decoction [426])

Dosage: 5-15g and up to 30g in severe cases

_____Salt Mix-fried *(Yan Zhi)*[1] _____

Names: *Yan Zhi Ze Xie, Yan Ze Xie, Yan Shui Ze Xie*

Flavors & nature: Sweet and slightly salty; cold tending to neutral

Functions: Eliminates dampness, supplements the kidneys, drains heat

Indications:

1. Spermatorrhea due to kidney yin vacuity involving vacuity fire with spermatorrhea accompanied by erotic dreams, premature ejaculation...

2. Low back pain and heaviness due to kidney vacuity and stagnation of cold dampness in the low back

3. Atony of the legs and feet due to kidney essence vacuity with pain in the heels...

Typical combinations:

1. With salt[-processed] Cortex Phellodendri (*Yan Huang Bai*), salt[-processed] Rhizoma Anemar-rhenae (*Yan Zhi Mu*), prepared Radix Rehmanniae (*Shu Di Huang*), and steamed Fructus Corni Officinalis (*Zheng Shan Zhu Yu*) as in *Zhi Bai Di Huang Wan* (Anemarrhena & Phellodendron Rehmannia Pills [431])

2. With salt[-processed] Cortex Eucommiae Ulmoidis (*Yan Du Zhong*) and Cortex Cinnamomi (*Rou Gui*) as in *Sheng Ji Ze Xie Tang* (Holy Relief Alisma Decoction [295])

3. With prepared Radix Rehmanniae (*Shu Di Huang*), steamed Fructus Corni Officinalis (*Zheng Shan Zhu Yu*), uncooked Sclerotium Poriae Cocos (*Sheng Fu Ling*), and uncooked Cortex Radicis Moutan (*Sheng Mu Dan Pi*) as in *Liu Wei Di Huang Wan* (Six Flavors Rehmannia Pills [204])

Dosage: 5-15g and up to 30g in severe cases

Note: 1. In fact, in supplementing prescriptions, Alisma should be prepared in both salt and rice wine.

8
Food Stagnation-dispersing Medicinals

Fructus Germinatus Oryzae Sativae (Gu Ya)

———————— Uncooked (Sheng) ————————

Names: *Sheng Gu Ya, Sheng Dao Ya*

Flavors & nature: Sweet; neutral

Functions: Fortifies the spleen, nourishes the stomach, stimulates the appetite

Indications:

1. Qi and yin vacuity of the stomach due to warm disease with dry lips and mouth, loss of appetite, chest and epigastric distention, constipation...

2. Lack of appetite due to spleen and stomach vacuity with nausea or vomiting after eating food, anorexia...

Typical combinations:

1. With Tuber Ophiopogonis Japonicae (*Mai Men Dong*), Radix Glehniae Littoralis (*Bei Sha Shen*), and uncooked Radix Dioscoreae Oppositae (*Sheng Shan Yao*)

2. With stir-fried Massa Medica Fermentata (*Chao Shen Qu*), Fructus Amomi (*Sha Ren*), and bran stir-fried Rhizoma Atractylodis Macrocephalae (*Fu Chao Bai Zhu*)

———————— Stir-fried (Chao) ————————

Names: *Chao Gu Ya, Chao Huang Gu Ya, Jiao Gu Ya, Xiang Gu Ya, Gu Ya*

Flavors & nature: Sweet; neutral tending to warm

Functions: Fortifies the spleen, disperses food stagnation

Indications:

1. Food stagnation[1] with epigastric and abdominal distention, disgust for eating, nausea, loss of appetite...

2. Lack of appetite[1] due to spleen and stomach vacuity with slow, difficult digestion, loose stools...

3. Diarrhea[2] due to stagnation of food with borborygmus, abdominal distention...

Typical combinations:

1. With stir-fried Fructus Crataegi (*Chao Shan Zha*), stir-fried Massa Medica Fermentata (*Chao Shen Qu*), stir-fried Semen Raphani Sativi (*Chao Lai Fu Zi*), and stir-fried Fructus Germinatus Hordei Vulgaris (*Chao Mai Ya*)

2. With bran stir-fried Rhizoma Atractylodis Macrocephalae (*Fu Chao Bai Zhu*), rice stir-fried Radix Codonopsis Pilosulae (*Mi Chao Dang Shen*), bran stir-fried Radix Dioscoreae Oppositae (*Fu Chao Shan Yao*), and Fructus Amomi (*Sha Ren*)

Fructus Germinatus Oryzae Sativae continued . . .

3. With stir-fried [till] scorched Fructus Germinatus Hordei Vulgaris (*Chao Jiao Mai Ya*), stir-fried [till] scorched Fructus Crataegi (*Chao Jiao Shan Zha*), stir-fried [till] scorched Massa Medica Fermentata (*Chao Jiao Shen Qu*), and stir-fried [till] scorched Radix Et Rhizoma Rhei (*Chao Jiao Da Huang*)

Dosage: 10-20g and up to 30-60g in severe cases

Notes: 1. For this indication, one should prescribe stir-fried [till] yellow *Gu Ya* (*Chao Huang Gu Ya*). 2. For this indication, one should prescribe stir-fried [till] scorched *Gu Ya* (*Chao Jiao Gu Ya*).

Endothelium Corneum Gigeriae Galli *(Ji Nei Jin)*

Uncooked *(Sheng)*

Names: *Sheng Ji Nei Jin, Sheng Ji Jin, Sheng Ji Zhun Pi*

Flavors & nature: Sweet; neutral

Functions: Disperses food stagnation, transforms stones, frees strangury

Indications:

1. Food stagnation with accumulation (*ji*) A) with abdominal masses, epigastric distention, epigastric pain aggravated by pressure, loss of appetite, B) with severe abdominal pain and distention, or C) with constipation

2. Strangury with stones (*shi lin*) due to a combination of dampness and heat, which produce stones with dysuria, piercing pain in the ureter, reddish urine with gravel, occasionally interrupted urination...

3. Abdominal distention[1] due to stagnation of liver qi and spleen vacuity

Typical combinations:

1. A) With bran stir-fried Fructus Immaturus Citri Seu Ponciri (*Fu Chao Zhi Shi*), stir-fried Fructus Crataegi (*Chao Shan Zha*), and stir-fried Fructus Germinatus Hordei Vulgaris (*Chao Mai Ya*)
B) With uncooked Radix Saussureae Seu Vladimiriae (*Sheng Mu Xiang*) and ginger[-processed] Cortex Magnoliae Officinalis (*Jiang Hou Po*)
C) With uncooked Radix Et Rhizoma Rhei (*Sheng Da Huang*) and stir-fried Semen Arecae Catechu (*Chao Bing Lang*)

2. With Spora Lygodii (*Hai Jin Sha*), Folium Pyrrosiae (*Shi Wei*), Herba Desmodii Seu Lysimachiae (*Jin Qian Cao*), and uncooked Radix Saussureae Seu Vladimiriae (*Sheng Mu Xiang*)

3. With bran stir-fried Rhizoma Atractylodis Macrocephalae (*Fu Chao Bai Zhu*), stir-fried Radix Albus Paeoniae Lactiflorae (*Chao Bai Shao Yao*), stir-fried Radix Bupleuri (*Chao Chai Hu*), and stir-fried Pericarpium Citri Reticulatae (*Chao Chen Pi*) as in *Ji Chi Tang* (Chicken Gizzard Membrane Decoction [164])

Dosage: 3-9g in decoction; 3-5g in powder

Note: 1. For this indication, vinegar-processed *Ji Nei Jin* (*Cu Zhi Ji Nei Jin*) can also be equally prescribed.

_____ Stir-fried _(Chao)_ _____

Names: _Chao Ji Nei Jin, Sha Chao Ji Nei Jin, Jiao Chao Jin Nei Jin, Jiao Jin Nei Jin_

Flavors & nature: Sweet and slightly astringent; neutral

Functions: Disperses food stagnation, stops diarrhea, secures the essence, controls urination

Indications:

1. Food stagnation[1] with epigastric and abdominal distention, vomiting, diarrhea...

2. Enuresis, urinary incontinence[1] due to kidney qi vacuity with nocturia, abundant, clear urination...

3. Spermatorrhea[1] due to kidney qi not securing

4. Diarrhea[2] due to either A) food stagnation with loss of appetite, epigastric and abdominal distention or B) spleen vacuity with chronic diarrhea, lack of appetite...

Typical combinations:

1. With stir-fried Fructus Germinatus Hordei Vulgaris (_Chao Mai Ya_), stir-fried Fructus Germinatus Oryzae Sativae (_Chao Gu Ya_), stir-fried Massa Medica Fermentata (_Chao Shen Qu_), and fermented Rhizoma Pinelliae Ternatae (_Ban Xia Qu_)

2. With salt[-processed] Os Sepiae Seu Sepiellae (_Yan Hai Piao Xiao_), salt[-processed] Fructus Alpiniae Oxyphyllae (_Yan Yi Zhi Ren_), and uncooked Semen Euryalis Ferocis (_Sheng Qian Shi_)

3. With salt[-processed] Semen Cuscutae (_Yan Tu Si Zi_), stir-fried Semen Nelumbinis Nuciferae (_Chao Lian Zi_), uncooked Semen Euryalis Ferocis (_Sheng Qian Shi_), and Fructus Rubi (_Fu Pen Zi_)

4. A) With stir-fried Fructus Crataegi (_Chao Shan Zha_), stir-fried Massa Medica Fermentata (_Chao Shen Qu_), and earth stir-fried Rhizoma Atractylodis Macrocephalae (_Tu Chao Bai Zhu_)
B) With earth stir-fried Rhizoma Atractylodis Macrocephalae (_Tu Chao Bai Zhu_), earth stir-fried Radix Dioscoreae Oppositae (_Chao Shan Yao_), and honey mix-fried Radix Codonopsis Pilosulae (_Mi Zhi Dang Shen_)

Dosage: 5-10g in decoction; 3-5g in powder

Notes: 1. For this indication, sand stir-fried _Ji Nei Jin_ (_Sha Chao Ji Nei Jin_) should be prescribed. 2. For this indication, stir-fried [till] yellow (_Chao Huang_) or stir-fried [till] scorched _Ji Nei Jin_ (_Chao Jiao Ji Nei Jin_) should be prescribed.

Semen Raphani Sativi (*Lai Fu Zi*)

Uncooked (*Sheng*)

Names: *Sheng Lai Fu Zi, Lai Fu Zi, Luo Bo Zi*

Flavors & nature: Acrid and sweet; neutral

Functions: Transforms phlegm, downbears counterflow qi

Indications:

1. Cough due to accumulation of qi and phlegm with asthmatic breathing, chest oppression, abundant mucus...

2. Asthma of the cold type with thin, clear, liquid phlegm...

Typical combinations:

1. With processed Rhizoma Typhonii (*Zhi Bai Fu Zi*) and uncooked Fructus Perillae Frutescentis (*Sheng Zi Su Zi*) as in *San Zi Yang Xin Tang* (Three Seeds Nourish the Aged Decoction [274])

2. With stir-fried Semen Sinapis Albae (*Chao Bai Jie Zi*), honey mix-fried Herba Cum Radice Asari (*Mi Zhi Xi Xin*), dry Rhizoma Zingiberis (*Gan Jiang*), honey mix-fried Herba Ephedrae (*Mi Zhi Ma Huang*), and clear Rhizoma Pinelliae Ternatae (*Qing Ban Xia*)

Dosage: 10-15g and up to 20g in severe cases

Stir-fried [till] Yellow (*Chao Huang*)

Name: *Chao Lai Fu Zi*

Flavors & nature: Slightly acrid and sweet; slightly warm

Functions: Disperses food stagnation, eliminates distention, transforms phlegm

Indications:

1. Food stagnation with fullness in the chest and epigastrium, pain and distention of the abdomen, fetid eructations, acid vomiting or vomiting of undigested food...

2. Abdominal distention due to chronic stagnation of qi and food with fullness in the epigastrium

and abdomen, eructation, borborygmus, flatulence, lack of appetite, slow digestion...

Typical combinations:

1. With stir-fried Fructus Crataegi (*Chao Shan Zha*), fermented Rhizoma Pinelliae Ternatae (*Ban Xia Qu*), and stir-fried Massa Medica Fermentata (*Chao Shen Qu*) as in *Bao He Wan* (Protecting Harmony Pills [29])

2. With uncooked Radix Saussureae Seu Vladimiriae (*Sheng Mu Xiang*), ginger[-processed] Cortex Magnoliae Officinalis (*Jiang Hou Po*), and Semen Arecae Catechu (*Bing Lang*)

Dosage: 10-15g and up to 20g in severe cases

Fructus Germinatus Hordei Vulgaris (Mai Ya)

Uncooked (Sheng)

Name: *Sheng Mai Ya*

Flavors & nature: Salty and sweet; neutral tending to cool

Functions: Soothes the liver, disperses food stagnation, disinhibits the flow of milk

Indications:

1. Mammary nodules (*ru pi*) due to liver qi stagnation and accumulation of phlegm in the network vessels of the breast with multiple, hard, not painful, and mobile nodular masses in the breast which vary with emotional fluctuations (*e.g.* cysts, adenomas, fibroadenomas, and benign breast tumors)

2. Mastitis due to liver qi stagnation and stagnation of milk with distention and pain of the breasts with possible hardness to palpation and possible fever, chills...

3. Food stagnation which has transformed into heat with epigastric and abdominal fullness, a sensation of heat in the chest and limbs, fetid vomiting, bad breath...

Typical combinations:

1. With Folium Citri Reticulatae (*Ju Ye*), vinegar[-processed] Radix Bupleuri (*Cu Chai Hu*), vinegar[-processed] Rhizoma Cyperi Rotundi (*Cu Xiang Fu*), stir-fried Pericarpium Citri Reticulatae (*Chao Chen Pi*), and Fasciculus Vascularis Luffae (*Si Gua Lou*)

2. With Herba Cum Radice Taraxaci Mongolici (*Pu Gong Ying*), Flos Lonicerae Japonicae (*Jin Yin Hua*), uncooked Fructus Forsythiae Suspensae (*Sheng Lian Qiao*), vinegar[-processed] Radix Bupleuri (*Cu Chai Hu*), vinegar[-processed] Pericarpium Viridis Citri Reticulatae (*Cu Qing Pi*), and Semen Vaccariae Segetalis (*Wang Bu Liu Xing*)

3. With stir-fried Fructus Germinatus Hordei Vulgaris (*Chai Mai Ya*), stir-fried Massa Medica Fermentata (*Chao Shen Qu*), stir-fried Rhizoma Coptidis Chinensis (*Chao Huang Lian*), uncooked Pericarpium Viridis Citri Reticulatae (*Qing Pi*), and uncooked Fructus Forsythiae Suspensae (*Sheng Lian Qiao*)

Dosage: 10-15g

Stir-fried (Chao)

Names: *Chao Mai Ya, Jiao Ma Ya, Ma Ya*

Flavors & nature: Salty, sweet, and slightly astringent; neutral; tending to neutral

Functions: Disperses food stagnation, harmonizes the stomach, stops diarrhea, stops lactation

Indications:

1. Food stagnation[1] with epigastric and abdominal distention, fetid eructations, loss of appetite, nausea, disgust for eating...

2. Loss of appetite[1] due to spleen and stomach vacuity, slow digestion, a tasteless mouth...

3. Galactorrhea or maternal weaning[1]

4. Diarrhea[2] due to either A) food stagnation with borborygmus, epigastric and abdominal distention or B) spleen and stomach yang vacuity with loss of appetite, fatigue, a pale complexion, cold limbs...

Fructus Germinatus Hordei Vulgaris continued . . .

Typical combinations:

1. With uncooked Endothelium Corneum Gigeriae Galli (*Sheng Ji Nei Jin*), stir-fried Fructus Crataegi (*Chao Shan Zha*), and stir-fried Pericarpium Citri Reticulatae (*Chao Chen Pi*)

2. With bran stir-fried Radix Dioscoreae Oppositae (*Fu Chao Shan Yao*), honey mix-fried Radix Codonopsis Pilosulae (*Mi Zhi Dang Shen*), bran stir-fried Rhizoma Atractylodis Macrocephalae (*Fu Chao Bai Zhu*), and uncooked Radix Saussureae Seu Vladimiriae (*Sheng Mu Xiang*)

3. Used alone in decoction. If the breasts are painful and distended, apply locally a plaster made from Mirabilitum (*Pi Xiao*).

4. A) With stir-fried [till] scorched Massa Medica Fermentata (*Chao Jiao Shen Qu*), stir-fried [till] scorched Fructus Crataegi (*Chao Jiao Shan Zha*), stir-fried Pericarpium Citri Reticulatae (*Chao Chen Pi*), and earth stir-fried Rhizoma Atractylodis Macrocephalae (*Tu Chao Bai Zhu*)
B) With bran stir-fried Rhizoma Atractylodis Macrocephalae (*Fu Chao Bai Zhu*), rice stir-fried Radix Codonopsis Pilosulae (*Mi Chao Dang Shen*), and dry Rhizoma Zingiberis (*Gan Jiang*)

Dosage: 10-15g; 15-30g for diarrhea; 30-120g for stopping lactation

Notes: 1. For this indication, one should prescribe stir-fried [till] yellow *Mai Ya* (*Chao Huang Mai Ya*). 2. For this indications, one should prescribe stir-fried [till] scorched *Mai Ya* (*Chao Jiao Mai Ya*).

Fructus Crataegi *(Shan Zha)*

Uncooked *(Sheng)*

Names: *Sheng Shan Zha, Zha Rou*

Flavors & nature: Sour and sweet; slightly warm

Functions: Quickens the blood, dispels stasis, scatters nodulations

Indications:

1. Postpartum abdominal pain due to blood stasis with retention of the lochia, pain aggravated by pressure...

2. Amenorrhea due to A) blood stasis, B) blood stasis caused by cold, or C) blood stasis caused by heat

3. Heart pain due to heart qi vacuity and blood stasis with palpitations, shortness of breath, pain in the chest, a purple tongue, a choppy (*se*) pulse...

4. Inguinal hernia, maladies of the scrotum or testicles due to qi stagnation with hernia which tends to fall downward, swollen, painful scrotum...

Typical combinations:

1. With wine[-processed] Radix Angelicae Sinensis (*Jiu Dang Gui*), wine[-processed] Herba Leonuri Heterophylli (*Jiu Yi Mu Cao*), and wine[-processed] Radix Cyathulae (*Jiu Chuan Niu Xi*)

2. A) With wine[-processed] Radix Cyathulae (*Jiu Chuan Niu Xi*), Herba Lycopi Lucidi (*Ze Lan*), and Caulis Millettiae Seu Spatholobi (*Ji Xue Teng*)

Fructus Crataegi continued . . .

B) With stir-fried Ramulus Cinnamomi (*Chao Gui Zhi*), blast-fried Rhizoma Zingiberis (*Pao Jiang*), and Flos Carthami Tinctorii (*Hong Hua*)
C) With wine[-processed] Cortex Radicis Moutan (*Jiu Mu Dan Pi*), wine[-processed] Radix Et Rhizoma Rhei (*Jiu Da Huang*), and uncooked Semen Pruni Persicae (*Sheng Tao Ren*)

3. With wine[-processed] Radix Salviae Miltiorrhizae (*Jiu Dan Shen*), mix-fried Radix Glycyrrhizae (*Zhi Gan Cao*), and stir-fried Ramulus Cinnamomi (*Chao Gui Zhi*)

4. With salt[-processed] Fructus Foeniculi Vulgaris (*Yan Xiao Hui Xiang*) and salt[-processed] Semen Litchi Chinensis (*Yan Li Zhi He*)

Dosage: 15-30g and up to 80g in case of a uterus that does not return to its normal position after birthing

_____ Stir-fried *(Chao)* _____

Names: *Chao Shan Zha, Chao Huang Shan Zha, Jiao Shan Zha, Shan Zha Tan*

Flavors & nature: Sweet, sour, and slightly astringent; warm

Functions: Disperses food stagnation, regulates the intestines, stops diarrhea

Indications:

1. Food stagnation[1] with epigastric and abdominal pain and distention, loss of appetite, disgust at eating, diarrhea...

2. Loss of appetite[1] due to spleen and stomach vacuity with loss of taste, loose stools...

3. Diarrhea[2] due to food stagnation with borborygmus, abdominal pain or distention...

4. Dysentery[2] due to either A) damp heat generated by food stagnation with abdominal pain during defecation, fetid stools, epigastric and abdominal fullness or B) food stagnation due to overeating meat, with pussy, bloody stools, abdominal pain and distention...

Typical combinations:

1. With stir-fried Massa Medica Fermentata (*Chao Shen Qu*), stir-fried Semen Raphani Sativi (*Chao Lai Fu Zi*), and stir-fried Fructus Germinatus Hordei Vulgaris (*Chao Mai Ya*) as in *Bao He Wan* (Protect Harmony Pills [29])

2. With bran stir-fried Rhizoma Atractylodis Macrocephalae (*Fu Chao Bai Zhu*), stir-fried Massa Medica Fermentata (*Chao Shen Qu*), and uncooked Sclerotium Poriae Cocos (*Sheng Fu Ling*) as in *Xiao Bao He Wan* (Minor Protect Harmony Pills [373])

3. With earth stir-fried Rhizoma Atractylodis Macrocephalae (*Tu Chao Bai Zhu*), roasted Radix Puerariae (*Wei Ge Gen*), and stir-fried Fructus Germinatus Hordei Vulgaris (*Chao Mai Ya*)

4. A) With uncooked Rhizoma Coptidis Chinensis (*Sheng Huang Lian*), stir-fried Radix Scutellariae Baicalensis (*Chao Huang Qin*), and roasted Radix Saussureae Seu Vladimiriae (*Wei Mu Xiang*)
B) With uncooked Pericarpium Viridis Citri Reticulatae (*Sheng Qing Pi*) and roasted Radix Saussureae Seu Vladimiriae (*Wei Mu Xiang*)

Dosage: 5-20g and up to 30g in severe cases; 10-15g to stop diarrhea

Notes: 1. For this indication, one should prescribe stir-fried [till] yellow Crataegus (*Chao Huang Shan Zha*).
2. For this indication, one should prescribe stir-fried [till] scorched (*Chao Jiao*) or stir-fried [till] carbonized Crataegus (*Chao Tan Shan Zha*).

Massa Medica Fermentata *(Shen Qu)*

_____ Uncooked *(Sheng)*[1] _____

Names: *Sheng Shen Qu, Sheng Jian Qu, Sheng Liu Qu*

Flavors & nature: Acrid and sweet; warm

Functions: Disperses food stagnation, resolves the exterior, promotes the absorption of minerals

Indications:

1. Food stagnation accompanying a cold or flu[2] due to wind cold with indigestion, epigastric and abdominal distention, loss of appetite, nausea, aversion to cold, fever...

2. Promotes digestion and the assimilation of mineral medicinals. This remedy is included in pills which contain large quantities of minerals as in *Ci Zhu Wan* (Magnetite & Cinnabar Pills)

Typical combinations:

1. With Folium Perillae Frutescentis (*Zi Su Ye*), Herba Agastachis Seu Pogostemi (*Huo Xiang*), and stir-fried Fructus Crataegi (*Chao Shan Zha*)

Dosage: 5-10g and up to 12-20g in severe cases

Notes: 1. *Shen Qu*, also called *Liu Qu* or literally six [ingredient] ferment, is a fermented [product] made from flour, wheat bran, Semen Pruni Armeniacae (*Xing Ren*) paste, powdered Semen Phaseoli Calcarati (*Chi Xiao Dou*), the juice of Herba Artemisiae Apiaceae (*Qing Hao*), Herba Xanthii (*Cang Er Cao*), and Herba Polygoni Lapathifolii (*La Liao Cao*). 2. Another type of Massa Medica Fermentata called *Jian Qu* is a fermented [product] made from 15 ingredients. *Jian Qu* possesses the same functions as *Shen Qu* (*i.e., Liu Qu*) but, in addition, it dispels external wind. It is, therefore, preferred for treating food stagnation when there is an external affection.

_____ Stir-fried *(Chao)* _____

Names: *Chao Shen Qu, Jiao Shen Qu, Fu Chao Shen Qu, Chao Liu Qu, Chao Liu Shen Qu*

Flavors & nature: Sweet and slightly astringent; warm

Functions: Transforms food stagnation, stimulates the appetite, harmonizes the stomach, stops diarrhea

Indications:

1. Lack of appetite due to either A) food stagnation and spleen vacuity with epigastric and abdominal distention, a bland mouth, loss of taste[1] or B) spleen and stomach vacuity with loose stools, shortness of breath, fatigue[2]

2. Abdominal mass[1] due to food stagnation and phlegm

3. Diarrhea[3] due to either A) food stagnation with epigastric and abdominal distention, loss of appetite or B) food stagnation and spleen vacuity

Typical combinations:

1. A) With stir-fried Fructus Germinatus Hordei Vulgaris (*Chao Mai Ya*), bran stir-fried Rhizoma Atractylodis Macrocephalae (*Fu Chao Bai Zhu*), Herba Eupatorii (*Pei Lan*), and uncooked Sclerotium Poriae Cocos (*Sheng Fu Ling*)
B) With rice stir-fried Radix Codonopsis Pilosulae (*Mi Chao Dang Shen*), bran stir-fried Radix Dioscoreae Oppositae (*Fu Chao Shan Yao*), and bran stir-fried Rhizoma Atractylodis Macrocephalae (*Fu Chao Bai Zhu*)

Massa Medica Fermentata continued . . .

2. With ginger[-processed] Cortex Magnoliae Officinalis (*Jiang Hou Po*), vinegar[-processed] Rhizoma Sparganii (*Cu San Leng*), vinegar[-processed] Rhizoma Curcumae Zedoariae (*Cu E Zhu*), and stir-fried Pericarpium Citri Reticulatae (*Chao Chen Pi*)

3. A) With stir-fried [till] scorched Fructus Crataegi (*Chao Jiao Shan Zha*), stir-fried Fructus Germinatus Hordei Vulgaris (*Chao Mai Ya*), and stir-fried Semen Raphani Sativi (*Chao Lai Fu Zi*) as in *Bao He Wan* (Protect Harmony Pills [29]) B) With earth stir-fried Rhizoma Atractylodis

Macrocephalae (*Tu Chao Bai Zhu*), uncooked Sclerotium Poriae Cocos (*Sheng Fu Ling*), and stir-fried [till] scorched Fructus Crataegi (*Chao Jiao Shan Zha*) as in *Da An Wan* (Great Quieting Pills [62])

Dosage: 5-10g and up to 12-20g in severe cases

Notes: 1. For this indication, one should prescribe stir-fried [till] yellow *Shen Qu* (*Chao Huang Shen Qu*). 2. For this indication, one should prescribe bran stir-fried *Shen Qu* (*Fu Chao Shen Qu*). 3. For this indication, one should prescribe stir-fried [till] scorched *Shen Qu* (*Chao Jiao Shen Qu*).

9
Qi-rectifying Medicinals

Semen Arecae Catechu (Bing Lang)

Uncooked (Sheng)

Names: *Bing Lang, Hua Bing Lang, Da Fu Zi, Sheng Bing Lang*

Flavors & nature: Acrid, bitter and slightly astringent; warm

Functions: Kills parasites, disperses accumulation of parasites, disinhibits urination, disperses swelling

Indications:

1. Intestinal parasites[1] A) with abdominal pain or B) with severe accumulation of parasites, abdominal pain aggravated by pressure, constipation...

2. Edema due to internal accumulation of dampness with generalized edema, shortness of breath, constipation, oliguria...

3. Beriberi due to accumulation of cold dampness with pain of the lower extremities, heavy, swollen feet...

4. Malaria

Typical combinations:

1. A) With Omphalia (*Lei Wan*) and uncooked Fructus Quisqualis Indicae (*Sheng Shi Jun Zi*) as in *Hua Chong Wan* (Transform Parasites Pills [147])

B) With uncooked Radix Et Rhizoma Rhei (*Sheng Da Huang*) and Cortex Radicis Meliae Azardach (*Ku Lian Pi*) as in *Wan Ying Wan* (Ten Thousand Responses Pills [336])

2. With Cortex Sclerotii Poriae Cocos (*Fu Ling Pi*) and uncooked Cortex Rhizomatis Zingiberis (*Sheng Jiang Pi*) as in *Shu Zao Yin Zi* (Coursing & Chiselling Drink [305])

3. With steamed Fructus Chaenomelis Lagenariae (*Zheng Mu Gua*) and processed Fructus Evodiae Rutecarpae (*Zhi Wu Zhu Yu*) as in *Ji Ming San* (Cock Crow Powder [167])

4. With bran stir-fried Radix Dichroae Febrifugae (*Fu Chao Chang Shan*) and uncooked Fructus Amomi Tsao-ko (*Sheng Cao Guo*) as in *Jie Nue Qi Bao Yin* (Resolve *Nue* Seven Treasures Drink [178])

Dosage: 5-15g; 30-60g for parasites; 60-120g for severe parasites

Note: 1. Semen Arecae Catechu treats all types of intestinal parasites but especially taenia or tapeworm. It notably suppresses the head and hook of taenia. It also has an anesthetic effect on parasites, which is particularly interesting in case of abdominal pain caused by parasitosis.

Semen Arecae Catechu continued . . .

_____ Stir-fried [till] Scorched *(Chao Jiao)* _____

Names: *Chao Bing Lang, Chao Da Fu Zi*

Flavors & nature: Bitter, acrid and slightly astringent; warm

Functions: Moves the qi, disperses food stagnation, disperses distention

Indications:

1. Food stagnation with epigastric distention, nausea, vomiting, fetid smelling eructations, possible abdominal pain and distention, constipation...

2. Dysentery with tenesmus due to accumulation of internal damp heat damaging the stomach and intestines

3. Inguinal hernia, maladies of the scrotum or testicles due to stagnation of qi and cold in the liver channel with pain in the lower abdomen radiating to the testicles...

Typical combinations:

1. With uncooked Radix Saussureae Seu Vladimiriae (*Sheng Mu Xiang*), uncooked Pericarpium Viridis Citri Reticulatae (*Sheng Qing Pi*), and uncooked Radix Et Rhizoma Rhei (*Sheng Da Huang*) as in *Mu Xiang Bing Lang Wan* (Saussurea & Areca Pills [225])

2. With stir-fried Radix Albus Paeoniae Lactiflorae (*Chao Bai Shao Yao*), uncooked Rhizoma Coptidis Chinensis (*Sheng Huang Lian*), and roasted Radix Saussureae Seu Vladimiriae (*Wei Mu Xiang*) as in *Shao Yao Tang* (Peony Decoction [285])

3. With salt[-processed] Radix Linderae Strychnifoliae (*Wu Yao*) and salt[-processed] Fructus Foeniculi Vulgaris (*Yan Xiao Hui Xiang*) as in *Tian Tai Wu Yao San* (Tian Tai Lindera Powder [325])

Dosage: 10-30g

Pericarpium Citri Reticulatae *(Chen Pi)*[1]

_____ Uncooked *(Sheng)* _____

Names: *Chen Pi, Ju Pi*[2], *Guan Chen Pi, Xin Hui Pi*

Flavors & nature: Acrid and bitter; warm

Functions: Dries dampness, transforms phlegm

Indications:

1. Cough due to either A) stagnation of phlegm dampness in the lungs with chest oppression, whitish, abundant phlegm or B) stagnation of phlegm heat in the lungs with yellow, thick, sticky phlegm...

2. Epigastric distention due to qi stagnation in the middle burner with epigastric pain and possible anuria and constipation...

Typical combinations:

1. A) With clear Rhizoma Pinelliae Ternatae (*Qing Ban Xia*) and uncooked Sclerotium Poriae Cocos (*Sheng Fu Ling*) as in *Er Chen Tang* (Two Aged [Ingredients] Decoction[3] [95])
B) With Lumbricus (*Di Long*) and Fel Agkistrodonis (*She Dan*) as in *She Dan Chen Pi Mo* (Snake Gall & Orange Peel Powder [286])

Pericarpium Citri Reticulatae continued . . .

2. With bran stir-fried Rhizoma Atractylodis Macrocephalae (*Fu Chao Bai Zhu*) and uncooked Radix Saussureae Seu Vladimiriae (*Sheng Mu Xiang*)

Dosage: 3-10g and up to 30g in severe cases

Notes: 1. All Chinese materia medicas in Western languages give the name Pericarpium Citri Reticulatae for *Chen Pi*. However, the pericarpium corresponds to the entire part of the fruit which encircles any seed or, in other words, the skin (epicarpium), the pulp (mesocarpium), and sometimes the kernel which protects the seed, the endocarpium. *Chen Pi* corresponds only to the exocarpium or skin. Thus its true name should be Epicarpium Citri Reticulatae. [The editors have elected to retain the name Pericarpium in order to maintain consistency with the rest of the English literature.] 2. *Ju Pi* and *Chen Pi* are the skins of the same fruit. However, *Ju Pi* is the fresh skin, while *Chen Pi* is the preserved, aged skin. *Ju Pi* is more irritating to the stomach, more dispersing, and more drying. *Chen Pi* is more moderate and therefore preferred in clinic. 3. Certain medicinals are preserved and aged in order to lessen their secondary effects and to strengthen their therapeutic actions. Traditionally, one lists six preserved remedies: Epicarpium Citri Reticulatae (*Chen Pi*), Rhizoma Pinelliae Ternatae (*Ban Xia*), Fructus Citri Seu Ponciri (*Zhi Ke*), Herba Ephedrae (*Ma Huang*), Fructus Evodiae Rutecarpae (*Wu Zhu Yu*), and Radix Stellaerae Chamaejasmi Seu Rhizoma Alocasiae Seu Radix Euphorbiae Pallasii (*Lang Du*).

Stir-fried (Chao)

Names: *Chao Chen Pi, Chao Ju Pi*

Flavors & nature: Bitter and slightly acrid; warm

Functions: Rectifies the qi, harmonizes the center

Indications:

1. Disharmony of the liver and spleen with epigastric and abdominal distention, loss of taste, lack of appetite, vomiting, diarrhea...

2. Nausea, vomiting due to cold which disturbs the stomach's function of downbearing with vomiting of clear liquids, eructation, regurgitation, cold hands and feet...

3. Food stagnation[1] due to spleen and stomach vacuity with anorexia, nausea, vomiting, loose stools...

Typical combinations:

1. With ginger[-processed] Cortex Magnoliae Officinalis (*Jiang Hou Po*), bran stir-fried Rhizoma Atractylodis (*Fu Chao Cang Zhu*), and uncooked Rhizoma Zingiberis (*Sheng Jiang*) as in *Ping Wei San* (Level the Stomach Powder [231])

2. With uncooked Rhizoma Zingiberis (*Sheng Jiang*) as in *Ju Pi Tang* (Orange Peel Decoction [190])

3. With bran stir-fried Rhizoma Atractylodis Macrocephalae (*Fu Chao Bai Zhu*), Radix Panacis Ginseng (*Ren Shen*), and uncooked Sclerotium Poriae Cocos (*Sheng Fu Ling*) as in *Yi Gong San* (Extraordinary Merit Powder [399])

Dosage: 3-10g and up to 30g in severe cases

Note: 1. Stir-fried Orange Peel stimulates the appetite and promotes digestion.

Addendum: Orange Peel is often added to formulas which supplement the qi, blood, or yin in order to facilitate the assimilation of such rich substances which tend to be heavy, thus digesting them while avoiding any qi stagnation.

Fructus Meliae Toosendan (Chuan Lian Zi)

Uncooked (Sheng)

Names: Chuan Lian Zi, Jin Ling Zi, Lian Shi

Flavors & nature: Bitter; cold

Functions: Kills parasites, treats xian

Indications:

1. Parasites: A) ascariasis with abdominal and periumbilical pain; B) oxyurosis or pinworm infestation

2. Tinea capitis

Typical combinations:

1. A) With Omphalia (Lei Wan), uncooked Semen Arecae Catechu (Sheng Bing Lang), Semen Cucurbitae (Nan Gua Zi), and uncooked Fructus Pruni Mume (Sheng Wu Mei)
B) With uncooked Semen Arecae Catechu (Sheng Bing Lang), Cortex Radicis Meliae Azerdach (Ku Lian Pi), and Rhizoma Dryopteridis (Guan Zhong)

2. Used locally as a paste made from finely powdered Melia Toosendan.

Dosage: 5-10g and up to 15g in severe cases

Stir-fried [till] Scorched (Chao Jiao)[1]

Names: Chao Chuan Lian Zi, Chao Jin Ling Zi, Jiao Chuan Lian Zi

Flavors & nature: Bitter; cold tending to neutral

Functions: Moves the qi, stops pain

Indications:

1. Lateral costal and epigastric distention and pain due to A) liver depression, qi stagnation, B) depressive heat in the liver channel, or C) liver qi and blood stagnation

2. Inguinal hernia, maladies of the scrotum or testicles[2] due to stagnation of qi and cold in the liver channel

Typical combinations:

1. A) With vinegar[-processed] Rhizoma Cyperi Rotundi (Cu Xiang Fu), vinegar[-processed] Radix Bupleuri (Cu Chai Hu), and vinegar[-processed] Pericarpium Viridis Citri Reticulatae (Cu Qing Pi)
B) With vinegar[-processed] Rhizoma Corydalis Yanhusuo (Cu Yan Hu Suo) as in Jin Ling Zi San (Melia Powder [181])
C) With vinegar[-processed] Tuber Curcumae (Cu Yu Jin) and vinegar[-processed] Rhizoma Corydalis Yanhusuo (Cu Yan Hu Suo)

2. With salt[-processed] Fructus Foeniculi Vulgaris (Yan Xiao Hui Xiang) and processed Fructus Evodiae Rutecarpae (Zhi Wu Zhu Yu) as in Dao Qi Tang (Abduct the Qi Decoction [80])

Dosage: 5-10g and up to 15g in severe cases

Notes: 1. Other methods of processing Melia include bran stir-frying (Fu Chao), wine mix-frying (Jiu Zhi), vinegar mix-frying (Cu Zhi), and stir-frying [till] carbonized (Chao Tan). However, these methods are not actually used much. 2. For this indication, salt mix-fried Melia (Yan Zhi Chuan Lian Zi) is most often prescribed.

Cortex Magnoliae Officinalis (Hou Po)

Uncooked (Sheng)

Names: *Sheng Hou Po, Sheng Chuan Po*

Flavors & nature: Bitter and acrid; warm

Functions: Downbears counterflow qi, calms cough and asthma

Indications:

1. Cough, asthma due to A) wind cold which attacks the lungs with fever, aversion to wind and cold, B) phlegm cold which transforms into heat with stertorous breathing, chest oppression, vexation, fever, C) lung qi vacuity which follows a counterflow of qi with spontaneous perspiration, cough or asthma aggravated by exertion, shortness of breath, fatigue, D) phlegm cold and kidney vacuity with abundant clear, liquid phlegm, chest oppression, dyspnea on exertion, low back and knee weakness and pain, fatigue, vertigo, tinnitus...

2. Plum pit qi (*mei he qi*) due to stagnation of qi and phlegm with dysphagia, a sensation of a pit in the throat, hysteria...

Typical combinations:

1. A) With uncooked Ramulus Cinnamomi (*Sheng Gui Zhi*) and uncooked Semen Pruni Armeniacae (*Sheng Xing Ren*) as in *Gui Zhi Jia Hou Po Xing Ren Tang* (Cinnamon Twig, Magnolia & Armeniaca Decoction [126])
B) With honey mix-fried Herba Ephedrae (*Mi Zhi Ma Huang*), honey mix-fried Herba Cum Radice Asari (*Mi Zhi Xi Xin*), and uncooked Gypsum Fibrosum (*Sheng Shi Gao*) as in *Hou Po Ma Huang Tang* (Magnolia & Ephedra Decoction [137])
C) With honey mix-fried Fructus Perillae Frutescentis (*Mi Zhi Zi Su Zi*), Lignum Aquilariae Agallochae (*Chen Xiang*), and Radix Panacis Ginseng (*Ren Shen*) as in *Chuan Si Jun Zi Tang* (Dyspnea Four Gentleman Decoction [51])
D) With stir-fried Fructus Perillae Frutescentis (*Chao Zi Su Zi*), stir-fried Radix Peucedani (*Chao Qian Hu*), and clear Rhizoma Pinelliae Ternatae (*Qing Ban Xia*) as in *Su Zi Jiang Qi Tang* (Perilla Seed Downbear Qi Decoction [316])

2. With clear Rhizoma Pinelliae Ternatae (*Qing Ban Xia*) as in *Ban Xia Hou Po Tang* (Pinellia & Magnolia Decoction [27])

Dosage: 3-10g and up to 30g in severe cases

Ginger Mix-fried (Jiang Zhi)

Names: *Jiang Zhi Hou Po, Jiang Hou Po, Zhi Hou Po*

Flavors & nature: Bitter and acrid; drying; warm

Functions: Dries dampness, relieves distention, harmonizes the stomach

Indications:

1. Epigastric and/or abdominal pain and distention due to A) qi stagnation and cold dampness in the middle burner, B) accumulation of cold dampness in the middle burner with constipation or irregular stools or alternating constipation and loose stools, or C) spleen qi vacuity

2. Vomiting, nausea due to either A) stomach vacuity with regurgitation, acid vomiting, epigastric distention or B) stagnation of damp turbidity in the middle burner with chest and abdominal oppression, lack of appetite, diarrhea, a sensation of heaviness...

Cortex Magnoliae Officinalis continued . . .

3. Constipation due to either A) stagnation of qi with epigastric and abdominal pain and distention, flatulence or B) heat with abdominal pain aggravated by pressure, dry, hard stools...

Typical combinations:

1. A) With roasted Semen Alpiniae Katsumadai (*Wei Cao Dou Kou*) and uncooked Pericarpium Citri Reticulatae (*Sheng Chen Pi*) as in *Hou Po Wen Zhong Tang* (Magnolia Warm the Center Decoction [140])
B) With bran stir-fried Fructus Immaturus Citri Seu Ponciri (*Fu Chao Zhi Shi*) and uncooked Radix Saussureae Seu Vladimiriae (*Sheng Mu Xiang*)
C) With Rhizoma Pinelliae Ternatae (*Fa Ban Xia*) and Radix Panacis Ginseng (*Ren Shen*) as in *Hou Po Sheng Jiang Ban Xia Gan Cao Ren Shen Tang* (Magnolia, Uncooked Ginger, Pinellia, Licorice & Ginseng Decoction [139]

2. A) With processed Fructus Evodiae Rutecarpae (*Zhi Wu Zhu Yu*) and bran stir-fried Rhizoma Atractylodis Macrocephalae (*Fu Chao Bai Zhu*)
B) With bran stir-fried Rhizoma Atractylodis (*Fu Chao Cang Zhu*) and stir-fried Pericarpium Citri Reticulatae (*Chao Chen Pi*) as in *Ping Wei San* (Level the Stomach Powder [231])

3. A) With bran stir-fried Fructus Immaturus Citri Seu Ponciri (*Fu Chao Zhi Shi*) and uncooked Radix Et Rhizoma Rhei (*Sheng Da Huang*) as in *Hou Po San Wu Tang* (Magnolia Three Materials Decoction [138])
B) With uncooked Radix Et Rhizoma Rhei (*Sheng Da Hvang*) and Mirabilitum (*Mang Xiao*) as in *Da Cheng Qi Tang* (Major Support Qi Decoction [61])

Dosage: 3-10g and up to 30g in severe cases

Radix Saussureae Seu Vladimiriae *(Mu Xiang)*

—————————— Uncooked *(Sheng)* ——————————

Names: *Guan Mu Xiang, Nan Mu Xiang, Tu Mu Xiang, Mu Xiang, Lao Mu Xiang, Yun Mu Xiang*

Flavors & nature: Acrid and bitter; warm

Functions: Warms the center, moves the qi, stops pain

Indications:

1. Epigastric pain due to either A) stagnation of cold, dampness, and qi in the stomach and intestines with epigastric and abdominal pain and distention or B) dysfunction in the spleen's transportation and transformation accompanied by qi stagnation with difficult, slow digestion, indigestion...

2. Lateral costal pain due to either A) damp heat in the liver and gallbladder accompanied by qi stagnation or B) liver qi stagnation with abdominal masses...

3. Vomiting due to spleen and stomach vacuity accompanied by qi stagnation and phlegm dampness in the middle burner with epigastric distention, loss of appetite...

4. Inguinal hernia, maladies of the scrotum or testicles due to qi stagnation and cold in the liver channel

5. Dysmenorrhea[1] due to liver qi stagnation with lower abdominal, lateral costal, and low back pain and distention...

Typical combinations:

1. A) With Fructus Cardamomi (*Bai Dou Kou*), Flos Caryophylli (*Ding Xiang*), and Fructus Amomi (*Sha Ren*) as in *Mu Xiang Tiao Qi San* (Saussurea Regulate the Qi Powder [227])

Radix Saussureae Seu Vladimiriae continued . . .

B) With stir-fried Fructus Crataegi (*Chao Shan Zha*) and vinegar[-processed] Pericarpium Viridis Citri Reticulatae (*Cu Qing Pi*) as in *Yun Qi San* (Move Qi Powder [425])

2. A) With Herba Desmodii Seu Lysimachiae (*Jin Qian Cao*), stir-fried Fructus Meliae Toosendan (*Chao Chuan Lian Zi*), vinegar[-processed] Tuber Curcumae (*Cu Yu Jin*), and uncooked Fructus Citri Seu Ponciri (*Sheng Zhi Ke*)
B) With vinegar[-processed] Pericarpium Viridis Citri Reticulatae (*Cu Qing Pi*), stir-fried Fructus Meliae Toosendan (*Chao Chuan Lian Zi*), vinegar[-processed] Rhizoma Sparganii (*Cu San Leng*), and vinegar[-processed] Rhizoma Curcumae Zedoariae (*Cu E Zhu*)

3. With ginger[-processed] Fructus Amomi (*Jiang Sha Ren*), stir-fried Pericarpium Citri Reticulatae (*Chao Chen Pi*), and uncooked Sclerotium Poriae Cocos (*Sheng Fu Ling*) as in *Xiang Sha Er Chen Tang* (Saussurea & Amomum Two Aged [Ingredients] Decoction [369])

4. With salt[-processed] Fructus Foeniculi Vulgaris (*Yan Xiao Hui Xiang*) and processed Fructus Evodiae Rutecarpae (*Zhi Wu Zhu Yu*) as in *Dao Qi Tang* (Abduct the Qi Decoction [80])

5. With stir-fried Fructus Meliae Toosendan (*Chao Chuan Lian Zi*), wine[-processed] Rhizoma Corydalis Yanhusuo (*Jiu Yan Hu Suo*), and vinegar[-processed] Tuber Curcumae (*Cu Yu Jin*)

Dosage: 3-10g and up to 15g in severe cases

Note: 1. For this indication, wine mix-fried Saussurea (*Jiu Zhi Mu Xiang*) is sometimes prescribed.

Addendum: Radix Saussureae Seu Vladimiriae is often added to formulas which supplement the qi, blood, or yin in order to facilitate the assimilation of these rich substances which are heavy, thus digesting [them] and preventing any stagnation of qi.

Roasted *(Wei)*[1]

Name: *Wei Mu Xiang*

Flavors & nature: Slightly acrid, bitter, and astringent; warm

Functions: Warms the center, stops diarrhea

Indications:

1. Dysentery due to damp heat in the large intestine with abdominal pain, tenesmus...

2. Diarrhea due to A) food stagnation which has transformed into damp heat with epigastric and abdominal distention and pain, tenesmus, indigestion, B) accumulation of cold dampness in the middle burner with borborygmus, abdominal pain, or C) spleen and stomach vacuity with chronic diarrhea...

Typical combinations:

1. With uncooked Rhizoma Coptidis Chinensis (*Sheng Huang Lian*) as in *Xiang Lian Wan* (Saussurea & Coptis Pills [367])

2. A) With stir-fried Semen Arecae Catechu (*Chao Bing Lang*), uncooked Pericarpium Viridis Citri Reticulatae (*Sheng Qing Pi*), and uncooked Rhizoma Coptidis Chinensis (*Sheng Huang Lian*) as in *Mu Xiang Bing Lang Wan* (Saussurea & Areca Pills [225])
B) With bran stir-fried Rhizoma Atractylodis (*Fu Chao Cang Zhu*), Fructus Amomi (*Sha Ren*), and roasted Semen Alpiniae Katsumadai (*Wei Cao Dou Kou*)
C) With rice stir-fried Radix Codonopsis Pilosulae

Radix Saussureae Seu Vladimiriae continued . . .

(*Mi Chao Dang Shen*), earth stir-fried Rhizoma Atractylodis Macrocephalae (*Tu Chao Bai Zhu*), stir-fried Pericarpium Citri Reticulatae (*Chao Chen Pi*), and roasted Radix Puerariae (*Wei Ge Gen*)

Dosage: 3-10g and up to 15g in severe cases

Note: 1. When prepared by roasting (*wei*), Saussurea is often wrapped in a paste of wheat bran before being grilled under coals. Thus it benefits from wheat bran's anti-diaphoretic action.

Pericarpium Viridis Citri Reticulatae *(Qing Pi)*

_____ Uncooked *(Sheng)* _____

Names: *Sheng Qing Pi, Xiao Qing Pi, Qing Pi*

Flavors & nature: Bitter and acrid; warm

Functions: Breaks qi stagnation, disperses food stagnation, dissipates accumulations

Indications:

1. Food stagnation[2] with epigastric distention, abdominal distension and pain, nausea, fetid eructation...

2. Abdominal masses due to qi stagnation, blood stasis with palpable, fixed abdominal masses, epigastric and abdominal distention...

3. Malaria[2] due to accumulation of phlegm with alternating fever and chills, a bitter taste in the mouth, dry throat, constipation, thoracic oppression, nausea, a thick, white [tongue] coating...

Typical combinations:

1. With stir-fried Massa Medica Fermentata (*Chao Shen Qu*), stir-fried Fructus Crataegi (*Chao Shan Zha*), and stir-fried Fructus Germinatus Hordei Vulgaris (*Chao Mai Ya*) as in *Qing Pi Wan*

(Green Orange Peel Pills [253a])

2. With uncooked Fructus Immaturus Citri Seu Ponciri (*Sheng Zhi Shi*), vinegar[-processed] Rhizoma Sparganii (*Cu San Leng*), vinegar[-processed] Rhizoma Curcumae Zedoariae (*Cu E Zhu*), and vinegar[-processed] Carapax Amydae Sinensis (*Cu Bie Jia*)

3. With uncooked Fructus Amomi Tsao-ko (*Sheng Cao Guo*), uncooked Radix Bupleuri (*Sheng Chai Hu*), and ginger[-processed] Rhizoma Pinelliae Ternatae (*Jiang Ban Xia*) as in *Qing Pi Tang* (Clear the Spleen Decoction [253])

Dosage: 3-10g and up to 30g in severe cases

Notes: 1. This refers to the entire fruit of the Mandarin orange. When it is small, it is called *Xiao Qing Pi* (small *Qing Pi*) or Pericarpium Viridis Citri Reticulatae. When the skin is thick, it is called *Qing Pi* or Epicarpium Viridis Citri Reticulatae. In both cases, it should be understood that the fruit is immature. *Ju Pi (Chen Pi)* and *Qing Pi* both come from the skin of the Citrus Reticulata. *Ju Pi (Chen Pi)* comes from the mature fruit and *Qing Pi* comes from the immature fruit. 2. For this indication, one can prescribe bran stir-fried *Qing Pi (Fu Chao Qing Pi)* if one wishes to moderate the dispersing action of *Qing Pi*.

_____ **Vinegar Mix-fried (Cu Zhi)** _____

Names: *Cu Zhi Qing Pi, Cu Qing Pi, Zhi Qing Pi*

Flavors & nature: Bitter, slightly acrid, and slightly sour; warm

Functions: Scatters cold, stops pain

Indications:

1. Lateral costal pain due to A) liver qi stagnation with lateral costal pain and distention, B) qi stagnation, blood stasis with splenomegaly, hepatomegaly, C) liver qi stagnation which has transformed into fire with irritability, a bitter taste in the mouth, or D) disharmony of the liver and stomach with nausea, eructation...

2. Inguinal hernia, maladies of the scrotum or testicles due to either A) qi stagnation in the liver channel with severe pain or B) stagnation of cold and qi in the liver channel with severe pain aggravated by cold...

3. Breast distention, mastitis due to liver qi stagnation with breast pain...

Typical combinations:

1. A) With vinegar[-processed] Radix Bupleuri (*Cu Chai Hu*) and vinegar[-processed] Rhizoma Cyperi Rotundi (*Cu Xiang Fu*)

B) With wine[-processed] Radix Salviae Miltiorrhizae (*Jiu Dan Shen*), vinegar[-processed] Carapax Amydae Sinensis (*Cu Bie Jia*), and vinegar[-processed] Rhizoma Curcumae Zedoariae (*Cu E Zhu*)

C) With vinegar[-processed] Radix Bupleuri (*Cu Chai Hu*), stir-fried Fructus Meliae Toosendan (*Chao Chuan Lian Zi*), Pulvis Indigonis (*Qing Dai*), and uncooked Cortex Radicis Moutan (*Sheng Mu Dan Pi*)

D) With uncooked Radix Saussureae Seu Vladimiriae (*Sheng Mu Xiang*) and vinegar[-processed] Rhizoma Cyperi Rotundi (*Cu Xiang Fu*) as in *Qi Wei Tiao Qi Tang* (Seven Flavors Regulate the Qi Decoction [238])

2. A) With salt[-processed] Semen Citri Reticulatae (*Yan Ju He*) and stir-fried Fructus Meliae Toosendan (*Chao Chuan Lian Zi*)

B) With salt[-processed] Radix Linderae Strychnifoliae (*Yan Wu Yao*) and salt[-processed] Fructus Foeniculi Vulgaris (*Yan Xiao Hui Xiang*) as in *Tian Tai Wu Yao San* (Tian Tai Lindera Powder [325])

3. With stir-fried Fasciculus Vascularis Luffae (*Chao Si Gua Lou*), Folium Citri Reticulatae (*Ju Ye*) and vinegar[-processed] Rhizoma Cyperi Rotundi (*Cu Xiang Fu*)

Dosage: 3-10g and up to 30g in severe cases

Radix Linderae Strychnifoliae (Wu Yao)

_____ **Wine Mix-fried (Jiu Zhi)** _____

Names: *Jiu Zhi Wu Yao, Jiu Wu Yao*

Flavors & nature: Acrid; warm

Functions: Moves the qi and stops pain

Indications:

1. Dyspnea, asthma due to inversion of lung qi caused by stagnation of cold and qi or a depression binding of the seven emotions (*qi qing yu jie*) with asthmatic breathing, chest distention and pain...

Radix Linderae Strychnifoliae continued . . .

2. Epigastric and abdominal pain[1] due to stagnation of cold and qi

3. Dysmenorrhea due to liver qi stagnation and blood stasis

Typical combinations:

1. With stir-fried Radix Saussureae Seu Vladimiriae (*Chao Mu Xiang*), Lignum Aquilariae Agallochae (*Chen Xiang*), and Radix Panacis Ginseng (*Ren Shen*) as in *Si Mo Yin Zi* (Four Grindings Drink [311]

2. With uncooked Radix Saussureae Seu Vladimiriae (*Sheng Mu Xiang*), Fructus Amomi (*Sha Ren*), and Semen Myristicae Fragrantis (*Rou Dou Kou*)

3. With wine[-processed] Radix Angelicae Sinensis (*Jiu Dang Gui*), wine[-processed] Radix Ligustici Wallichii (*Jiu Chuan Xiong*), and vinegar[-processed] Rhizoma Cyperi Rotundi (*Cu Xiang Fu*)

Dosage: 3-12g and up to 30g in severe cases

Note: 1. If pain is accompanied by epigastric or abdominal distention, one can prescribe bran stir-fried Lindera (*Fu Chao Wu Yao*).

Salt Mix-fried (*Yan Zhi*)

Names: *Yan Zhi Wu Yao, Yan Wu Yao*

Flavors & nature: Slightly acrid and slightly salty; warm

Functions: Warms the kidneys, scatters cold, controls urination

Indications:

1. Enuresis, urinary incontinence, abundant urination due to kidney yang vacuity

2. Inguinal hernia, maladies of the scrotum or testicles[1] due to stagnation of qi and cold in the liver channel

Typical combinations:

1. With salt[-processed] Fructus Alpiniae Oxy-

phyllae (*Yan Yi Zhi Ren*) and bran stir-fried Radix Dioscoreae Oppositae (*Fu Chao Shan Yao*) as in *Suo Quan Wan* (Shut the Spring Pills [319])

2. With salt[-processed] Fructus Foeniculi Vulgaris (*Yan Xiao Hui Xiang*), uncooked Radix Saussureae Seu Vladimiriae (*Sheng Mu Xiang*), and stir-fried Fructus Meliae Toosendan (*Chao Chuan Lian Zi*) as in *Tian Tai Wu Yao San* (Tian Tai Lindera Powder [325])[2]

Dosage: 3-12g and up to 30g in severe cases

Notes: 1. For this indication, one can prescribe wine mix-fried Lindera (*Jiu Zhi Wu Yao*). 2. Tian Tai is a place in Zhejiang Province where the best quality Lindera is grown.

Rhizoma Cyperi Rotundi (*Xiang Fu*)

___ Uncooked (*Sheng*) ___

Names: *Sheng Xiang Fu, Sheng Xiang Fu Zi, Sheng Jin Xiang Fu*

Flavors & nature: Acrid and slightly bitter; neutral

Functions: Rectifies the qi, resolves depression

Indications:

1. Chest and diaphragmatic oppression due to qi stagnation and dampness with lateral costal pain, loss of appetite, fetid-smelling eructation...

2. Common cold, flu due to wind cold with qi stagnation in the middle burner with headache, fever, chills, no sweating, chest and epigastric distention, loss of appetite...

Typical combinations:

1. With bran stir-fried Rhizoma Atractylodis (*Fu Chao Cang Zhu*) and stir-fried Massa Medica Fermentata (*Chao Shen Qu*) as in *Yue Ju Wan* (Escape Restraint Pills [424])

2. With Folium Perillae Frutescentis (*Zi Su Ye*) and uncooked Rhizoma Atractylodis (*Sheng Cang Zhu*) as in *Xiang Su San* (Cyperus & Perilla Powder [370])

Dosage: 5-12g and up to 30g in severe cases

___ Vinegar Mix-fried (*Cu Zhi*) ___

Names: *Xiang Fu, Xiang Fu Mi, Xiang Fu Zi, Jin Xiang Fu, Sha Cao Gen*

Flavors & nature: Slightly acrid, bitter, and slightly sour; neutral tending to warm

Functions: Drains the liver, regulates the menses, stops pain, disperses food stagnation

Indications:

1. Epigastric and abdominal pain due to stagnation of qi and cold

2. Inguinal hernia, maladies of the scrotum or testicles[1] due to qi stagnation and cold in the liver channel with swelling and distention of the scrotum, pain in the lower abdomen aggravated by cold and radiating to the testicles, inguinal hernia...

3. Dysmenorrhea, irregular menstruation[1] due to liver qi stagnation or disharmony between the qi and blood with menstrual irregularity, premenstrual syndrome...

4. Food stagnation with epigastric and abdominal distention, nausea, diarrhea, loss of appetite...

Typical combinations:

1. With roasted Rhizoma Alpiniae Officinari (*Wei Gao Liang Jiang*) as in *Liang Fu Wan* (Alpinia Officinarus & Cyperus Pills [197])

2. With salt[-processed] Radix Linderae Strychnifoliae (*Yan Wu Yao*), salt[-processed] Semen Citri Reticulatae (*Yan Ju He*), and salt[-processed] Fructus Foeniculi Vulgaris (*Yan Xiao Hui Xiang*)

3. With wine[-processed] Rhizoma Corydalis Yanhusuo (*Jiu Yan Hu Suo*), wine[-processed] Radix Angelicae Sinensis (*Jiu Dang Gui*), and wine[-processed] Radix Ligustici Wallichii (*Jiu Chuan Xiong*)

Rhizoma Cyperi Rotundi continued . . .

4. With stir-fried Massa Medica Fermentata (*Chao Shen Qu*), stir-fried Fructus Germinatus Hordei Vulgaris (*Chao Mai Ya*), roasted Radix Saussureae Seu Vladimiriae (*Wei Mu Xiang*), and Fructus Amomi (*Sha Ren*)

Dosage: 5-12g and up to 30g in severe cases

Note: 1. For these indications, *Si Zhi Xiang Fu* can be prescribed, particularly in case of qi stagnation accompanied by cold or blood stasis. *Si* means four; *zhi* means process of preparation. Thus Cyperus is processed with the aid of four adjuvants: vinegar (*cu*), wine (*jiu*), salt (*yan*), and ginger (*jiang*).

Stir-fried [till] Carbonized (*Chao Tan*)

Name: *Xiang Fu Tan*

Flavors & nature: Slightly acrid, bitter, and astringent; neutral tending to warm

Functions: Harmonizes the blood, stops bleeding

Indications:

1. Metrorrhagia, menorrhagia due to disharmony of the *chong* and *ren* with scanty but incessant bleeding...

2. Hemorrhage due to qi stagnation with hematemesis, hematuria, melena, or metrorrhagia...

Typical combinations:

1. With carbonized Radix Rubiae Cordifoliae (*Qian Cao Tan*), carbonized Radix Angelicae Sinensis (*Dang Gui Tan*), Radix Albus Paeoniae Lactiflorae (*Bai Shao Yao*), and stir-fried Os Sepiae Seu Sepiellae (*Chao Hai Piao Xiao*)

2. With wine[-processed] Radix Angelicae Sinensis (*Jiu Dang Gui*), wine[-processed] Radix Ligustici Wallichii (*Jiu Chuan Xiong*), and carbonized Folium Artemisiae Argyii (*Ai Ye Tan*)

Dosage: 5-10g and up to 30g in severe cases

Fructus Citri Seu Ponciri (*Zhi Ke*)

Uncooked (*Sheng*)

Name: *Sheng Zhi Ke*

Flavors & nature: Acrid and bitter; cool

Functions: Breaks qi stagnation, scatters nodulations, disperses distention

Indications:

1. Epigastric and abdominal pain due to qi stagnation with epigastric and abdominal distention, oliguria, constipation...

2. Lateral costal pain and distention due to liver qi stagnation with chest and lateral costal pain and

distention, slow digestion, constipation, oliguria...

3. Abdominal masses due to qi stagnation, blood stasis with fixed, palpable abdominal masses which are sometimes painful...

Typical combinations:

1. With stir-fried Semen Arecae Catechu (*Chao Bing Lang*), uncooked Radix Saussureae Seu Vladimiriae (*Sheng Mu Xiang*), vinegar[-processed] Pericarpium Viridis Citri Reticulatae (*Cu Qing Pi*), and uncooked Radix Et Rhizoma Rhei (*Sheng Da Huang*)

Fructus Citri Seu Ponciri continued . . .

2. With vinegar[-processed Rhizoma Cyperi Rotundi (*Cu Xiang Fu*), stir-fried Fructus Meliae Toosendan (*Chao Chuan Lian Zi*), and vinegar[-processed] Radix Bupleuri (*Cu Chai Hu*)

3. With wine[-processed] Feces Trogopterori Seu Pteromi (*Jiu Wu Ling Zhi*), uncooked Semen Pruni Persicae (*Sheng Tao Ren*), vinegar[-processed] Rhizoma Cyperi Rotundi (*Cu Xiang Fu*), and vinegar[-processed] Rhizoma Corydalis Yan

husuo (*Cu Yan Hu Suo*) as in *Ge Xia Zhu Yu Tang* (Below the Diaphragm Dispel Stasis Decoction [114])

Dosage: 5-10g and up to 15-60g in severe cases

Addendum: *Zhi Ke* and *Zhi Shi* come from the same fruit, Citrus Seu Poncirus. *Zhi Ke* is the large (*da*), ripe fruit, called *Da Zhi Ke*. *Zhi Shi* is the small (*xiao*), immature fruit, called *Xiao Zhi Shi*. *Zhi Ke* and *Zhi Shi* have analogous actions. However, *Zhi Shi* is stronger and *Zhi Ke* is more moderate.

_____ Bran Stir-fried (*Fu Chao*) _____

Names: *Zhi Ke, Fu Chao Ke, Chao Ke*

Flavors & nature: Bitter and slightly acrid; neutral

Functions: Rectifies the qi, disperses food stagnation

Indications:

1. Food stagnation with epigastric and abdominal pain and distention, loss of appetite...

2. Regurgitation, eructation due to either A) disharmony of the stomach accompanied by deficiency in the spleen's function of transportation and transformation with loss of appetite or B) spleen and stomach vacuity

Typical combinations:

1. With stir-fried Pericarpium Citri Reticulatae

(*Chao Chen Pi*), uncooked Radix Saussureae Seu Vladimiriae (*Sheng Mu Xiang*), stir-fried Fructus Crataegi (*Chao Shan Zha*), stir-fried Fructus Germinatus Hordei Vulgaris (*Chao Mai Ya*), and stir-fried Massa Medica Fermentata (*Chao Shen Qu*)

2. A) With uncooked Radix Saussureae Seu Vladimiriae (*Sheng Mu Xiang*), Fructus Cardamomi (*Bai Dou Kou*), and ginger[-processed] Fructus Amomi (*Jiang Sha Ren*)
B) With bran stir-fried Rhizoma Atractylodis Macrocephalae (*Fu Chao Bai Zhu*), honey mix-fried Radix Codonopsis Pilosulae (*Mi Zhi Dang Shen*), and mix-fried Radix Glycyrrhizae (*Zhi Gan Cao*)

Dosage: 5-10g and up to 15-60g in severe cases

_____ Honey Mix-fried (*Mi Zhi*) _____

Names: *Mi Zhi Zhi Ke, Zhi Zhi Ke*

Flavors & nature: Acrid, bitter, and slightly sweet; cool tending to warm; tending to moistening

Functions: Rectifies the lung qi, eliminates phlegm, raises the fallen

Indications:

1. Chest pain or distention due to lung qi stagnation or accumulation of phlegm in the lungs

2. Cough due to A) disharmony of the lung qi with abundant phlegm, chest oppression, B) disharmony of the lung qi with phlegm heat, or C) disharmony of the lung qi with phlegm dampness

Fructus Citri Seu Ponciri continued . . .

3. Uterine or rectal prolapse due to fall of qi with a sensation of heaviness of the uterus or anus, fatigue, shortness of breath...

Typical combinations:

1. With uncooked Radix Platycodi Grandiflori (*Sheng Jie Geng*)

2. A) With uncooked Pericarpium Trichosanthis Kirlowii (*Sheng Gua Lou Pi*), uncooked Fructus Perillae Frutescentis (*Sheng Zi Su Zi*), and uncooked Semen Pruni Armeniacae (*Sheng Xing Ren*)

B) With Bulbus Fritillariae Thunbergii (*Zhe Bei Mu*), wine[-processed] Radix Scutellariae Baicalensis (*Jiu Huang Qin*), and uncooked Fructus Gardeniae Jasminoidis (*Sheng Shan Zhi Zi*)
C) With clear Rhizoma Pinelliae Ternatae (*Qing Ban Xia*), uncooked Pericarpium Citri Reticulatae (*Chen Pi*), and uncooked Sclerotium Poriae Cocos (*Sheng Fu Ling*)

3. With honey mix-fried Radix Astragali Membranacei (*Mi Zhi Huang Qi*), honey mix-fried Radix Codonopsis Pilosulae (*Mi Zhi Dang Shen*), honey mix-fried Rhizoma Cimicifugae (*Mi Zhi Sheng Ma*), and stir-fried Radix Bupleuri (*Chao Chai Hu*)

Dosage: 5-10g and up to 15-60g in severe cases

Fructus Immaturus Citri Seu Ponciri *(Zhi Shi)*

—————————————————— Uncooked *(Sheng)* ——————————————————

Names: *Zhi Shi, Sheng Zhi Shi, Chuan Zhi Shi, Jiang Zhi Shi*

Flavors & nature: Bitter; slightly cold

Functions: Breaks qi stagnation, transforms phlegm

Indications:

1. Chest pain (*xiong bi*) due to stagnation of qi and phlegm in the chest at the same time as a deficiency of yang in the chest with chest pain radiating to the back...

2. Phlegm rheum (*tan yin*), *i.e.*, accumulation of phlegm in the chest with asthmatic breathing, cough, thick, sticky saliva, possible syncope due to an excess of phlegm (*tan jue*, phlegm inversion) with cold limbs, loss of consciousness, vertigo...

3. Wind stroke (*zhong feng*) due to phlegm wind misting the clear portals of the heart with loss of consciousness, a rigid tongue, aphasia...

4. Abdominal masses due to qi stagnation, blood stasis with fixed, palpable, painful abdominal masses...

Typical combinations:

1. With Bulbus Allii Macrostemi (*Xie Bai*), stir-fried Pericarpium Trichosanthis Kirlowii (*Chao Gua Lou Pi*), and stir-fried Ramulus Cinnamomi (*Chao Gui Zhi*) as in *Zhi Shi Xie Bai Gui Zhi Tang* (Immature Citrus, Allium Macrostemum & Cinnamon Twig Decoction [436])

2. With clear Rhizoma Pinelliae Ternatae (*Qing Ban Xia*), processed Rhizoma Arisaematis (*Zhi Tian Nan Xing*), and stir-fried Exocarpium Rubrum Citri Reticulatae (*Ju Hong*) as in *Dao Tan Tang* (Abduct Phlegm Decoction [81])

3. With bile[-processed] Rhizoma Arisaematis (*Dan Nan Xing*), Rhizoma Acori Graminei (*Shi Chang Pu*), stir-fried Exocarpium Rubrum Citri Reticulatae (*Chao Ju Hong*), and clear Rhizoma Pinelliae Ternatae (*Qing Ban Xia*) as in *Di Tan Tang* (Scour Phlegm Decoction [85])

Fructus Immaturus Citri Seu Ponciri continued . . .

4. With vinegar[-processed] Rhizoma Curcumae Zedoariae (*Cu E Zhu*), vinegar[-processed] Rhi-zoma Sparganii (*Cu San Leng*), and vinegar[-pro-cessed] Pericarpium Viridis Citri Reticulatae (*Cu Qing Pi*)

Dosage: 3-10g and up to 30g in severe cases

Bran Stir-fried *(Fu Chao)*

Names: *Fu Chao Zhi Shi, Chao Zhi Shi*

Flavors & nature: Bitter and slightly astringent; neutral

Functions: Disperses accumulations, relieves distention

Indications:

1. Epigastric and abdominal distention and pain due to qi and food stagnation and spleen and stomach vacuity with loss of appetite...

2. Diarrhea, dysentery due to food stagnation and damp heat with abdominal pain...

3. Constipation due to heat in the large intestine with abdominal distention, dry, hard stools...

Typical combinations:

1. With bran stir-fried Rhizoma Atractylodis Macrocephalae (*Fu Chao Bai Zhu*), stir-fried Fructus Germinatus Hordei Vulgaris (*Chao Mai Ya*), ginger[-processed] Cortex Magnoliae Offi-cinalis (*Jiang Hou Po*), and uncooked Sclerotium Poriae Cocos (*Sheng Fu Ling*) as in *Zhi Shi Xiao Pi Wan* (Immature Citrus Disperse Glomus Pills [435])

2. With uncooked Radix Et Rhizoma Rhei (*Sheng Da Huang*), stir-fried [till] scorched Massa Med-ica Fermentata (*Chao Jiao Shen Qu*), stir-fried Radix Scutellariae Baicalensis (*Chao Huang Qin*), and uncooked Rhizoma Coptidis Chinensis (*Sheng Huang Lian*) as in *Zhi Shi Dao Zhi Wan* (Imma-ture Citrus Abduct Stagnation Pills [434])

3. With uncooked Radix Et Rhizoma Rhei (*Da Huang*), Mirabilitum (*Mang Xiao*), and ginger[-processed] Cortex Magnoliae Officinalis (*Jiang Hou Po*) as in *Da Cheng Qi Tang* (Mahor Support the Qi Decoction [61])

Dosage: 3-10g and up to 30g in severe cases

10
Blood-quickening, Stasis-dispelling Medicinals

Radix Cyathulae *(Chuan Niu Xi)*[1]
_____Uncooked *(Sheng)* _____

Names: *Sheng Chuan Niu Xi, Chuan Niu Xi*

Flavors & nature: Sweet and slightly bitter; neutral

Functions: Dispels wind, eliminates dampness, disinhibits the joints

Indications:

1. Rheumatic complaints due to wind dampness with joint pain accompanied by a sensation of heaviness and numbness...

2. Knee and foot pain due to stagnation of damp heat in the lower burner with pain, redness, and swelling of the knees and feet...

Typical combinations:

1. With steamed Fructus Chaenomelis Lagenariae (*Zheng Mu Gua*), Radix Et Rhizoma Notopterygii (*Qiang Huo*), Radix Angelicae Pubescentis (*Du Huo*), and wine[-processed] Radix Clematidis Chinensis (*Jiu Wei Ling Xian*)

2. With salt[-processed] Cortex Phellodendri (*Yan Huang Bai*) and uncooked Rhizoma Atractylodis (*Sheng Cang Zhu*) as in *San Miao San* (Three Marvels Powder [273])

Dosage: 10-15g and up to 30g in severe cases; 5-10g if used as a messenger medicinal[2]

Notes: 1. Radix Cyathulae (*Chuan Niu Xi*) and Radix Achyranthis Bidentatae (*Huai Niu Xi*) possess similar functions and indications. However, Cyathula is superior for quickening the blood and dispelling stasis, disinhibiting the joints and dispersing swelling. On the other hand, Achyranthes is better for supplementing the liver and kidneys and strengthening the sinews and bones. In addition, *Tu Niu Xi* (Radix Achyranthis), also called *Ye Niu Xi* (wild Achyranthes) drains fire, resolves toxins, dispels stasis, eliminates dampness, and frees strangury. It favorably treats diphtheria, sore throat, aphthae, amenorrhea, strangury, hematuria, etc. 2. Both Cyathula and Achyranthes downbear the blood to the lower body. This allows them to A) treat bleeding in the upper body, such as hematemesis and epistaxis, B) downbear vacuity heat in the upper body, such as aphthae, glossitis, toothache, sore throat, etc., and C) lead the action of other medicinals to the lower body to treat diseases located below the knees.

_____ Wine Mix-fried *(Jiu Zhi)* _____

Names: *Jiu Zhi Chuan Niu Xi, Jiu Chuan Niu Xi*

Flavors & nature: Sweet and slightly bitter; neutral tending to warm

Functions: Quickens the blood, dispels stasis, free strangury

Radix Cyathulae continued . . .

Indications:

1. Dysmenorrhea, amenorrhea due to qi stagnation, blood stasis

2. Abdominal masses due to blood stasis

3. Retention of the placenta or retention of the fetus with pain and distention of the lower abdomen...

4. Strangury (*lin*)[1] of all types with blood stasis in the urinary pathways with piercing pain in the urethra, blood clots in the urine...

Typical combinations:

1. With wine[-processed] Radix Angelicae Sinensis (*Jiu Dang Gui*), wine[-processed] Rhizoma Corydalis Yanhusuo (*Jiu Yan Hu Suo*), and uncooked Semen Pruni Persicae (*Sheng Tao Ren*) as in *Niu Xi San* (Cyathula Powder [228])

2. With vinegar[-processed] Rhizoma Curcumae Zedoariae (*Cu E Zhu*), vinegar[-processed] Rhizoma Sparganii (*Cu San Leng*), vinegar[-processed] Carapax Amydae Sinensis (*Cu Bie Jia*), and uncooked Pericarpium Viridis Citri Reticulatae (*Sheng Qing Pi*)

3. With wine[-processed] Radix Angelicae Sinensis (*Jiu Dang Gui*), Semen Malvae Seu Abutilonis (*Dong Kui Zi*), Herba Dianthi (*Qu Mai*), and Talcum (*Hua Shi*) as in *Niu Xi Tang* (Cyathula Decoction [229])

4. With Folium Pyrrosiae (*Shi Wei*), Spora Lygodii (*Hai Jin Sha*), Succinum (*Hu Po*), wine[-processed] Radix Rubrus Paeoniae Lactiflorae (*Jiu Chi Shao Yao*), and wine[-processed] Cortex Radicis Moutan (*Jiu Mu Dan Pi*)

Dosage: 10-15g and up to 30g in severe cases; 5-10g when used as a messenger medicinal (see note 2 under on the preceding page)

Note: 1. For this indication, Radix Achyranthis (*Tu Niu Xi*) can be prescribed advantageously.

Squama Manitis Pentadactylis (*Chuan Shan Jia*)

Sand Stir-fried (*Sha Chao*)

Names: *Sha Chao Shan Jia, Chao Chuan Shan Jia, Chao Jia Pian, Shan Jia Pian*

Flavors & nature: Salty; slightly cold

Functions: Disperses swelling, evacuates pus, dispels wind, and eliminates dampness

Indications:

1. Pyogenic inflammation (such as abscesses, acute appendicitis, mastitis, furuncles, etc.) due to either A) heat toxins and blood stasis or B) qi and blood vacuity

2. Rheumatic complaints due to wind dampness and blood stasis with severe, fixed joint pain, loss of mobility...

Typical combinations:

1. A) With uncooked Flos Lonicerae Japonicae (*Sheng Jin Yin Hua*), Radix Trichosanthis Kirlowii (*Tian Hua Fen*), and uncooked Radix Rubrus Paeoniae Lactiflorae (*Sheng Chi Shao Yao*) as in *Xian Fang Huo Ming Yin* (Immortal Formula for Saving Life Drink [364])
B) With uncooked Radix Astragali Membranacei (*Sheng Huang Qi*), wine[-processed] Radix Ligustici Wallichii (*Jiu Chuan Xiong*), wine[-processed] Radix Angelicae Sinensis (*Jiu Dang Gui*), and Spina Gleditschiae Chinensis (*Zao Jiao Ci*) as in *Tou Nong San* (Outthrust Pus Powder [334])

Squama Manitis Pentadactylis continued . . .

2. With Radix Et Rhizoma Notopterygii (*Qiang Huo*), uncooked Radix Ledebouriellae Sesloidis (*Sheng Fang Feng*), Lignum Sappanis (*Su Mu*), and wine[-processed] Radix Clematidis Chinensis (*Jiu Wei Ling Xian*)

Dosage: 5-15g in decoction; 1-5g in powder

_____ **Vinegar-dipped Calcination (*Cu Cui*)[1]** _____

Names: *Cu Shan Jia, Cu Jia Pian, Cu Chuan Shan Jia*

Flavors & nature: Salty and sour; neutral

Functions: Quickens the blood, dispels stasis, stops pain, promotes lactation

Indications:

1. Amenorrhea due to blood stasis with fixed, palpable abdominal masses, lower abdominal pain...

2. Traumatic injury with blood stasis, swelling, pain...

3. Agalactia due to qi and blood stagnation with swollen, hard, painful breasts...

4. Abdominal masses due to blood stasis which are palpable, fixed, and possibly painful...

Typical combinations:

1. With uncooked Semen Pruni Persicae (*Sheng Tao Ren*), wine[-processed] Radix Angelicae Sinensis (*Jiu Dang Gui*), and Flos Carthami Tinctorii (*Hong Hua*)

2. With Lignum Sappanis (*Su Mu*), wine[-processed] Radix Dipsaci (*Jiu Xu Duan*), vinegar-dipped calcined Pyritum (*Cu Cui Zi Ran Tong*), vinegar[-processed] Resina Olibani (*Cu Ru Xiang*), and vinegar[-processed] Resina Myrrhae (*Cu Mo Yao*)

3. With uncooked Semen Vaccariae Segetalis (*Sheng Wang Bu Liu Xing*), stir-fried Radix Astragali Membranacei (*Chao Huang Qi*), Medulla Tetrapanacis Papyriferi (*Tong Cao*), and Fructus Liquidambaris Taiwaniae (*Lu Lu Tong*)

4. With wine[-processed] Radix Angelicae Sinensis (*Jiu Dang Gui*), vinegar[-processed] Carapax Amydae Sinensis (*Cu Bie Jia*), and wine[-processed] Radix Ligustici Wallichii (*Jiu Chuan Xiong*) as in *Chuan Shan Jia San* (Squama Manitis Powder [50])

Dosage: 5-15g in decoction; 1-1.5g in powder

Note: 1. This refers to a method of calcining (*cui fa*). The pangolin scales are heated and dipped while hot in vinegar. This operation is repeated several times. This process facilitates the pulverization of the pangolin scales and strengthens their action of quickening the blood so as to relieve pain.

Radix Ligustici Wallichii (Chuan Xiong)

Uncooked (Sheng)

Names: *Chuan Xiong, Sheng Chuan Xiong, Xiong Qiong, Fu Xiong, Da Chuan Xiong*

Flavors & nature: Acrid; warm

Functions: Dispels wind, stops pain

Indications:

1. Headache due to A) wind cold with pain in the whole head, fever, chills, nasal congestion, neck pain; B) wind heat with pain and distention of the head, fever, slight aversion to wind, sore throat; or C) wind dampness with a sensation of heaviness in the head, joint pain, fever, chills...

2. Rheumatic complaints due to wind dampness with headache, backache, and low back pain accompanied by a sensation of heaviness, generalized pain, chills, slight fever...

3. Skin inflammations (abscess) due to either A) heat toxins or B) qi and blood vacuity

Typical combinations:

1. A) With uncooked Herba Cum Radice Asari (*Sheng Xi Xin*) and Radix Angelicae Dahuricae (*Bai Zhi*) as in *Chuan Xiong Cha Tiao San* (Ligusticum Wallichium & Tea Regulating Powder [52])
B) With uncooked Flos Chrysanthemi Morifolii (*Sheng Ju Hua*), uncooked Fructus Viticis (*Sheng Man Jing Zi*), and uncooked Bombyx Batryticatus (*Sheng Jiang Can*)
C) With Radix Et Rhizoma Ligustici Chinensis (*Gao Ben*) and uncooked Fructus Viticis (*Sheng Man Jing Zi*) as in *Qiang Huo Sheng Shi Tang* (Notopterygium Overcome Dampness Decoction [247])

2. With Radix Et Rhizoma Notopterygii (*Qiang Huo*) and Radix Angelicae Pubescentis (*Du Huo*) as in *Qiang Huo Sheng Shi Tang* (Notopterygium Overcome Dampness Decoction [247])

3. A) With Herba Cum Radice Taraxaci Mongolici (*Pu Gong Ying*) and Herba Violae Yedoensis (*Zi Hua Di Ding*)
B) With wine[-processed] Radix Angelicae Sinensis (*Jiu Dang Gui*) and uncooked Radix Astragali Membranacei (*Sheng Huang Qi*)

Dosage: 3-10g and up to 30g in severe cases

Wine Mix-fried (Jiu Zhi)

Names: *Jiu Zhi Chuan Xiong, Jiu Chuan Xiong, Jiu Fu Xiong, Zhi Chuan Xiong*

Flavors & nature: Acrid; warm; drying

Functions: Moves the qi, quickens the blood, frees the channels, stops pain

Indications:

1. Menstrual irregularity due to either A) blood vacuity and blood stasis or B) blood stasis and cold in the uterus...

2. Lateral costal pain due to qi stagnation possibly accompanied by blood stasis with chest and epigastric oppression, lateral costal distention...

3. Rheumatic complaints due to cold dampness with severe, fixed joint pain aggravated by cold and dampness, cold feet and knees...

Typical combinations:

1. A) With wine[-processed] Radix Angelicae Sinensis (*Jiu Dang Gui*), wine[-processed] Radix Albus Paeoniae Lactiflorae (*Jiu Bai Shao Yao*), and prepared Radix Rehmanniae (*Shu Di Huang*) as in *Si Wu Tang* (Four Materials Decoction [315])

Radix Ligustici Wallichii continued . . .

B) With stir-fried Ramulus Cinnamomi (*Chao Gui Zhi*), wine[-processed] Radix Angelicae Sinensis (*Jiu Dang Gui*), blast-fried Rhizoma Zingiberis (*Pao Jiang*), uncooked Pollen Typhae (*Sheng Pu Huang*), and wine[-processed] Feces Trogopterori Seu Pteromi (*Jiu Wu Ling Zhi*)

2. With uncooked Radix Bupleuri (*Sheng Chai Hu*), uncooked Fructus Citri Seu Ponciri (*Sheng Zhi Ke*), and wine[-processed] Radix Rubrus Paeoniae Lactiflorae (*Jiu Chi Shao Yao*) as in *Xue Fu Zhu Yu Tang* (Blood Mansion Dispel Stasis Decoction [393])

3. With processed Radix Lateralis Praeparatus Aconiti Carmichaeli (*Zhi Fu Zi*), uncooked Ramulus Cinnamomi (*Sheng Gui Zhi*), Radix Et Rhizoma Notopterygii (*Qiang Huo*), and Radix Angelicae Pubescentis (*Du Huo*)

Dosage: 3-10g and up to 30g in severe cases

Radix Salviae Miltiorrhizae *(Dan Shen)*
—————————— Uncooked *(Sheng)* ——————————

Names: *Sheng Dan Shen, Dan Shen, Zi Dan Shen*

Flavors & nature: Bitter; slightly cold

Functions: Clears heat, resolves vexation, cools the blood, disperses swelling

Indications:

1. Vexation with a warm disease due to heat in the constructive level or in the blood level with agitation, irritability, agitated sleep, macules, fever...

2. Mastitis (inflammatory stage) with redness, pain, heat, swelling...

3. Erysipelas due to heat toxins in the blood level with pruritus...

Typical combinations:

1. With uncooked Radix Rehmanniae (*Sheng Di Huang*), Radix Scrophulariae Ningpoensis (*Xuan Shen*), and uncooked Rhizoma Coptidis Chinensis (*Sheng Huang Lian*) as in *Qing Ying Tang* (Clear the Constructive Decoction [259])

2. With stir-fried Resina Olibani (*Chao Ru Xiang*), stir-fried Resina Myrrhae (*Chao Mo Yao*), uncooked Fructus Forsythiae Suspensae (*Sheng Lian Qiao*), uncooked Flos Lonicerae Japonicae (*Sheng Jin Yin Hua*), and sand stir-fried Squama Manitis Pentadactylis (*Sha Chao Chuan Shan Jia*) as in *Xiao Ru Tang* (Disperse the Breasts Decoction [378])

3. With uncooked Radix Rubrus Paeoniae Lactiflorae (*Sheng Chi Shao Yao*), uncooked Cortex Radicis Moutan (*Sheng Mu Dan Pi*), Herba Violae Yedoensis (*Zi Hua Di Ding*), Herba Cum Radice Taraxaci Mongolici (*Pu Gong Ying*), uncooked Flos Lonicerae Japonicae (*Sheng Jin Yin Hua*), and uncooked Fructus Forsythiae Suspensae (*Sheng Lian Qiao*)

Dosage: 10-15g and up to 30-60g in severe cases

Radix Salviae Miltiorrhizae continued . . .

———————— Pork Blood [Processed] (Zhu Xue)[1] ————————

Names: *Zhu Xue Ban Dan Shen, Xue Ban Dan Shen*

Flavors & nature: Bitter and slightly sweet; neutral

Functions: Nourishes the blood, quiets the spirit

Indications:

1. Insomnia due to heart blood vacuity

2. Heart palpitations due to heart blood vacuity

3. Hysteria, mental confusion due to heart yin vacuity and depressed liver qi

Typical combinations:

1. With processed Radix Polygalae Tenuifoliae (*Zhi Yuan Zhi*), defatted Semen Biotae Orientalis (*Bai Zi Ren Shuang*), and uncooked Semen Zizyphi Spinosae (*Sheng Suan Zao Ren*)

2. With Cinnabar[-processed] Tuber Ophiopogonis Japonicae (*Zhu Sha Ban Mai Men Dong*), uncooked Semen Zizyphi Spinosae (*Sheng Suan Zao Ren*), defatted Semen Biotae Orientalis (*Bai Zi Ren Shuang*), Arillus Euphoriae Longanae (*Long Yan Rou*), and Caulis Polygoni Multiflori (*Ye Jiao Teng*)

3. With uncooked Bulbus Lilii (*Sheng Bai He*), Cinnabar[-processed] Tuber Ophiopogonis Japonicae (*Zhu Sha Ban Mai Men Dong*), Cinnabar[-processed] Tuber Asparagi Cochinensis (*Zhu Sha Ban Tian Men Dong*), and uncooked Radix Bupleuri (*Sheng Chai Hu*)

Dosage: 15-30g

Note: 1. *Zhu Xue* is pork blood which is mixed with the Salvia. Pork blood's flavor is sweet and its nature is neutral. Its principal function is to nourish the blood.

———————————— Wine Mix-fried (Jiu Zhi) ————————————

Names: *Jiu Zhi Dan Shen, Jiu Dan Shen, Zhi Dan Shen*

Flavors & nature: Bitter and slightly acrid; neutral

Functions: Quickens the blood, dispels stasis, stops pain

Indications:

1. Menstrual irregularity due to blood stasis with long or short cycles, abundant or scanty periods, severe dysmenorrhea...

2. Retention of the lochia due to blood stasis in the uterus with postpartum abdominal pain...

3. Heart pain due to either A) heart blood stasis with severe pain or B) heart blood stasis and heart

qi vacuity with severe pain, palpitations, shortness of breath...

4. Epigastric pain due to qi stagnation, blood stasis in the middle burner

5. Lateral costal pain due to liver qi and blood stagnation

6. Abdominal masses due to qi stagnation, blood stasis with abdominal pain and distention...

Typical combinations:

1. With Herba Lycopi Lucidi (*Ze Lan*), vinegar[-processed] Rhizoma Cyperi Rotundi (*Cu Xiang Fu*), wine[-processed] Radix Ligustici Wallichii (*Jiu Chuan Xiong*), uncooked Semen Pruni Persicae (*Sheng Tao Ren*), and Flos Carthami Tinctorii (*Hong Hua*)

Radix Salviae Miltiorrhizae continued . . .

2. With wine[-processed] Herba Leonuri Heterophylli (*Jiu Yi Mu Cao*), wine[-processed] Radix Ligustici Wallichii (*Jiu Chuan Xiong*), and uncooked Semen Pruni Persicae (*Sheng Tao Ren*)

3. A) With stir-fried Resina Olibani (*Chao Ru Xiang*) and stir-fried Resina Myrrhae (*Chao Mo Yao*) as in *Huo Luo Xiao Ling Dan* (Quicken the Network Vessels Fantastically Effective Elixir [162])
B) With Flos Carthami Tinctorii (*Hong Hua*), stir-fried Resina Olibani (*Chao Ru Xiang*), stir-fried Resina Myrrhae (*Chao Mo Yao*), Radix Panacis Ginseng (*Ren Shen*), and honey mix-fried Radix Astragali Membranacei (*Mi Zhi Huang Qi*)

4. With Lignum Santali Albi (*Tan Xiang*) and Fructus Amomi (*Sha Ren*) as in *Dan Shen Yin* (Salvia Drink)

5. With vinegar[-processed] Tuber Curcumae (*Cu Yu Jin*), vinegar[-processed] Radix Bupleuri (*Cu Chai Hu*), vinegar[-processed] Rhizoma Sparganii (*Cu San Leng*), and vinegar[-processed] Rhizoma Corydalis Yanhusuo (*Cu Yan Hu Suo*)

6. With vinegar[-processed] Rhizoma Curcumae Zedoariae (*Cu E Zhu*), vinegar[-processed] Rhizoma Sparganii (*Cu San Leng*), vinegar[-processed] Carapax Amydae Sinensis (*Cu Bie Jia*), and vinegar[-processed] Pericarpium Viridis Citri Reticulatae (*Cu Qing Pi*)

Dosage: 10-15g and up to 30-60g in severe cases

Rhizoma Curcumae Zedoariae (*E Zhu*)

—————————— Uncooked (*Sheng*) ——————————

Names: *Sheng E Zhu, E Zhu, Peng E Zhu*

Flavors & nature: Bitter and acrid; warm

Functions: Moves the qi, disperses food stagnation, stops pain

Indications:

1. Food stagnation with severe abdominal pain and distention, acid vomiting...

2. Dysentery due to qi stagnation and damp heat in the stomach and intestines with abdominal pain, tenesmus...

Typical combinations:

1. With stir-fried [till] yellow Fructus Germinatus Hordei Vulgaris (*Chao Huang Mai Ya*), uncooked Rhizoma Sparganii (*Sheng San Leng*), Semen Arecae Catechu (*Bing Lang*), and Pericarpium Viridis Citri Reticulatae (*Sheng Qing Pi*) as in *E Zhu Wan* (Zedoaria Pills [94])

2. With Semen Arecae Catechu (*Bing Lang*), roasted Radix Saussureae Seu Vladimiriae (*Wei Mu Xiang*), and uncooked Rhizoma Coptidis Chinensis (*Sheng Huang Lian*) as in *Mu Xiang Bing Lang Wan* (Saussurea & Arecae Pills [225])

Dosage: 5-10g and up to 20g in severe cases

—————————— Vinegar Mix-fried (*Cu Zhi*) ——————————

Names: *Cu Zhi E Zhu, Cu E Zhu, Zhi E Zhu*

Flavors & nature: Bitter, slightly acrid, and slightly sour; warm

Functions: Breaks blood stasis, dissipates abdominal masses, stops pain

Rhizoma Curcumae Zedoariae continued . . .

Indications:

1. Amenorrhea due to either A) blood stasis with pain in the lower abdomen or B) blood vacuity and stasis

2. Abdominal masses due to blood stasis with fixed, palpable masses which may be painful under the lateral costal region

Typical combinations:

1. A) With wine[-processed] Radix Ligustici Wallichii (*Jiu Chuan Xiong*), vinegar[-processed] Rhizoma Sparganii (*Cu San Leng*), wine[-processed] Cortex Radicis Moutan (*Jiu Mu Dan Pi*), and wine[-processed] Radix Cyathulae (*Jiu Chuan Niu Xi*) as in *San Leng Wan* (Sparganium Pills [272])

B) With wine[-processed] Radix Angelicae Sinensis (*Jiu Dang Gui*), wine[-processed] Radix Albus Paeoniae Lactiflorae (*Jiu Bai Shao Yao*), wine[-processed] Radix Ligustici Wallichii (*Jiu Chuan Xiong*), and prepared Radix Rehmanniae (*Shu Di Huang*) as in *E Zhu San* (Zedoaria Powder [93])

2. With vinegar[-processed] Rhizoma Sparganii (*Cu San Leng*), vinegar[-processed] Carapax Amydae Sinensis (*Cu Bie Jia*), vinegar[-processed] Squama Manitis Pentadactylis (*Cu Chuan Shan Jia*), wine[-processed] Radix Salviae Miltiorrhizae (*Jiu Dan Shen*), and Flos Carthami Tinctorii (*Hong Hua*) as in *E Leng Zhu Yu Tang* (Zedoaria & Sparganium Dispel Stasis Decoction [92])

Dosage: 5-10g and up to 30g in severe cases

Radix Achyranthis Bidentatae (Huai Niu Xi)[1]

Uncooked (Sheng)

Names: *Sheng Huai Niu Xi, Huai Niu Xi, Niu Xi[2], Sheng Niu Xi*

Flavors & nature: Bitter and sour; neutral

Functions: Quickens the blood, downbears the blood

Indications:

1. Gingivitis[3] due to stomach fire with swollen, red, painful gums, aphthae, glossitis...

2. Vertigo due to liver yang rising followed by accumulation of blood and heat in the upper body with ocular distention, tinnitus, dizziness, headache...

3. Rheumatic complaints[4] due to wind dampness with joint, bone, tendinous, and muscular pain, loss of mobility...

Typical combinations:

1. With uncooked Radix Rehmanniae (*Sheng Di Huang*) and uncooked Gypsum Fibrosum (*Sheng Shi Gao*) as in *Yu Nu Jian* (Jade Maiden Decoction [416])

2. With uncooked Haematitum (*Sheng Dai Zhe Shi*), uncooked Plastrum Testudinis (*Sheng Gui Ban*), and uncooked Radix Albus Paeoniae Lactiflorae (*Sheng Bai Shao Yao*) as in *Zhen Gan Xi Feng Tang* (Settle the Liver & Extinguish Wind Decoction [428])

3. With Caulis Millettiae Seu Spatholobi (*Ji Xue Teng*), uncooked Fasciculus Vascularis Luffae (*Sheng Si Gua Luo*), Radix Angelicae Pubescentis (*Du Huo*), and Radix Et Rhizoma Notopterygii (*Qiang Huo*)

Radix Achyranthis Bidentatae continued . . .

Dosage: 10-15g and up to 30g in severe cases; 5-10g if used as a messenger medicinal[5]

Notes: 1. See note 1 under uncooked Radix Cyathulae (*Sheng Chuan Niu Xi*) in this same chapter. 2. The abbreviation *Niu Xi* in particular always corresponds to Radix Achyranthis Bidentatae (*Huai Niu Xi*). In prescriptions where it is necessary to use Radix Cyathulae (*Chuan Niu Xi*) or Radix Achyranthis (*Tu Niu Xi*), one should not write *Niu Xi* but either *Chuan Niu Xi* or *Tu Niu Xi*. 3. For this indication, one can prescribe Radix Achyranthis (*Tu Niu Xi*). 4. For this indication, one can prescribe Radix Cyathulae (*Chuan Niu Xi*). 5. See note 2 under uncooked Radix Cyathulae (*Sheng Chuan Niu Xi*) in this same chapter.

Wine Mix-fried (Jiu Zhi)

Names: *Jiu Zhi Huai Niu Xi, Jiu Huai Niu Xi, Jiu Niu Xi*

Flavors & nature: Bitter and sour; neutral tending to warm

Functions: Quickens the blood, dispels stasis, stops pain

Indications:

1. Amenorrhea, dysmenorrhea due to blood stasis with menstrual irregularity, severe pain in the lower abdomen, clots in the menses...

2. Retention of the placenta, retention of the fetus due to blood stasis with lower abdominal distention and pain...

Typical combinations:

1. With wine[-processed] Radix Angelicae Sinensis (*Jiu Dang Gui*), wine[-processed] Radix Rubrus Paeoniae Lactiflorae (*Jiu Chi Shao Yao*), Flos Carthami Tinctorii (*Hong Hua*), uncooked Semen Pruni Persicae (*Sheng Tao Ren*), wine[-processed] Radix Ligustici Wallichii (*Jiu Chuan Xiong*), and wine[-processed] Rhizoma Corydalis Yanhusuo (*Jiu Yan Hu Suo*)

2. With Secretio Moschi Moschiferi (*She Xiang*), wine[-processed] Herba Leonuri Heterophylli (*Jiu Yi Mu Cao*), vinegar[-processed] Rhizoma Sparganii (*Cu San Leng*), wine[-processed] Radix Et Rhizoma Rhei (*Jiu Da Huang*), and uncooked Pollen Typhae (*Sheng Pu Huang*)

Dosage: 10-15g and up to 30g in severe cases

Salt Mix-fried (Yan Zhi)

Names: *Yan Zhi Huai Niu Xi, Yan Huai Niu Xi, Yan Niu Xi*

Flavors & nature: Bitter, sour, and slightly salty; neutral

Functions: Supplements the liver and kidneys, strengthens the sinews and bones, disinhibits urination

Indications:

1. Low back pain due to either A) liver/kidney vacuity with weakness, stiffness, or pain of the limbs, weakness or pain of the knees or B) kidney vacuity associated with cold dampness in the lumbar region with a sensation of heaviness and numbness of the low back, weak knees...

2. Atony of the lower extremities due to liver/-kidney vacuity

3. Rheumatic complaints due to either A) liver/-kidney vacuity with weakness of the sinews and bones, loss of mobility, weakness of the lower extremities or B) damp heat in the lower burner with pain and weakness in the lower extremities and low back, pain in the feet...

Radix Achyranthis Bidentatae continued . . .

4. Strangury with hematuria[1] due to damp heat in the bladder with dysuria, urgent urination, frequent but scant urination, reddish urine with the possible presence of blood clots or stones...

Typical combinations:

1. A) With salt[-processed] Cortex Eucommiae Ulmoidis (*Yan Du Zhong*), salt[-processed] Radix Dipsaci (*Yan Xu Duan*), Ramus Loranthi Seu Visci (*Sang Ji Sheng*), and wine[-processed] Cortex Radicis Acanthopanacis (*Jiu Wu Jia Pi*)
B) With salt[-processed] Cortex Eucommiae Ulmoidis (*Yan Du Zhong*), Ramulus Loranthi Seu Visci (*Sang Ji Sheng*), Radix Angelicae Pubescentis (*Du Huo*), Cortex Cinnamomi (*Rou Gui*), and uncooked Herba Cum Radice Asari (*Sheng Xi Xin*) as in *Du Huo Ji Sheng Tang* (*Du Huo & Loranthus Decoction* [88])

2. With Os Tigridis (*Hu Gu*) [substitute pig bone][2], Herba Cynomorii (*Suo Yang*), prepared Radix Rehmanniae (*Shu Di Huang*), and vinegar dip calcined Plastrum Testudinis (*Cu Cui Gui Ban*) as in *Hu Qian Wan* (Hidden Tiger Pills [144])

3. A) With wine[-processed] Cortex Radicis Acanthopanacis (*Jiu Wu Jia Pi*), Os Tigridis (*Hu Gu*) [substitute pig bone], Ramus Loranthi Seu Visci (*Sang Ji Sheng*), salt[-processed] Radix Dipsaci (*Yan Xu Duan*), and salt[-processed] Cortex Eucommiae Ulmoidis (*Yan Du Zhong*)

B) With uncooked Rhizoma Atractylodis (*Sheng Cang Zhu*) and salt[-processed] Cortex Phellodendri (*Yan Huang Bai*) as in *San Miao Wan* (Three Marvels Pills [273])

4. With carbonized Herba Cirsii Japonici (*Da Ji Tan*), carbonized Herba Cephalanoploris Segeti (*Xiao Ji Tan*), Folium Pyrrosiae (*Shi Wei*), and salt[-processed] Semen Plantaginis (*Yan Che Qian Zi*)

Dosage: 10-15g and up to 30g in severe cases; 5-10g when used as a messenger medicinal[3]

Notes: 1. For this indication, if there is severe hematuria, one can prescribe carbonized Radix Achyranthis Bidentatae (*Huai Niu Xi Tan*). Radix Achyranthis (*Tu Niu Xi*) can also be used. 2. Editor's note: Tigers are an extremely endangered species primarily due to their bones being used in Chinese medicine. It requires 50 tigers per year to supply 1 Chinese or Taiwanese factory manufacturing Tiger Bone medicines, and there are a number of such factories in those two countries. The most famous Indian tiger refuge only counted 16 tigers in their last census. Although most Chinese pharmacies sell pig bone under the name *Hu Gu*, because the name Tiger Bone is used, it fosters the desire in some people to continue to poach this species. Therefore, it is Blue Poppy Press' editorial position that Tiger Bone should be stricken from the Chinese materia medica to be replaced with *Zhu Gu*, Pig Bone. 3. See note 2 under uncooked Radix Cyathulae (*Sheng Chuan Niu Xi*) in this same chapter.

Addendum: Carbonized Radix Achyranthis Bidentatae (*Huai Niu Xi Tan*) is sometimes used for hematemesis, hematuria, or epistaxis due to blood heat.

Resina Myrrhae (*Mo Yao*)

————————— Uncooked (*Sheng*)[1] —————————

Names: *Sheng Mo Yao, Mo Yao*

Flavors & nature: Bitter; neutral

Functions: Quickens the blood, promotes the engenderment of new tissue, stops pain

Indications: Skin inflammation with ulceration

Typical combinations: With Resina Olibani (*Ru Xiang*).[2] These two substances are reduced to a fine powder and then applied locally.

Resina Myrrhae continued . . .

Dosage: Used externally, whatever quantity is needed. There is no overdosage when used topically.

Notes: 1. Uncooked Resina Myrrhae is irritating to the stomach. It is, therefore, reserved for external usage only. 2. Resina Olibani and Resina Myrrhae have nearly the same actions and indications and they are often prescribed together. In this case in this prescription, one might simply write [in Chinese] *Ru* *Mo*, meaning *Ru (Xiang) + Mo (Yao)*. Li Shi-zhen said, "*Ru Xiang* quickens the blood and *Mo Yao* breaks the blood." Yang Qing-yu said: "If the patient cannot extend their joints, it is necessary to add the remedies *Ru Mo* which deploy the sinews." These two medicinals quicken the blood, stop pain, disperse swelling, and promote tissue regeneration. However, Resina Myrrhae is superior for quickening the blood, breaking blood stasis, and stopping pain, while Resina Olibani is superior for quickening the blood and freeing the network vessels for treating *bi* with loss of joint mobility and contracture of the sinews.

_____ Stir-fried *(Chao)*[1] _____

Names: *Chao Mo Yao, Zhi Mo Yao*

Flavors & nature: Bitter and slightly acrid; neutral or slightly warm

Functions: Quickens the blood, dispels stasis, disperses swelling, stops pain

Indications:

1. Skin inflammation due to heat toxins with redness, pain, swelling, pus...

2. Traumatic injury[2] with blood stasis, pain, hematoma...

3. Abdominal masses due to blood stasis and qi stagnation with palpable, fixed, possibly painful masses...

Typical combinations:

1. With stir-fried Resina Olibani (*Chao Ru Xiang*), Realgar (*Xiong Huang*), and Secretio Moschi Moschiferi (*She Xiang*) as in *Xing Xiao* *Wan* (Move & Disperse Pills [385])

2. With vinegar[-processed] Resina Olibani (*Cu Ru Xiang*), wine[-processed] Radix Angelicae Sinensis (*Jiu Dang Gui*), Lignum Sappanis (*Su Mu*), and wine[-processed] Radix Dipsaci (*Jiu Xu Duan*)

3. With vinegar[-processed] Carapax Amydae Sinensis (*Cu Bie Jia*), vinegar[-processed] Rhizoma Curcumae Zedoariae (*Cu E Zhu*), uncooked Pericarpium Viridis Citri Reticulatae (*Sheng Qing Pi*), and vinegar[-processed] Rhizoma Sparganii (*Cu San Leng*)

Dosage: 5-10g[3]

Notes: 1. Stir-frying allows one to lessen the side effects of uncooked Resina Myrrhae, such as irritation to the stomach's mucosa. 2. For this indication, one can prescribe vinegar mix-fried Resina Myrrhae (*Cu Zhi Mo Yao*) if the pain is severe. 3. This dosage should be strictly respected since Resina Myrrhae is very aromatic and, in case of overdosage, nausea and vomiting will occur.

_____ Vinegar Mix-fried *(Cu Zhi)*[1] _____

Names: *Cu Zhi Mo Yao, Cu Mo Yao, Zhi Mo Yao*

Flavors & nature: Bitter, slightly sour, and slightly acrid; neutral

Functions: Moves the qi, quickens the blood, dispels stasis, disperses swelling, stops pain

Indications:

1. Chest pain due to qi stagnation, blood stasis with piercing pain in the chest, a purple tongue, a choppy (*se*) pulse...

Resina Myrrhae continued . . .

2. Epigastric or abdominal pain due to qi stagnation and blood stasis

3. Amenorrhea due to blood stasis and cold with pain in the lower abdomen aggravated by pressure and cold...

Typical combinations:

1. With vinegar[-processed] Resina Olibani (*Cu Zhi Ru Xiang*), wine[-processed] Radix Salviae Miltiorrhizae (*Jiu Dan Shen*), Radix Pseudo-ginseng (*San Qi*), and Lignum Santali Albi (*Tan Xiang*)

2. With vinegar mix-fried Rhizoma Cyperi Rotundi (*Cu Zhi Xiang Fu*), vinegar[-processed] Rhizoma Corydalis Yanhusuo (*Cu Yan Hu Suo*), and vinegar[-processed] Feces Trogopterori Seu Pteromi (*Cu Wu Ling Zhi*)

3. With dry Rhizoma Zingiberis (*Gan Jiang*), stir-fried Ramulus Cinnamomi (*Chao Gui Zhi*), wine[-processed] Radix Ligustici Wallichii (*Jiu Chuan Xiong*), Fructus Foeniculi Vulgaris (*Xiao Hui Xiang*), and wine[-processed] Radix Angelicae Sinensis (*Jiu Dang Gui*)

Dosage: 5-10g[2]

Notes: 1. Vinegar mix-fried Resina Myrrhae is preferred over stir-fried Resina Myrrhae when pain is the major complaint of the patient. 2. This dosage should be strictly respected since Resina Myrrhae is very aromatic and, in case of overdosage, nausea and vomiting will occur.

Resina Olibani *(Ru Xiang)*

———————————— Uncooked *(Sheng)*[1] ————————————

Names: *Sheng Ru Xiang, Ming Ru Xiang, Di Ru Xiang, Sheng Xun Lu Xiang*

Flavors & nature: Acrid and bitter; warm

Functions: Quickens the blood, disperses swelling, promotes the engenderment of new tissue

Indications:

1. Skin inflammations which will not heal over[1]

2. *Yong* which will not heal[1] due to qi stagnation and blood stasis

3. Traumatic injury[1] with blood stasis, pain, swelling, hematoma...

Typical combinations:

1. With uncooked Resina Myrrhae (*Sheng Mo Yao*), Calcitum (*Han Shui Shi*), and Borneol (*Bing Pian*)

2. With Radix Pseudoginseng (*San Qi*), uncooked Resina Myrrhae (*Sheng Mo Yao*), Borneol (*Bing Pian*), Radix Trichosanthis Kirlowii (*Tian Hua Fen*), uncooked Cortex Radicis Moutan (*Sheng Mu Dan Pi*), and uncooked Radix Rubrus Paeoniae Lactiflorae (*Sheng Chi Shao Yao*)

3. With Sanguis Draconis (*Xue Jie*), uncooked Resina Myrrhae (*Sheng Mo Yao*), and Flos Carthami Tinctorii (*Hong Hua*) as in *Qi Li San* (Seven *Li* Powder [236])

Dosage: Used externally, as much as needed. There is no overdosage when used topically.

Note: 1. Uncooked Resina Olibani is irritating to the stomach. Therefore, it is reserved for external use only.

Addendum: See note 2 under Uncooked Resina Myrrhae (*Sheng Mo Yao*) in this same chapter.

Resina Olibani continued . . .

_____ **Stir-fried** *(Chao)*[1] _____

Names: *Chao Ru Xiang, Zhi Ru Xiang, Xun Lu Xiang*

.8Functions: Quickens the blood, dispels stasis, stops pain, disperses swelling

Indications:

1. Pyogenic skin inflammation due to heat toxins with redness, pain, swelling, pus...

2. Rheumatic complaints[2] due to wind dampness with joint pain, numbness or contracture of the sinews, loss of mobility...

3. Traumatic injury[2] with blood stasis, hematoma, bone fracture, or torn ligaments which will not heal...

4. Abdominal masses due to qi stagnation and blood stasis with palpable, hard, fixed, possibly painful masses...

Typical combinations:

1. With Radix Angelicae Dahuricae (*Bai Zhi*), Radix Trichosanthis Kirlowii (*Tian Hua Fen*), and Squama Manitis Pentadactylis (*Chuan Shan Jia*) as in *Xiang Fang Huo Ming Yin* (Immortal

Formula for Saving Life Drink [364])

2. With Radix Et Rhizoma Notopterygii (*Qiang Huo*) and wine[-processed] Ramulus Mori Albi (*Jiu Sang Zhi*) as in *Cheng Shi Juan Bi Tang* (Master Cheng's Alleviate *Bi* Decoction [47])

3. With Rhizoma Drynariae (*Gu Sui Bu*), wine[-processed] Radix Dipsaci (*Jiu Xu Duan*), vinegar dip calcined Pyritum (*Cu Cui Zi Ran Tong*), and vinegar[-processed] Resina Myrrhae (*Cu Mo Yao*)

4. With vinegar[-processed] Rhizoma Sparganii (*Cu San Leng*), vinegar[-processed] Rhizoma Curcumae Zedoariae (*Cu E Zhu*), vinegar[-processed] Carapax Amydae Sinensis (*Cu Bie Jia*), and stir-fried Resina Myrrhae (*Cu Mo Yao*)

Dosage: 3-9g[3]

Notes: 1. Stir-frying Resina Olibani allows one to lessen the side-effects of uncooked *Ru Xiang*, such as irritation to the stomach mucosa. 2. For this indication, vinegar mix-fried *Ru Xiang* (*Cu Zhi Ru Xiang*) can be prescribed if the pain is severe. 3. This dosage should be strictly respected since *Ru Xiang* is very aromatic and, in case of overdose, nausea and vomiting will occur.

_____ **Vinegar Mix-fried** *(Cu Zhi)*[1] _____

Names: *Cu Zhi Ru Xiang, Cu Ru Xiang*

Flavors & nature: Bitter, slightly acrid, and slightly sour; warm

Functions: Quickens the blood, dispels stasis, stops pain

Indications:

1. Epigastric pain due to blood stasis in the stomach with severe, fixed pain aggravated by pressure...

2. Heart pain due to heart blood stasis

3. Postpartum abdominal pain due to blood stasis with retention of the lochia...

4. Amenorrhea due to blood stasis with severe pain in the lower abdomen...

Typical combinations:

1. With vinegar[-processed] Rhizoma Corydalis Yanhusuo (*Cu Yan Hu Suo*), stir-fried Fructus

Blood-quickening, Stasis-dispelling Medicinals 137

Resina Olibani continued . . .

Meliae Toosendan (*Chao Chuan Lian Zi*), stir-fried Resina Myrrhae (*Chao Mo Yao*), and vinegar[-processed] Rhizoma Sparganii (*Cu San Leng*)

2. With uncooked Pollen Typhae (*Sheng Pu Huang*), stir-fried Resina Myrrhae (*Chao Mo Yao*), wine[-processed] Radix Salviae Miltiorrhizae (*Jiu Dan Shen*), and Radix Pseudoginseng (*San Qi*)

3. With uncooked Pollen Typhae (*Sheng Pu Huang*), wine[-processed] Feces Trogopterori Seu Pteromi (*Jiu Wu Ling Zhi*), vinegar[-processed] Resina Myrrhae (*Cu Mo Yao*), and wine[-

processed] Radix Cyathulae (*Jiu Chuan Niu Xi*)

4. With uncooked Semen Pruni Persicae (*Sheng Tao Ren*), wine[-processed] Radix Ligustici Wallichii (*Jiu Chuan Xiong*), wine[-processed] Radix Salviae Miltiorrhizae (*Jiu Dan Shen*), and wine[-processed] Radix Cyathulae (*Jiu Chuan Niu Xi*)

Dosage: 3-9g[2]

Notes: 1. Vinegar mix-fried Resina Olibani is preferable to stir-fried *Ru Xiang* if pain is the major complaint of the patient. 2. This dosage should be strictly respected. *Ru Xiang* is very aromatic and, in case of overdose, nausea and vomiting will appear.

Rhizoma Sparganii *(San Leng)*

———————————— Uncooked *(Sheng)* ————————————

Names: *Sheng San Leng, San Leng, Jing San Leng, Shan Leng*

Flavors & nature: Bitter; neutral

Functions: Moves the qi, transforms food stagnation, breaks blood stasis

Indications:

1. Food stagnation A) with severe epigastric and abdominal distention and pain, loss of appetite, indigestion of meat foods; B) the same pattern accompanied by constipation; or C) the same pattern accompanied by diarrhea...

2. Retention of the fetus due to blood stasis

Typical combinations:

1. A) With uncooked Rhizoma Curcumae Zedoariae (*Sheng E Zhu*), stir-fried Fructus Crataegi (*Chao Shan Zha*), stir-fried Fructus

Germinatus Hordei Vulgaris (*Chao Mai Ya*), and uncooked Radix Saussureae Seu Vladimiriae (*Sheng Mu Xiang*)
B) With uncooked Radix Et Rhizoma Rhei (*Sheng Da Huang*) and Semen Arecae Catechu (*Bing Lang*)
C) With stir-fried [till] scorched Massa Medica Fermentata (*Chao Jiao Shen Qu*) and earth stir-fried Rhizoma Atractylodis Macrocephalae (*Tu Chao Bai Zhu*)

2. With wine[-processed] Radix Cyathulae (*Jiu Chuan Niu Xi*), Secretio Moschi Moschiferi (*She Xiang*), uncooked Semen Pruni Persicae (*Sheng Tao Ren*), Flos Carthami Tinctorii (*Hong Hua*), wine[-processed] Feces Trogopterori Seu Pteromi (*Jiu Wu Ling Zhi*), and uncooked Pollen Typhae (*Sheng Pu Huang*)

Dosage: 5-10g and up to 20g in severe cases

Rhizoma Sparganii continued . . .

_____ Vinegar Mix-fried *(Cu Zhi)* _____

Names: *Cu Zhi San Leng, Cu San Leng, Zhi San Leng*

Flavors & nature: Bitter and slightly sour; slightly warm

Functions: Breaks blood stasis, dissipates abdominal masses, stops pain

Indications:

1. Amenorrhea due to blood stasis with pain in the lower abdomen aggravated by pressure...

2. Abdominal masses of all types (*i.e.*, splenomegaly, hepatomegaly, abdominal tumors, etc.) due to blood stasis

3. Pain in the abdomen, epigastrium, or lateral costal regions due to qi and blood stagnation

Typical combinations:

1. With wine[-processed] Radix Ligustici

Wallichii (*Jiu Chuan Xiong*), vinegar[-processed] Rhizoma Curcumae Zedoariae (*Cu E Zhu*), wine[-processed] Cortex Radicis Moutan (*Jiu Mu Dan Pi*), and wine[-processed] Radix Cyathulae (*Jiu Chuan Niu Xi*) as in *San Leng Wan* (Sparganium Pills [272])

2. With vinegar[-processed] Rhizoma Curcumae Zedoariae (*Cu E Zhu*), wine[-processed] Radix Angelicae Sinensis (*Jiu Dang Gui*), vinegar[-processed] Carapax Amydae Sinensis (*Cu Bie Jia*), and wine[-processed] Radix Salviae Miltiorrhizae (*Jiu Dan Shen*) as in *E Leng Zhu Yu Tang* (Zedoaria & Sparganium Dispel Stasis Decoction [92])

3. With vinegar[-processed] Rhizoma Corydalis Yanhusuo (*Cu Yan Hu Suo*) and vinegar[-processed] Rhizoma Curcumae Zedoariae (*Cu E Zhu*) as in *San Leng Wan* (Sparganium Pills [272])

Dosage: 6-12g and up to 20g in severe cases

Fasciculus Vascularis Luffae *(Si Gua Luo)*

_____ Uncooked *(Sheng)* _____

Names: *Sheng Si Gua Luo, Si Gua Luo*

Flavors & nature: Sweet; slightly cold

Functions: Dispels wind, transforms phlegm, clears heat

Indications:

1. Rheumatic complaints of the heat type (*re bi*) with pain, heat, redness, and swelling of the muscles or joints...

2. Cough due to lung heat and phlegm heat with expectoration of yellow, thick phlegm, chest oppression, pain in the chest and lateral costal region...

3. Chest pain due to qi stagnation and phlegm with chest oppression and pain...

Typical combinations:

1. With uncooked Radix Aristolochiae Fangchi (*Sheng Mu Fang Ji*), uncooked Ramulus Mori

Fasciculus Vascularis Luffae continued . . .

Albi (*Sheng Sang Zhi*), and uncooked Radix Cyathulae (*Sheng Chuan Niu Xi*) as in *Sang Zhi Tang* (Morus Twig Decoction [280])

2. With honey mix-fried Herba Ephedrae (*Mi Zhi Ma Huang*), uncooked Semen Pruni Armeniacae (*Sheng Xing Ren*), uncooked Gypsum Fibrosum (*Sheng Shi Gao*), stir-fried Semen Benincasae

Hispidae (*Chao Dong Gua Ren*), and Rhizoma Phragmitis Communis (*Lu Gen*)

3. With uncooked Fructus Citri Seu Ponciri (*Sheng Zhi Ke*), stir-fried Semen Trichosanthis Kirlowii (*Chao Gua Lou Ren*), uncooked Radix Platycodi Grandiflori (*Sheng Jie Geng*), and Fasciculus Vascularis Citri Reticulatae (*Ju Luo*)

Dosage: 5-15g and up to 60g in severe cases

_____ **Stir-fried [till] Yellow (Chao Huang)** _____

Name: *Chao Si Gua Luo*

Flavors & nature: Sweet; neutral

Functions: Quickens the blood, moves the qi, frees the network vessels, stops pain

Indications:

1. Traumatic injury with hematoma, swelling...

2. Amenorrhea, dysmenorrhea due to qi stagnation and blood stasis with pain in the lower abdomen, scanty menstruation accompanied by clots...

3. Mastitis, agalactia due to qi stagnation in the network vessels of the breasts

4. Lateral costal pain due to liver qi stagnation with lateral costal distention, pain aggravated by stress or anger...

Typical combinations:

1. With vinegar[-processed] Resina Olibani (*Cu Ru Xiang*), vinegar[-processed] Resina Myrrhae (*Cu Mo Yao*), uncooked Fructus Citri Seu Ponciri

(*Sheng Zhi Ke*), and Fasciculus Vascularis Citri Reticulatae (*Ju Luo*) as in *Tong Luo Zhi Tong Tang* (Open the Network Vessels & Stop Pain Decoction [331])

2. With Flos Carthami Tinctorii (*Hong Hua*), uncooked Semen Pruni Persicae (*Sheng Tao Ren*), wine[-processed] Radix Ligustici Wallichii (*Jiu Chuan Xiong*), and wine[-processed] Radix Angelicae Sinensis (*Jiu Dang Gui*)

3. With uncooked Semen Vaccariae Segetalis (*Sheng Wang Bu Liu Xing*), vinegar[-processed] Squama Manitis Pentadactylis (*Cu Chuan Shan Jia*), and Medulla Tetrapanacis Papyriferi (*Tong Cao*)

4. With vinegar[-processed] Radix Bupleuri (*Cu Chai Hu*), vinegar[-processed] Tuber Curcumae (*Cu Yu Jin*), uncooked Fructus Citri Seu Ponciri (*Sheng Zhi Ke*), and wine[-processed] Radix Albus Paeoniae Lactiflorae (*Jiu Bai Shao Yao*)

Dosage: 5-15g and up to 60g in severe cases

Semen Pruni Persicae *(Tao Ren)*

————————— Uncooked *(Sheng)* —————————

Names: *Tao Ren, Guang Tao Ren, Sheng Tao Ren*

Flavors & nature: Bitter and sweet; neutral

Functions: Moves the blood, dispels stasis

Indications:

1. Amenorrhea due to blood stasis with lower abdominal pain aggravated by pressure...

2. Abdominal masses due to blood stasis with abdominal pain aggravated by pressure, fixed, palpable abdominal masses, scanty metrorrhagia...

3. Traumatic injury with pain, hematoma, swelling...

Typical combinations:

1. With wine[-processed] Radix Et Rhizoma Rhei *(Jiu Da Huang)* and stir-fried Ramulus Cinnamomi *(Chao Gui Zhi)* as in *Tao He Cheng Qi Tang* (Persica Seed Support the Qi Decoction [320])

2. With stir-fried Ramulus Cinnamomi *(Chao Gui Zhi)*, wine[-processed] Cortex Radicis Moutan *(Jiu Mu Dan Pi)*, and wine[-processed] Radix Rubrus Paeoniae Lactiflorae *(Jiu Chi Shao Yao)* as in *Gui Zhi Fu Ling Wan* (Cinnamon Twig & Poria Pills [123])

3. With vinegar[-processed] Resina Olibani *(Cu Ru Xiang)*, vinegar[-processed] Resina Myrrhae *(Cu Mo Yao)*, Lignum Sappanis *(Su Mu)*, and wine[-processed] Radix Dipsaci *(Jiu Xu Duan)*

Dosage: 5-10g and up to 60g in severe cases

————————— Scalded *(Dan)*[1] —————————

Name: *Dan Tao Ren*

Flavors & nature: Bitter and sweet; neutral

Functions: Downbears counterflow qi, stops cough, dissipates abscesses

Indications:

1. Cough, asthma due to counterflow lung qi and stagnant phlegm with asthmatic breathing, shortness of breath, fullness in the chest...

2. Appendicitis due to accumulation of heat toxins and qi and blood stagnation with abdominal pain aggravated by pressure...

3. Pulmonary abscess due to accumulation of heat toxins and qi and blood stagnation with chest pain, cough, pussy, bloody expectoration...

Typical combinations:

1. With uncooked Semen Pruni Armeniacae *(Sheng Xing Ren)*, stir-fried Flos Tussilaginis Farfarae *(Chao Kuan Dong Hua)*, Bulbus Fritillariae Thunbergii *(Zhe Bei Mu)*, and uncooked Folium Eriobotryae Japonicae *(Sheng Pi Pa Ye)*

2. With uncooked Radix Et Rhizoma Rhei *(Sheng Da Huang)*, uncooked Cortex Radicis Moutan *(Sheng Mu Dan Pi)*, and uncooked Semen Benincasae Hispidae *(Sheng Dong Gua Ren)* as in *Da Huang Mu Dan Pi Tang* (Rhubarb & Moutan Decoction [64])

3. With Semen Coicis Lachryma-jobi *(Yi Yi Ren)*, Rhizoma Phragmitis Communis *(Lu Gen)*, and uncooked Semen Benincasae Hispidae *(Sheng Dong Gua Ren)* as in *Wei Jing Tang* (Phragmites Decoction [338])

Semen Pruni Persicae continued . . .

Dosage: 5-10g and up to 60g in severe cases

Note: 1. This refers to a method which consists of scalding or par-boiling the Persica. See the chapter on "Methods of Preparing the Chinese Materia Medica".

_____ **Stir-fried [till] Yellow (Chao Huang)** _____

Name: *Chao Tao Ren*

Flavors & nature: Bitter and sweet; neutral tending to slightly warm

Functions: Moistens dryness, quickens the blood

Indications:

1. Constipation due to blood vacuity occasioning dryness of the large intestine especially in the elderly or postpartum women...

2. Inflammatory processes with redness, swelling, heat, pain...

Typical combinations:

1. With stir-fried Semen Cannabis Sativae (*Chao Huo Ma Ren*), uncooked Radix Angelicae Sinensis (*Sheng Dang Gui*), and prepared Radix Rehmanniae (*Shu Di Huang*) as in *Run Zao Tang* (Moisten Dryness Decoction [270])

2. With uncooked Flos Lonicerae Japonicae (*Sheng Jin Yin Hua*), Radix Trichosanthis Kirlowii (*Tian Hua Fen*), sand stir-fried Squama Manitis Pentadactylis (*Sha Chao Chuan Shan Jia*), and uncooked Fructus Forsythiae Suspensae (*Sheng Lian Qiao*)

Dosage: 5-10g and up to 60g in severe cases

Semen Vaccariae Segetalis *(Wang Bu Liu Xing)*

_____ **Uncooked (Sheng)** _____

Names: *Wang Bu Liu Xing, Sheng Liu Xing Zi, Liu Xing Zi, Wang Bu Liu*

Flavors & nature: Bitter; neutral

Functions: Disinhibits lactation, disperses swelling and abscesses

Indications:

1. Agalactia, hypogalactia due either to A) liver qi stagnation or B) qi vacuity and stagnation

2. Mastitis due to stagnation of qi which has transformed into heat at the A) inflammatory stage or B) pus production stage

Typical combinations:

1. A) With Medulla Tetrapanacis Papyriferi (*Tong Cao*), stir-fried Fasciculus Vascularis Luffae (*Chao Si Gua Luo*), vinegar[-processed] Pericarpium Viridis Citri Reticulatae (*Cu Qing Pi*), and Semen Malvae Seu Abutilonis (*Dong Kui Zi*) B) With stir-fried Radix Astragali Membranacei (*Chao Huang Qi*), vinegar[-processed] Squama Manitis Pentadactylis (*Cu Chuan Shan Jia*), and Fructus Liquidambaris Taiwaniae (*Lu Lu Tong*) as in *Tong Ru Tang* (Open the Breasts Decoction [332])

2. A) With uncooked Flos Lonicerae Japonicae (*Sheng Jin Yin Hua*), uncooked Fructus Forsythiae Suspensae (*Sheng Lian Qiao*), and Herba Cum Radice Taraxaci Mongolici (*Pu Gong Ying*)

Semen Vaccariae Segetalis continued . . .

B) With Spina Gleditschiae Chinensis (*Zao Jiao Ci*), Herba Cum Radice Taraxaci Mongolici (*Pu Gong Ying*), Radix Angelicae Dahuricae (*Bai Zhi*), and Radix Semiaquilegiae (*Tian Kui Zi*)

Dosage: 5-10g and up to 30g in severe cases

_____ **Stir-fried [till] Yellow (Chao Huang)** _____

Names: *Chao Wang Bu Liu Xing, Chao Liu Xing Zi*

Flavors & nature: Bitter; neutral tending to warm

Functions: Moves the blood, frees the channels, disinhibits strangury

Indications:

1. Amenorrhea, oligomenorrhea due to blood stasis with lower abdominal pain aggravated by pressure, scanty menstruation with dark, purple blood clots...

2. Retention of the fetus due to qi stagnation and blood stasis with foul breath, abdominal pain...

3. Strangury with hematuria (*xue lin*) due to damp heat in the bladder with urgent need to urinate, frequent, painful urination, blood and blood clots in the urine...

Typical combinations:

1. With wine[-processed] Radix Angelicae Sinensis (*Jiu Dang Gui*), wine[-processed] Radix Ligustici Wallichii (*Chuan Xiong*), uncooked Semen Pruni Persicae (*Sheng Tao Ren*), and Flos Carthami Tinctorii (*Hong Hua*)

2. With wine[-processed] Radix Cyathulae (*Jiu Chuan Niu Xi*), vinegar[-processed] Rhizoma Sparganii (*Cu San Leng*), wine[-processed] Herba Leonuri Heterophylli (*Jiu Yi Mu Cao*), uncooked Pollen Typhae (*Sheng Pu Huang*), and wine[-processed] Feces Trogopterori Seu Pteromi (*Jiu Wu Ling Zhi*)

3. With Folium Pyrrosiae (*Shi Wei*), uncooked Rhizoma Imperatae Cylindricae (*Sheng Bai Mao Gen*), carbonized Herba Cirsii Japonici (*Da Ji Tan*), and carbonized Herba Cephalanoploris Segeti (*Xiao Ji Tan*)

Dosage: 5-10g and up to 30g in severe cases

Feces Trogopterori Seu Pteromi *(Wu Ling Zhi)*

_____ **Stir-fried [till] Scorched (Chao Jiao)** _____

Names: *Chao Wu Ling Zhi, Chao Wu Ling*

Flavors & nature: Salty, slightly sweet, and astringent; warm

Functions: Harmonizes the blood, stops bleeding

Indications:

1. Metrorrhagia due to blood stasis with lower abdominal pain, loss of dark, purplish colored blood...

2. Bloody dysentery due to damp heat in the large intestine accompanied by qi stagnation and blood stasis with abdominal pain, pain in the anus, tenesmus...

Feces Trogopterori Seu Pteromi continued . . .

Typical combinations:

1. With carbonized Pollen Typhae (*Pu Huang Tan*), Crinis Carbonisatus (*Xue Yu Tan*), wine[-processed] Herba Leonuri Heterophylli (*Jiu Yi Mu Cao*), and carbonized Radix Angelicae Sinensis (*Dang Gui Tan*)

2. With uncooked Rhizoma Coptidis Chinensis (*Sheng Huang Lian*), Radix Pulsatillae Chinensis (*Bai Tou Weng*), uncooked Herba Agrimoniae Pilosae (*Sheng Xian He Cao*), uncooked Cacumen Biotae Orientalis (*Sheng Ce Bai Ye*), and roasted Radix Saussureae Seu Vladimiriae (*Wei Mu Xiang*)

Dosage: 6-10g and up to 60g in severe cases

Wine Mix-fried *(Jiu Zhi)*

Names: *Jiu Zhi Wu Ling Zhi, Jiu Wu Ling Zhi, Jiu Wu Ling*

Flavors & nature: Salty, slightly sweet, and slightly acrid; warm

Functions: Moves the blood, dispels stasis

Indications:

1. Amenorrhea, dysmenorrhea due to blood stasis with severe lower abdominal pain, scanty, dark colored menstruation with clots...

2. Retention of the lochia due to blood stasis with severe lower abdominal pain...

Typical combinations:

1. With uncooked Pollen Typhae (*Sheng Pu Huang*) as in *Shi Xiao San* (Sudden Smile Powder [301])

2. With wine[-processed] Herba Leonuri Heterophylli (*Jiu Yi Mu Cao*), wine[-processed] Radix Ligustici Wallichii (*Jiu Chuan Xiong*), and wine[-processed] Radix Angelicae Sinensis (*Jiu Dang Gui*)

Dosage: 6-10g and up to 60g in severe cases

Vinegar Mix-fried *(Cu Zhi)*

Names: *Cu Zhi Wu Ling Zhi, Cu Wu Ling Zhi, Cu Wu Ling*

Flavors & nature: Salty, slightly sweet, and slightly sour; warm

Functions: Moves the blood, stops pain

Indications:

1. Epigastric pain due to qi stagnation and blood stasis in the stomach with severe pain, vomiting fluids and acid...

2. Lateral costal pain due to liver qi stagnation and blood stasis with piercing pain, chest oppression...

3. Chest pain due to heart blood stasis with precordial pain, lateral costal pain...

Typical combinations:

1. With dry Rhizoma Zingiberis (*Gan Jiang*), vinegar[-processed] Rhizoma Corydalis Yanhusuo (*Cu Yan Hu Suo*), uncooked Radix Saussureae Seu Vladimiriae (*Sheng Mu Xiang*), and stir-fried Rhizoma Coptidis Chinensis (*Chao Huang Lian*)

Feces Trogopterori Seu Pteromi continued . . .

2. With vinegar[-processed] Radix Bupleuri (*Cu Chai Hu*), vinegar[-processed] Rhizoma Cyperi Rotundi (*Cu Xiang Fu*), and vinegar[-processed] Tuber Curcumae (*Cu Yu Jin*)

3. With stir-fried Resina Olibani (*Chao Ru Xiang*), vinegar[-processed] Rhizoma Corydalis Yanhusuo (*Cu Yan Hu Suo*), wine[-processed] Radix Salviae Miltiorrhizae (*Jiu Dan Shen*), uncooked Pollen Typhae (*Sheng Pu Huang*), and Radix Pseudoginseng (*San Qi*)

Dosage: 6-10g and up to 60g in severe cases

Rhizoma Corydalis Yanhusuo *(Yan Hu Suo)*
Wine Mix-fried *(Jiu Zhi)*[1]

Names: *Jiu Zhi Yan Hu Suo, Jiu Yan Hu Suo, Jiu Xuan Hu Suo, Jiu Yuan Hu Suo*

Flavors & nature: Acrid and bitter; warm

Functions: Moves the blood, dispels stasis, stops pain

Indications:

1. Heart pain due to heart blood stasis and heart yang vacuity with chest pain and oppression, palpitations...

2. Amenorrhea, dysmenorrhea due to blood stasis with severe lower abdominal pain aggravated by pressure...

3. Pain in the four limbs due to blood stasis in the limbs with incessant pain...

4. Traumatic injury with hematoma, pain, swelling...

5. Abdominal masses due to qi stagnation and blood stasis with palpable, fixed, painful masses...

Typical combinations:

1. With stir-fried Fructus Trichosanthis Kirlowii (*Chao Gua Lou*), Bulbus Allii Macrostemi (*Xie Bai*), wine[-processed] Radix Salviae Miltiorrhizae (*Jiu Dan Shen*), and Radix Pseudoginseng (*San Qi*)

2. With wine[-processed] Radix Angelicae Sinensis (*Jiu Dang Gui*) and vinegar[-processed] Rhizoma Sparganii (*Cu San Leng*)

3. With stir-fried Ramulus Cinnamomi (*Chao Gui Zhi*), wine[-processed] Radix Angelicae Sinensis (*Jiu Dang Gui*), and wine[-processed] Radix Albus Paeoniae Lactiflorae (*Jiu Bai Shao Yao*)

4. With vinegar[-processed] Resina Olibani (*Cu Ru Xiang*) and vinegar[-processed] Resina Myrrhae (*Cu Mo Yao*)

5. With vinegar[-processed] Rhizoma Sparganii (*Cu San Leng*), and uncooked Pericarpium Viridis Citri Reticulatae (*Sheng Qing Pi*)

Dosage: 5-10g, and in case of severe pain, up to 20-50g in decoction, 10g in powder

Note: 1. Wine mix-fried Corydalis is commonly replaced with uncooked Corydalis (*Sheng Yan Hu Suo*). However, it is less powerful.

Vinegar Mix-fried (Cu Zhi)

Names: *Cu Zhi Yan Hu Suo, Cu Yan Hu Suo, Cu Xuan Hu Suo, Cu Yuan Hu Suo*

Flavors & nature: Bitter, slightly acrid, and slightly sour; warm

Functions: Moves the qi, stops pain

Indications:

1. Lateral costal pain due to liver qi stagnation

2. Epigastric pain due to stomach qi stagnation and vacuity cold in the middle burner

3. Inguinal hernia, maladies of the scrotum or testicles due to qi stagnation and cold in the liver channel

Typical combinations:

1. With stir-fried Fructus Meliae Toosendan (*Chao Chuan Lian Zi*) as in *Jin Ling Zi San* (Melia Powder [181])

2. With vinegar[-processed] Rhizoma Cyperi Rotundi (*Cu Xiang Fu*), Rhizoma Alpiniae Officinari (*Gao Liang Jiang*), and uncooked Radix Saussureae Seu Vladimiriae (*Sheng Mu Xiang*)

3. With salt[-processed] Fructus Foeniculi Vulgaris (*Yan Xiao Hui Xiang*), salt[[-processed] Semen Citri Reticulatae (*Yan Ju He*), salt[-processed] Semen Litchi Chinensis (*Yan Li Zhi He*), and salt[-processed] Radix Linderae Strychnifoliae (*Yan Wu Yao*)

Dosage: 5-10g, and in case of severe pain, up to 20-50g in decoction, 10g in powder

Herba Leonuri Heterophylli (Yi Mu Cao)

Uncooked (Sheng)

Names: *Sheng Yi Mu Cao, Yi Mu Cao*

Flavors & nature: Acrid and bitter; slightly cold

Functions: Disinhibits urination, disperses swelling, resolves toxins

Indications:

1. Edema[1] due to A) kidney vacuity, B) spleen vacuity, or C) accumulation of dampness

2. Skin inflammation, abscess, erysipelas[1] due to heat toxins

Typical combinations:

1. A) With stir-fried Ramulus Cinnamomi (*Chao Gui Zhi*), processed Radix Lateralis Praeparatus Aconiti Carmichaeli (*Zhi Fu Zi*), Sclerotium Polypori Umbellati (*Zhu Ling*), and salt[-processed] Semen Plantaginis (*Yan Che Qian Zi*)
B) With uncooked Sclerotium Poriae Cocos (*Sheng Fu Ling*), uncooked Rhizoma Atractylodis Macrocephalae (*Sheng Bai Zhu*), uncooked Radix Astragali Membranacei (*Sheng Huang Qi*), and uncooked Cortex Rhizomatis Zingiberis (*Sheng Jiang Pi*)
C) With Pericarpium Arecae Catechu (*Da Fu Pi*), uncooked Rhizoma Alismatis (*Sheng Ze Xie*), Cortex Sclerotii Poriae Cocos (*Fu Ling Pi*), uncooked Cortex Rhizomatis Zingiberis (*Sheng Jiang Pi*), and Radix Stephaniae Tetrandrae (*Fang Ji*)

Herba Leonuri Heterophylli continued . . .

2. With Herba Violae Yedoensis (*Zi Hua Di Ding*), Herba Cum Radice Taraxaci Mongolici (*Pu Gong Ying*), uncooked Flos Lonicerae Japonicae (*Sheng Jin Yin Hua*), and uncooked Fructus Forsythiae Suspensae (*Sheng Lian Qiao*)

Dosage: 30-60g and up to 120g in severe cases

Note: 1. For these two indications, Leonurus is not very powerful and not often prescribed. It is only used as an auxiliary remedy.

_____ **Wine Mix-fried (*Jiu Zhi*)** _____

Names: *Jiu Zhi Yi Mu Cao, Jiu Yi Mu Cao*

Flavors & nature: Acrid and bitter; cool tending to neutral

Functions: Quickens the blood, dispels stasis, regulates the menses, stops pain

Indications:

1. Menstrual irregularity, dysmenorrhea due to blood stasis

2. Retention of the lochia due to blood stasis

3. Retention of the placenta

4. Metrorrhagia due to blood vacuity and stasis

5. Traumatic injury with pain, hematoma, swelling...

Typical combinations:

1. With wine[-processed] Radix Ligustici Wallichii (*Jiu Chuan Xiong*) and wine[-processed] Radix Angelicae Sinensis (*Jiu Dang Gui*) as in *Yi Mu Wan* (Leonurus Pills [402])

2. With wine[-processed] Feces Trogopterori Seu Pteromi (*Jiu Wu Ling Zhi*), uncooked Pollen Typhae (*Sheng Pu Huang*), and wine[-processed] Radix Cyathulae (*Jiu Chuan Niu Xi*)

3. With Secretio Moschi Moschiferi (*She Xiang*), wine[-processed] Radix Cyathulae (*Jiu Chuan Niu Xi*), and vinegar[-processed] Rhizoma Sparganii (*Cu San Leng*)

4. With wine[-processed] Radix Angelicae Sinensis (*Jiu Dang Gui*), wine[-processed] Radix Ligustici Wallichii (*Jiu Chuan Xiong*), and wine[-processed] Radix Albus Paeoniae Lactiflorae (*Jiu Bai Shao Yao*) as in *Yi Mu Si Wu Tang* (Leonurus Four Materials Decoction [401])

5. With vinegar[-processed] Resina Olibani (*Cu Ru Xiang*) and vinegar[-processed] Resina Myrrhae (*Cu Mo Yao*)

Dosage: 15-30g and up to 100g in severe cases

11
Stop Bleeding Medicinals

Folium Artemisiae Argyii *(Ai Ye)*[1]
Uncooked *(Sheng)*

Names: *Sheng Ai Ye, Ai Ye, Ai Rong, Ai Tiao*

Flavors & nature: Bitter and acrid; warm

Functions: Dispels wind, eliminates dampness, moves the qi and blood

Indications:

1. Pain, such as rheumatic, epigastric, abdominal, gynecological, etc., due to cold dampness

2. Eczema due to cold dampness with itching...

Typical combinations:

1. Used in the form of a moxa cone *(Ai Rong)* or a moxa roll *(Ai Tiao)* for warming an acupuncture point or a larger area, such as the stomach, abdomen, joints...

2. With Realgar *(Xiong Huang)* and uncooked Sulfur *(Sheng Liu Huang)*. These three substances are prepared in decoction. Then the decoction is applied locally.

Dosage: Used externally as much as is necessary

Note: 1. The uncooked form of Artemisia Argyium is irritating to the stomach. It is therefore reserved for external application.

Vinegar Mix-fried *(Cu Zhi)*

Names: *Cu Zhi Ai Ye, Cu Ai Ye, Cu Chen Ai Ye, Cu Dan Ai Ye*

Flavors & nature: Bitter, slightly acrid, and slightly sour; warm

Functions: Warms the channels, scatters cold, stops pain

Indications:

1. Epigastric pain due to vacuity cold

2. Abdominal pain due to accumulation of cold yin in the lower burner

3. Dysmenorrhea due to cold in the uterus

4. Threatened abortion due to vacuity cold in the lower burner, as that of the spleen and stomach

Typical combinations:

1. With roasted Rhizoma Alpiniae Officinari *(Wei Gao Liang Jiang)*, Fructus Amomi *(Sha Ren)*, and uncooked Fructus Foeniculi Vulgaris *(Sheng Xiao Hui Xiang)*

2. With dry Rhizoma Zingiberis *(Gan Jiang)*, processed Fructus Evodiae Rutecarpae *(Zhi Wu Zhu Yu)*, and stir-fried Ramulus Cinnamomi *(Chao Gui Zhi)*

Folium Artemisiae Argyii continued . . .

3. With Cortex Cinnamomi (*Rou Gui*), wine[-processed] Radix Angelicae Sinensis (*Jiu Dang Gui*), vinegar[-processed] Rhizoma Cyperi Rotundi (*Cu Xiang Fu*), and blast-fried Rhizoma Zingiberis (*Pao Jiang*)

4. With bran stir-fried Rhizoma Atractylodis Macrocephalae (*Fu Chao Bai Zhu*), salt[-processed] Radix Dipsaci (*Yan Xu Duan*), salt[-processed] Cortex Eucommiae Ulmoidis (*Yan Du Zhong*), Fructus Amomi (*Sha Ren*), and Radix Panacis Ginseng (*Ren Shen*)

Dosage: 5-10g and up to 30g in severe cases

_____ **Stir-fried [till] Carbonized (Chao Tan)** _____

Names: *Ai Ye Tan, Ai Tan, Chen Ai Tan, Dan Ai Tan*

Flavors & nature: Bitter, slightly acrid, and slightly astringent; warm

Functions: Warms the channels, stops bleeding

Indications:

1. Hemoptysis, epistaxis, hematemesis, melena[1]

2. Menorrhagia, metrorrhagia during pregnancy or postpartum due to vacuity cold and blood vacuity

Typical combinations:

1. For hemoptysis: With carbonized Nodus Nelumbinis Nuciferae (*Ou Jie Tan*) and carbonized Folium Et Petiolus Trachycarpi (*Zong Lu Tan*)

For epistaxis: With uncooked Cacumen Biotae Orientalis (*Sheng Ce Bai Ye*)
For hematemesis: With Radix Pseudoginseng (*San Qi*) and Terra Flava Usta (*Fu Long Gan*)
For rectal bleeding: With carbonized Fructus Immaturus Sophorae Japonicae (*Huai Jiao Tan*) and uncooked Radix Sanguisorbae (*Sheng Di Yu*)

2. With carbonized Radix Angelicae Sinensis (*Dang Gui Tan*), Radix Albus Paeoniae Lactiflorae (*Bai Shao Yao*), and Pollen Typhae stir-fried Gelatinum Corii Asini (*Pu Huang Chao E Jiao*) as in *Jiao Ai Tang* (Donkey Skin Glue & Artemisia Argyium Decoction [173])

Dosage: 2-5g and up to 15g in severe cases

Note: 1. When hemorrhaging is accompanied by pain, one can prescribe carbonized vinegar mix-fried Artemisiae Argyii (*Cu Zhi Ai Ye Tan*).

Rhizoma Imperatae Cylindricae *(Bai Mao Gen)*

_____ **Uncooked (Sheng)** _____

Names: *Bai Mao Gen, Mao Gen*

Flavors & nature: Sweet; cold

Functions: Clears heat, cools the blood, disinhibits urination, disperses swelling

Indications:

1. Heat in the blood level[1] with fever aggravated at night, a dry mouth but without thirst, vexation, abundant bleeding (hematemesis, epistaxis)...

2. Cough, asthma[1] due to replete lung heat...

3. Fetid vomiting[1] due to replete stomach heat with malodorous eructations...

Rhizoma Imperatae Cylindricae continued . . .

4. Edema due to accumulation of damp heat

5. Jaundice due to accumulation of damp heat

6. Strangury (*re lin*) of the heat type due to damp heat in the bladder

Typical combinations:

1. With uncooked Cortex Radicis Moutan (*Sheng Mu Dan Pi*) and uncooked Radix Rehmanniae (*Sheng Di Huang*)

2. With honey mix-fried Cortex Radicis Mori Albi (*Mi Zhi Sang Bai Pi*) as in *Ru Shen Tang* (Like Magic Decoction [267])

3. With ginger[-processed] Caulis In Taeniis Bambusae (*Jiang Zhu Ru*), Rhizoma Phragmitis Communis (*Lu Gen*), and stir-fried Folium Eriobotryae Japonicae (*Chao Pi Pa Ye*)

4. With uncooked Rhizoma Alismatis (*Sheng Ze Xie*), salt[-processed] Semen Plantaginis (*Yan Che Qian Zi*), Talcum (*Hua Shi*), and uncooked Semen Benincasae Hispidae (*Sheng Dong Gua Ren*)

5. With Herba Artemisiae Capillaris (*Yin Chen Hao*), Herba Desmodii Seu Lysimachiae (*Jin Qian Cao*), and Radix Et Rhizoma Polygoni Cuspidati (*Hu Zhang*)

6. With Herba Dianthi (*Qu Mai*) and Talcum (*Hua Shi*) as in *Qu Mai Tang* (Dianthus Decoction [263])

Dosage: 30-60g and up to 100g in severe cases. In case of acute nephritis, Imperata is commonly prescribed alone at a dosage of 250-500g.

Note: 1. As long as the pattern or the heat is replete, it is preferable to prescribe the crude, fresh form of Imperata (*Xian Bai Mao Gen*). Dosage: 100g and up to 250g in severe cases.

_____ Stir-fried [till] Carbonized (Chao Tan)¹ _____

Name: *Mao Gen Tan*

Flavors & nature: Sweet and slightly astringent; cold tending to neutral

Functions: Clears heat, stops bleeding

Indications:

1. Hemoptysis due to heat damaging the network vessels of the lungs with hemoptysis of fresh red blood or expectoration of blood-streaked phlegm...

2. Epistaxis due to depressive heat (*yu re*) in the liver and lungs which has transformed into fire, this fire damaging the network vessels of the nose...

3. Hematemesis due to depressive heat (*yu re*) in the liver and stomach which has damaged the

network vessels of the stomach with vomiting of abundant blood which is purple and dark in color and contains clots...

4. Hematuria due to accumulation of dampness and fire damaging the network vessels of the urethra...

Typical combinations:

1. With Herba Agrimoniae Pilosae (*Xian He Cao*), uncooked Cacumen Biotae Orientalis (*Sheng Ce Bai Ye*), uncooked Concha Cyclinae (*Sheng Hai Ge Ke*), and honey mix-fried Fructus Aristolochiae (*Mi Zhi Ma Dou Ling*)

2. With Herba Ecliptae Prostratae (*Han Lian Cao*), carbonized Radix Rubiae Cordifoliae (*Qian Cao Gen Tan*), and uncooked Cacumen Biotae Orientalis (*Sheng Ce Bai Ye*)

Rhizoma Imperatae Cylindricae continued . . .

3. With Rhizoma Bletillae Striatae (*Bai Ji*), uncooked Radix Et Rhizoma Rhei (*Sheng Da Huang*), Crinis Carbonisatus (*Xue Yu Tan*), and calcined Haematitum (*Cui Dai Zhe Shi*)

4. With carbonized Herba Cephalanoploris Segeti (*Xiao Ji Tan*), carbonized Nodus Nelumbinis Nuciferae (*Ou Jie Tan*), uncooked Radix Rehmanniae (*Sheng Di Huang*), and carbonized Herba Cirsii Japonici (*Da Ji Tan*)

Dosage: 30-60g and up to 100g in severe cases

Note: 1. Although Imperata has been traditionally carbonized in order to stop bleeding, modern research has shown that its hemostatic effects are superior when used in its uncooked (*sheng*) form.

Cacumen Biotae Orientalis (*Ce Bai Ye*)

———————————— Uncooked (*Sheng*)————————————

Names: *Sheng Ce Bai Ye, Ce Bai Ye*

Flavors & nature: Bitter and astringent; slightly cold

Functions: Clears heat, cools the blood, eliminates phlegm, stops cough, stimulates hair [growth]

Indications:

1. Heat in the blood level with dry throat and mouth but without thirst, vexation, hematemesis, epistaxis, a scarlet red tongue, a rapid (*shu*) pulse...

2. Cough, asthma due to accumulation of phlegm heat in the lungs

3. Abnormal vaginal discharge due to damp heat in the lower burner with heavy limbs, yellowish, foul-smelling, possibly bloody discharge...

4. Premature whitening of the hair due to liver/-kidney essence vacuity

5. Alopecia areata

Typical combinations:

1. With uncooked Radix Rehmanniae (*Sheng Di Huang*), uncooked Folium Nelumbinis Nuciferae (*Sheng He Ye*), and uncooked Folium Artemisiae Argyii (*Sheng Ai Ye*) as in *Si Sheng Wan* (Four Uncooked [Ingredients] Pills [314])

2. With uncooked Semen Pruni Armeniacae (*Sheng Xing Ren*), uncooked Radix Peucedani (*Sheng Qian Hu*), and uncooked Folium Eriobotryae Japonicae (*Sheng Pi Pa Ye*)

3. With stir-fried Cortex Ailanthi Altissimi (*Chao Chun Gen Pi*) and uncooked Cortex Phellodendri (*Sheng Huang Bai*) as in *Ce Bai Chu Gen Wan* (Cacumen Biotae & Ailanthus Pills [41])

4. With processed Radix Polygoni Multiflori (*Zhi He Shou Wu*) and wine-steamed Fructus Ligustri Lucidi (*Jiu Zheng Nu Zhen Zi*) as in *Wu Fa Wan* (Blacken the Hair Pills [344])

5. Soak 60g of fresh Cacumen Biotae Orientalis (*Xian Ce Bai Ye*) in 100g of rice wine for two weeks. Apply locally with cotton. Massage until there is a sensation of heat. 3 times per day

Dosage: 10-15g and up to 30g in severe cases

Cacumen Biotae Orientalis continued . . .

_____ Stir-fried [till] Carbonized (Chao Tan)_____

Names: *Ce Bai Ye Tan, Ce Bai Tan*

Flavors & nature: Bitter and astringent; tending to neutral

Functions: Astringes the blood, stops bleeding

Indications:

1. Hematemesis[1] due to either A) heat in the blood or B) cold in the blood

2. Hemoptysis[1] due to heat damaging the network vessels of the lungs

3. Epistaxis due to lung heat damaging the network vessels of the nose

4. Bloody stools, bleeding hemorrhoids[1] due to damp heat damaging the network vessels of the intestines

5. Hematuria[1] due to damp heat damaging the network vessels of the bladder

6. Metrorrhagia[1] due to heat disturbing the *chong* and *ren*

Typical combinations:

1. A) With uncooked Radix Rehmanniae (*Sheng Di Huang*) as in *Si Sheng Wan* (Four Uncooked [Ingredients] Pills [314])

B) With blast-fried Rhizoma Zingiberis (*Pao Jiang*), carbonized Folium Artemisiae Argyii (*Ai Ye Tan*) as in *Bai Ye Tang* (Cacumen Biotae Decoction [20])

2. With carbonized Nodus Nelumbinis Nuciferae (*Ou Jie Tan*) and uncooked Rhizoma Imperatae Cylindricae (*Sheng Bai Mao Gen*)

3. With carbonized Pollen Typhae (*Pu Huang Tan*) and Flos Imperatae Cylindricae (*Bai Mao Hua*)

4. With carbonized Flos Immaturus Sophorae Japonicae (*Huai Hua Tan*) as in *Ce Bai San* (Cacumen Biotae Powder [42])

5. With carbonized Herba Cephalanoploris Segeti (*Xiao Ji Tan*), Talcum (*Hua Shi*), and uncooked Rhizoma Imperatae Cylindricae (*Sheng Bai Mao Gen*)

6. With carbonized Radix Albus Paeoniae Lactiflorae (*Bai Shao Yao Tan*) as in *Zong Lu Bai Shao Tang* (General Collection Peony Decoction [450])

Dosage: 5-12g and up to 30g in severe cases

Note: 1. Although traditionally Cacumen Biotae Orientalis is carbonized (*Chao Tan*) for stopping bleeding, modern research has shown clearly that its hemostatic effects are superior when used uncooked (*Sheng Ce Bai Ye*).

Herba Cirsii Japonici *(Da Ji)*

_____Uncooked *(Sheng)*_____

Names: *Sheng Da Ji, Da Ji Cao, Da Ji*

Flavors & nature: Sweet and bitter; cool

Functions: Dispels blood stasis, disperses swelling

Indications:

1. Appendicitis[1] due to blood stasis with abdominal pain and swelling...

Herba Circii Japonici continued . . .

2. Skin inflammation,[1] such as folliculitis, furuncles, and *yong*, due to heat toxins and blood stasis with pain, redness, swelling, itching...

Typical combinations:

1. With uncooked Radix Sanguisorbae (*Sheng Di Yu*), wine[-processed] Radix Cyathulae (*Jiu Chuan Niu Xi*), uncooked Flos Lonicerae Japonicae (*Sheng Jin Yin Hua*), and uncooked Radix Rubiae Cordifoliae (*Sheng Qian Cao Gen*)

2. With Herba Violae Yedoensis (*Zi Hua Di Ding*), Alumen (*Ming Fan*), stir-fried Resina Olibani (*Chao Ru Xiang*), and Flos Chrysanthemi Indici (*Ye Ju Hua*)

Dosage: 10-15g and up to 50g in severe cases

Note: 1. The fresh, crude form of Herba Cirsii (*Xian Da Ji*) is more powerful for these indications. Dosage: 30-60g

Addendum: There exist both Herba Cirsii (*Da Ji* or *Da Ji Cao*) and Radix Cirsii (*Da Ji Gen*). These two remedies both cool the blood, dispel blood stasis, stop bleeding, and disperse swelling. However, Radix Cirsii is superior for dispelling stasis and dispersing swelling and, therefore, it should be prescribed in the form of uncooked Radix Cirsii (*Sheng Da Ji Gen*) for the treatment of appendicitis and skin inflammations. Herba Cirsii is better for cooling the blood and stopping bleeding. Therefore, it should be prescribed in the form of carbonized Herba Cirsii (*Da Ji Cao Tan*) for treating hemorrhages.

Stir-fried [till] Carbonized (*Chao Tan*)

Name: *Da Ji Tan*

Flavors & nature: Sweet and bitter; neutral

Functions: Cools the blood, stops bleeding

Indications:

1. Hematemesis, hemoptysis, epistaxis due to heat in the blood

2. Metrorrhagia, hematuria due to heat in the lower burner

3. Traumatic hemorrhages

Typical combinations:

1. With uncooked Cacumen Biotae Orientalis (*Sheng Ce Bai Ye*), uncooked Rhizoma Imperatae Cylindricae (*Sheng Bai Mao Gen*), and carbonized Cortex Radicis Moutan (*Mu Dan Pi Tan*) as in *Shi Hui San* (Ten Ashes Powder [299])

2. With carbonized Pollen Typhae (*Pu Huang Tan*), carbonized Folium Et Petiolus Trachycarpi (*Zong Lu Tan*, carbonized Herba Cephalanoploris Segeti (*Xiao Ji Tan*), and uncooked Cacumen Biotae Orientalis (*Sheng Ce Bai Ye*)

3. Applied locally as a powder

Dosage: 10-15g and up to 50g in severe cases

Radix Sanguisorbae (Di Yu)[1]

Uncooked (Sheng)

Names: *Sheng Di Yu, Di Yu*

Flavors & nature: Bitter and sour; slightly cold

Functions: Clears heat, resolves toxins, cools the blood

Indications:

1. Dysentery due to A) accumulation of damp heat in the large intestine with bloody stools, abdominal pain or B) incessant dysentery which will not heal

2. Abnormal vaginal discharge due to accumulation of damp heat

3. Furuncles on the face due to toxic heat

4. Localized burns[2]

Typical combinations:

1. A) With uncooked Rhizoma Coptidis Chinensis (*Sheng Huang Lian*), uncooked Radix Rubrus Paeoniae Lactiflorae (*Sheng Chi Shao Yao*), and uncooked Flos Lonicerae Japonicae (*Sheng Jin Yin Hua*)

B) With stir-fried Fructus Terminaliae Chebulae (*Chao He Zi*), carbonized Fructus Pruni Mume (*Wu Mei Tan*), and uncooked Rhizoma Coptidis Chinensis (*Sheng Huang Lian*), and stir-fried Radix Albus Paeoniae Lactiflorae (*Chao Bai Shao Yao*)

2. With stir-fried Cortex Ailanthi Altissimi (*Chao Chun Gen Pi*), uncooked Cortex Phellodendri (*Sheng Huang Bai*), and Rhizoma Smilacis Glabrae (*Tu Fu Ling*)

3. With uncooked Flos Lonicerae Japonicae (*Sheng Jin Yin Hua*), stir-fried Resina Olibani (*Chao Ru Xiang*), and stir-fried Resina Myrrhae (*Chao Mo Yao*)

4. With Borneol (*Bing Pian*) and uncooked Radix Et Rhizoma Rhei (*Sheng Da Huang*). Reduce these three medicinals to a powder and then mix with sesame oil. Apply locally.

Dosage: 10-20g

Notes: 1. Sanguisorba is contraindicated orally or locally for those suffering from hepatitis. 2. Sanguisorba should be used on small areas. In case of overdosage or application on large areas, there is a risk of toxic hepatitis.

Stir-fried [till] Carbonized (Chao Tan)

Name: *Di Yu Tan*

Flavors & nature: Bitter, slightly sour, and astringent; cool tending to neutral

Functions: Cools the blood, stops bleeding

Indications:

1. Bloody stools, bleeding hemorrhoids[1] due to heat in the blood or damp heat in the lower burner with bright red blood...

2. Hematuria, strangury with hematuria[1] due to accumulation of damp heat in the bladder

3. Metrorrhagia[1] due to heat disturbing the *chong* and *ren* with bleeding of bright red blood...

4. Chronic purulent eczema[1]

Typical combinations:

1. With carbonized Flos Immaturus Sophorae Japonicae (*Huai Hua Tan*), uncooked Cacumen

Radix Sanguisorbae continued . . .

Biotae Orientalis (*Sheng Ce Bai Ye*), carbonized Radix Scutellariae Baicalensis (*Huang Qin Tan*), and carbonized Herba Cirsii Japonici (*Da Ji Tan*)

2. With carbonized Herba Cephalanoploris Segeti (*Xiao Ji Tan*), uncooked Rhizoma Imperatae Cylindricae (*Sheng Bai Mao Gen*), uncooked Cortex Radicis Moutan (*Sheng Mu Dan Pi*), and Folium Pyrrosiae (*Shi Wei*)

3. With carbonized Radix Rubiae Cordifoliae (*Qian Cao Gen Tan*), carbonized Folium Et Petiolus Trachycarpi (*Zong Lu Tan*), carbonized uncooked Radix Rehmanniae (*Sheng Di Huang Tan*), and carbonized Radix Angelicae Sinensis (*Dang Gui Tan*)

4. With calcined Gypsum Fibrosum (*Duan Shi Gao*), calcined Alumen (*Ming Fan*), and uncooked Cortex Phellodendri (*Sheng Huang Bai*). Reduce these four medicinals to powder and apply locally.

Dosage: 5-10g

Note: 1. Although traditionally Sanguisorba should be carbonized (*Chao Tan*) for stopping bleeding, modern research has clearly shown that its hemostatic effects are superior when used in its uncooked form (*Sheng Di Yu*).

Flos Immaturus Sophorae Japonicae *(Huai Hua)*

————————— Uncooked *(Sheng)*—————————

Names: *Huai Hua, Huai Mi, Sheng Huai Hua*

Flavors & nature: Bitter; slightly cold

Functions: Clears heat, cools the blood, soothes the liver, brightens the eyes

Indications:

1. Heat in the blood level with epistaxis, bloody stools, fever aggravated at night, vexation, a scarlet red tongue, a fine (*xi*), rapid (*shu*) pulse...

2. Vertigo, headache, red eyes[1] due to liver yang rising

3. Skin inflammation due to heat toxins with heat, redness, pain, swelling...

Typical combinations:

1. With uncooked Cortex Radicis Moutan (*Sheng Mu Dan Pi*), uncooked Radix Rehmanniae (*Sheng Di Huang*), uncooked Radix Sanguisorbae (*Sheng Di Yu*), and uncooked Radix Rubrus Paeoniae Lactiflorae (*Sheng Chi Shao Yao*)

2. With Spica Prunellae Vulgaris (*Xia Ku Cao*), stir-fried Flos Chrysanthemi Morifolii (*Chao Ju Hua*), and uncooked Semen Cassiae Torae (*Sheng Jue Ming Zi*)

3. With uncooked Radix Salviae Miltiorrhizae (*Sheng Dan Shen*), Flos Lonicerae Japonicae (*Jin Yin Hua*), Herba Violae Yedoensis (*Zi Hua Di Ding*), and Herba Cum Radice Taraxaci Mongolici (*Pu Gong Ying*)

Dosage: 10-15g and up to 30g in severe cases

Notes: 1. Flos Sophorae is used to treat arterial hypertension (notably due to liver yang rising).

Flos Immaturus Sophorae Japonicae continued . . .

_____Stir-fried [till] Carbonized *(Chao Tan)*_____

Names: *Huai Hua Tan, Huai Mi Tan*

Flavors & nature: Bitter and slightly astringent; neutral

Functions: Cools the blood, stops bleeding

Indications:

1. Bloody stools, bleeding hemorrhoids due to accumulation of heat in the large intestine

2. Hematuria due to accumulation of heat in the bladder

3. Metrorrhagia due to heat in the blood

4. Hemoptysis, epistaxis[1] due to depressive heat (*yu re*) in the liver and lungs

Typical combinations:

1. With uncooked Cacumen Biotae Orientalis (*Sheng Ce Bai Ye*) and carbonized Schizonepetae Tenuifoliae (*Jing Jie Tan*) as in *Huai Hua San* (Flos Sophorae Powder [149])

2. With carbonized Herba Cephalanoploris Segeti (*Xiao Ji Tan*), carbonized Pollen Typhae (*Pu Huang Tan*), uncooked Rhizoma Imperatae Cylindricae (*Sheng Bai Mao Gen*), and carbonized uncooked Radix Rehmanniae (*Sheng Di Huang Tan*)

3. With uncooked Radix Sanguisorbae (*Sheng Di Yu*), uncooked Radix Rehmanniae (*Sheng Di Yu*), uncooked Cacumen Biotae Orientalis (*Sheng Ce Bai Ye*), and carbonized Cortex Radicis Moutan (*Mu Dan Pi Tan*)

4. With uncooked Rhizoma Imperatae Cylindricae (*Sheng Bai Mao Gen*), uncooked Cacumen Biotae Orientalis (*Sheng Ce Bai Ye*), and Herba Agrimoniae Pilosae (*Xian He Cao*)

Dosage: 5-12g

Note: 1. Flos Sophorae is less effective for bleeding in the upper body. It is advantageously prescribed for bleeding in the lower body.

Fructus Sophorae Japonicae *(Huai Jiao)*

_____Uncooked *(Sheng)*_____

Names: *Huai Jiao, Huai Shi*

Flavors & nature: Bitter; cold

Functions: Drains heat, cools the blood, soothes the liver, moistens dryness of the large intestine

Indications:

1. Heat in the blood level with bloody stools, epistaxis, bleeding gums, fever aggravated at night, vexations...

2. Vertigo, headache[1] due to liver yang rising

3. Red eyes[1] due to liver fire rising

4. Genital itching due to damp heat

5. Constipation[2] due to large intestine dryness

Typical combinations:

1. With uncooked Radix Rehmanniae (*Sheng Di Huang*), uncooked Cortex Radicis Moutan (*Mu Dan Pi*), and uncooked Radix Rubrus Paeoniae Lactiflorae (*Sheng Chi Shao Yao*)

Fructus Sophorae Japonicae continued . . .

2. With stir-fried Flos Chrysanthemi Morifolii (*Chao Ju Hua*), uncooked Radix Albus Paeoniae Lactiflorae (*Sheng Bai Shao Yao*), and stir-fried Rhizoma Gastrodiae Elatae (*Chao Tian Ma*)

3. With wine[-processed] Radix Gentianae Scabrae (*Jiu Long Dan Cao*), Spica Prunellae Vulgaris (*Xia Ku Cao*), and uncooked Semen Cassiae Torae (*Sheng Jue Ming Zi*)

4. With Radix Sophorae Flavescentis (*Ku Shen*), Fructus Cnidii Monnieri (*She Chuang Zi*), Fructus Kochiae Scopariae (*Di Fu Zi*), and uncooked Cortex Phellodendri (*Sheng Huang Bai*)

5. With stir-fried Semen Cannabis Sativae (*Chao Huo Ma Ren*), stir-fried Semen Pruni Persicae (*Chao Tao Ten*), and uncooked Semen Biotae Orientalis (*Sheng Bai Zi Ren*)

Dosage: 10-15g and up to 20g in severe cases

Notes: 1. For these indications, vinegar mix-fried Fructus Sophorae (*Cu Zhi Huai Jiao*) can be prescribed in order to guide the therapeutic action to the liver and thus clear liver fire better. 2. For this indication, honey mix-fried Fructus Sophorae (*Mi Zhi Huai Jiao*) can be prescribed in order to lessen its bitter flavor and cold nature and to reinforce its moistening character.

Stir-fried [till] Carbonized (*Chao Tan*)

Flavors & nature: Bitter and slightly astringent; cold tending to neutral

Functions: Cools the blood, stops bleeding

Indications:

1. Bloody stools, bleeding hemorrhoids due to damp heat damaging the network vessels of the large intestine

2. Dysentery due to accumulation of damp heat in the large intestine with bloody stools, abdominal pain, tenesmus...

Typical combinations:

1. With uncooked Radix Sanguisorbae (*Sheng Di Yu*), uncooked Cacumen Biotae Orientalis (*Sheng Ce Bai Ye*), carbonized Herba Cirsii Japonici (*Da Ji Tan*), and carbonized Cortex Radicis Moutan (*Mu Dan Pi Tan*)

2. With carbonized Herba Cirsii Japonici (*Da Ji Tan*), carbonized Herba Cephalanoploris Segeti (*Xiao Ji Tan*), carbonized Pollen Typhae (*Pu Huang Tan*), and Folium Pyrrosiae (*Shi Wei*)

Dosage: 5-12g and up to 20g in severe cases

Nodus Nelumbinis Nuciferae (*Ou Jie*)

Uncooked (*Sheng*)

Names: *Sheng Ou Jie, Ou Jie*

Flavors & nature: Sweet and astringent; neutral tending to cool

Functions: Cools the blood, stops bleeding, transforms blood stasis

Indications:

1. Acute, severe hematemesis[1] due to replete heat damaging the network vessels of the stomach with vomiting of purple blood...

2. Acute, severe hemoptysis[1] due to replete heat damaging the network vessels of the lungs with spitting up fresh blood...

Nodus Nelumbinis Nuciferae continued . . .

3. Acute, severe epistaxis[1] due to depressive fire in the liver and lungs damaging the network vessels of the nose...

4. Strangury with hematuria (*xue lin*)[1] due to damp heat damaging the network vessels of the bladder

Typical combinations:

1. With Folium Nelumbinis Nuciferae (*He Ye*) as in *Shuang He San* (Two Lotuses Powder [306])

2. With uncooked Cacumen Biotae Orientalis (*Sheng Ce Bai Ye*) and uncooked Rhizoma Imperatae Cylindricae (*Sheng Bai Mao Gen*) as in *Shu Xue Wan* (Course the Blood Pills [303])

3. With uncooked Rhizoma Imperatae Cylindricae (*Sheng Bai Mao Gen*), carbonized Cortex Radicis Moutan (*Mu Dan Pi Tan*), and Herba Agrimoniae Pilosae (*Xian He Cao*)

4. With Succinum (*Hu Po*), carbonized Herba Cephalanoploris Segeti (*Xiao Ji Tan*), carbonized Herba Cirsii Japonici (*Da Ji Tan*), and Folium Pyrrosiae (*Shi Wei*)

Dosage: 15-30g and up to 60-100g in severe cases

Note: 1. When this refers to hemorrhaging due to heat in the blood, it is preferable to use the fresh juice of Nodus Nelumbinis (*i.e.*, the juice of 100-250g of the fresh, crude plant). For other types of bleeding, carbonized Nodus Nelumbinis (*Ou Jie Tan*) can be used.

_____ Stir-fried [till] Carbonized *(Chao Tan)* _____

Name: *Ou Jie Tan*

Flavors & nature: Sweet and astringent; neutral tending to warm

Functions: Astringes the blood and stops bleeding

Indications:

1. Chronic, incessant hematemesis due to a lesion in the stomach network vessels

2. Chronic, incessant hemoptysis due to lung dryness

3. Bloody stools, bleeding hemorrhoids due to replete heat damaging the network vessels of the large intestine

Typical combinations:

1. With carbonized Folium Et Petiolus Trachycarpi (*Zong Lu Tan*), dip calcined Haematitum (*Cui Dai Zhe Shi*), Radix Pseudoginseng (*San Qi*), and Rhizoma Bletillae Striatae (*Bai Ji*)

2. Herba Agrimoniae Pilosae (*Xian He Cao*), uncooked Cacumen Biotae Orientalis (*Sheng Ce Bai Ye*), uncooked Gelatinum Corii Asini (*Sheng E Jiao*), and honey mix-fried Fructus Aristolochiae (*Mi Zhi Ma Dou Ling*)

3. With uncooked Radix Sanguisorbae (*Sheng Di Yu*) and carbonized Flos Immaturus Sophorae Japonicae (*Huai Hua Tan*)

Dosage: 15-30g and up to 60-100g in severe cases

Pollen Typhae (Pu Huang)

Uncooked (Sheng)[1]

Names: *Sheng Pu Huang, Pu Huang*

Flavors & nature: Sweet; neutral

Functions: Quickens the blood, dispels stasis, stops pain

Indications:

1. Amenorrhea, dysmenorrhea due to blood stasis with severe lower abdominal pain...

2. Retention of the lochia due to blood stasis with abdominal pain, scanty lochia...

3. Retention of the placenta due to blood stasis with abdominal pain...

4. Epigastric pain due to blood stasis in the stomach

5. Pain from traumatic injury with hematoma, swelling...

6. Dysuria due to accumulation of damp heat in the lower burner with hematuria...

Typical combinations:

1. With wine[-processed] Feces Trogopterori Seu Pteromi (*Jiu Wu Ling Zhi*) as in *Shi Xiao San* (Sudden Smile Powder [301])

2. With wine[-processed] Feces Trogopterori Seu Pteromi (*Jiu Wu Ling Zhi*), Radix Pseudoginseng (*San Qi*), and wine[-processed] Herba Leonuri Heterophylli (*Jiu Yi Mu Cao*)

3. With wine[-processed] Radix Cyathulae (*Jiu Chuan Niu Xi*) and wine[-processed] Herba Heterophylli (*Jiu Yi Mu Cao*)

4. With vinegar[-processed] Rhizoma Corydalis Yanhusuo (*Cu Yan Hu Suo*), vinegar[-processed] Feces Trogopterori Seu Pteromi (*Jiu Wu Ling Zhi*), and vinegar[-processed] Resina Olibani (*Cu Ru Xiang*)

5. With vinegar[-processed] Resina Myrrhae (*Cu Mo Yao*) and vinegar[-processed] Resina Olibani (*Cu Ru Xiang*)

6. With Talcum (*Hua Shi*), Semen Malvae Seu Abutilonis (*Dong Kui Zi*), and Folium Pyrrosiae (*Shi Wei*)

Dosage: 6-15g and up to 30g in severe cases

Note: 1. Traditionally the actions of uncooked Pollen Typhae (*Sheng Pu Huang*) and carbonized Pollen Typhae (*Pu Huang Tan*) are clearly distinguished. Thus, for example, the *Ri Hua Zi Ben Cao (Ri Hua-zi's Materia Medica)* states: "To break the blood and disperse swelling, it is necessary to use *Sheng Pu Huang*, while to supplement the blood and stop bleeding, it is necessary to use *Chao Pu Huang*." Nevertheless, clinical experience shows that uncooked Pollen Typhae gives equally good results for stopping hemorrhage.

Stir-fried [till] Carbonized (Chao Tan)

Name: *Pu Huang Tan*

Flavors & nature: Sweet and slightly astringent; neutral tending to warm

Functions: Harmonizes the blood, stops bleeding[1]

Indications:

1. Hematemesis due to a lesion in the network vessels of the stomach with vomiting blackish blood...

Pollen Typhae continued . . .

2. Hemoptysis due to heat damaging the network vessels of the lungs with spitting up of blood or phlegm streaked with blood...

3. Epistaxis due to heat in the liver and lungs

4. Bloody stools due to damp heat in the large intestine

5. Hematuria due to accumulation of damp heat in the bladder with dysuria...

6. Metrorrhagia due to *chong* and *ren* not securing

Typical combinations:

1. With carbonized Folium Et Petiolus Trachycarpi (*Zong Lu Tan*), carbonized Nodus Nelumbinis Nuciferae (*Ou Jie Tan*), and carbonized Radix Pseudoginseng (*San Qi*)

2. With Herba Ecliptae Prostratae (*Han Lian Cao*), carbonized Radix Rubiae Cordifoliae (*Qian Cao Gen Tan*), and uncooked Cacumen Biotae Orientalis (*Sheng Ce Bai Ye*)

3. With Herba Ecliptae Prostratae (*Han Lian Cao*), carbonized Radix Rubiae Cordifoliae (*Qian Cao Gen Tan*), and uncooked Cacumen Biotae Orientalis (*Sheng Ce Bai Ye*)

4. With carbonized Flos Immaturus Sophorae Japonicae (*Huai Hua Tan*) and uncooked Radix Sanguisorbae (*Sheng Di Yu*)

5. With Semen Malvae Seu Abutilonis (*Dong Kui Zi*) and uncooked Radix Rehmanniae (*Sheng Di Huang*) as in *Pu Huang San* (Pollen Typhae Powder [232])

6. With carbonized Folium Artemisiae Argyii (*Ai Ye Tan*) and calcined Os Draconis (*Duan Long Gu*) as in *Pu Huang Wan* (Pollen Typhae Pills [233])

Dosage: 5-10g and up to 20g in severe cases

Note: 1. Clinical experience shows that the uncooked form (*Sheng Pu Huang*) gives equally good results for stopping bleeding.

Radix Rubiae Cordifoliae *(Qian Cao Gen)*

Uncooked *(Sheng)*

Names: *Qian Cao, Qian Gen, Qian Cao Gen, Xue Qian Cao, Sheng Qian Cao*

Flavors & nature: Bitter; cold

Functions: Moves the blood, opens the channels, cools the blood

Indications:

1. Amenorrhea, dysmenorrhea due to blood stasis with severe lower abdominal pain...

2. Retention of the lochia due to blood stasis with

severe lower abdominal pain...

3. Traumatic injury with hematoma, swelling...

4. Rheumatic complaints due to wind cold dampness and blood stasis with severe joint pain, loss of mobility...

5. Pyogenic inflammation and *yong* of the inflammatory stage with redness, pain, heat, swelling...

Typical combinations:

1. With wine[-processed] Radix Angelicae Sinensis (*Jiu Dang Gui*), wine[-processed] Radix Ligus-

Radix Rubiae Cordifoliae continued . . .

tici Wallichii (*Jiu Chuan Xiong*), and vinegar[-processed] Rhizoma Cyperi Rotundi (*Cu Xiang Fu*)

2. With wine[-processed] Feces Trogopterori Seu Pteromi (*Jiu Wu Ling Zhi*), uncooked Pollen Typhae (*Sheng Pu Huang*), wine[-processed] Radix Cyathulae (*Jiu Chuan Niu Xi*), and wine[-processed] Herba Leonuri Heterophylli (*Jiu Yi Mu Cao*)

3. With vinegar[-processed] Resina Olibani (*Cu*

Ru Xiang), vinegar[-processed] Resina Myrrhae (*Cu Mo Yao*), and wine[-processed] Radix Salviae Miltiorrhizae (*Jiu Dan Shen*)

4. With wine[-processed] Radix Clematidis Chinensis (*Jiu Wei Ling Xian*), Caulis Millettiae Seu Spatholobi (*Ji Xue Teng*), and uncooked Cortex Radicis Acanthopanacis (*Sheng Wu Jia Pi*)

5. With Herba Cum Radice Taraxaci Mongolici (*Pu Gong Ying*), uncooked Cortex Radicis Moutan (*Sheng Mu Dan Pi*), and uncooked Radix Rubrus Paeoniae Lactiflorae (*Sheng Chi Shao Yao*)

Dosage: 10-15g and up to 30g in severe cases

_____Stir-fried [till] Carbonized (*Chao Tan*)_____

Names: *Qian Cao Gen Tan, Qian Cao Tan, Qian Gen Tan*

Flavors & nature: Bitter and astringent; cold tending to neutral

Functions: Cools the blood, moves the blood, and stops bleeding[1]

Indications:

1. Hemoptysis due to vacuity heat damaging the network vessels of the lungs with dry throat...

2. Dysentery, bloody hemorrhoids due to damp heat in the large intestine with bloody stools...

3. Hematuria due to replete heat damaging the network vessels of the uterus with clots and fresh blood in the urine...

4. Metrorrhagia due to either A) *chong* and *ren* vacuity or B) blood stasis caused by heat in the blood

5. Hematemesis, epistaxis due to heat in the blood

Typical combinations:

1. With uncooked Cacumen Biotae Orientalis (*Sheng Ce Bai Ye*) and uncooked Gelatinum Corii Asini (*Sheng E Jiao*) as in *Qian Gen San* (Rubia Root Powder [240])

2. With uncooked Rhizoma Coptidis Chinensis (*Sheng Huang Lian*) and uncooked Radix Sanguisorbae (*Sheng Di Yu*) as in *Qian Gen Tang* (Rubia Root Decoction [241])

3. With carbonized Herba Cephalanoploris Segeti (*Xiao Ji Tan*) and uncooked Rhizoma Imperatae Cylindricae (*Sheng Bai Mao Gen*) as in *Shi Hui San* (Ten Ashes Powder [299])

4. A) With stir-fried Os Sepiae Seu Sepiellae (*Chao Hai Piao Xiao*) and uncooked Radix Albus Paeoniae Lactiflorae (*Sheng Bai Shao Yao*) as in *Gu Chong Tang* (Secure the *Chong* Decoction [117])
B) With wine[-processed] Radix Rubrus Paeoniae Lactiflorae (*Jiu Chi Shao Yao*), wine[-processed] Cortex Radicis Moutan (*Jiu Mu Dan Pi*), and uncooked Pollen Typhae (*Sheng Pu Huang*)

Radix Rubiae Cordifoliae continued . . .

5. With carbonized Cortex Radicis Moutan (*Mu Dan Pi Tan*) and uncooked Cacumen Biotae Orientalis (*Sheng Ce Bai Ye*) as in *Shi Hui San* (Ten Ashes Powder [299])

Dosage: 5-10g and up to 20g in severe cases

Note: 1. Radix Rubiae is probably the best plant for treating hemorrhage due to blood stasis caused by heat in the blood.

Herba Cephalanoploris Segeti *(Xiao Ji)*

Uncooked *(Sheng)*

Names: *Xiao Ji, Xiao Ji Cao, Sheng Xiao Ji*

Flavors & nature: Sweet; cool

Functions: Dispels blood stasis, cools the blood, resolves toxins, disperses swelling

Indications:

1. Skin inflammations due to heat toxins in the blood

2. Mycoses, scabies with pruritus...

Typical combinations:

1. With uncooked Fructus Forsythiae Suspensae (*Sheng Lian Qiao*), uncooked Flos Lonicerae Japonicae (*Sheng Jin Yin Hua*), Herba Violae Yedoensis (*Zi Hua Di Ding*), and Herba Cum Taraxaci Mongolici (*Pu Gong Ying*)

2. With uncooked Resina Olibani (*Sheng Ru Xiang*), calcined Alumen (*Duan Ming Fan*), uncooked Agkistrodon Seu Bungarus (*Sheng Bai Hua She*), and Radix Sophorae Flavescentis (*Ku Shen*). Reduce these five medicinals to powder and apply locally.

Dosage: 10-15g and up to 60g in severe cases

Stir-fried [till] Carbonized *(Chao Tan)*

Name: *Xiao Ji Tan*

Flavors & nature: Sweet and slightly bitter

Functions: Cools the blood, stops bleeding

Indications:

1. Hemorrhages of all types due to heat in the blood, such as hematemesis, hemoptysis, epistaxis, metrorrhagia...

2. Hematuria, strangury with hematuria (*xue lin*) due to damp heat in the bladder

Typical combinations:

1. With carbonized Cortex Radicis Moutan (*Mu Dan Pi Tan*), uncooked Cacumen Biotae Orientalis (*Sheng Ce Bai Ye*), uncooked Rhizoma Imperatae Cylindricae (*Sheng Bai Mao Gen*), and carbonized Herba Cirsii Japonici (*Da Ji Tan*) as in *Shi Hui San* (Ten Ashes Powder [299])

2. With carbonized Pollen Typhae (*Pu Huang Tan*), Folium Pyrrosiae (*Shi Wei*), uncooked Nodus Nelumbinis Nuciferae (*Sheng Ou Jie*), uncooked Rhizoma Imperatae Cylindricae (*Sheng Bai Mao Gen*), and Succinum (*Hu Po*)

Dosage: 10-15g and up to 30g in severe cases

12
Phlegm Cold Warming
& Transforming Medicinals

Rhizoma Typhonii *(Bai Fu Zi)*

_____ Uncooked *(Sheng)* _____

Names: *Sheng Bai Fu Zi, Sheng Yun Bai Fu Zi*

Flavors & nature: Acrid and sweet; warm; toxic

Functions: Dispels phlegm wind, stops spasms and convulsions, stops pruritus, scatters nodulations

Indications:

1. Deviated mouth and eyes, hemiplegia due to phlegm wind in the channels with facial neuralgia, deviated tongue, aphasia...

2. Convulsions, spasms due to phlegm wind with vomiting of phlegmy fluids, convulsions of the four limbs...

3. Pruritus due to damp type eczema

4. Subcutaneous nodules, scrofula due to phlegm

Typical combinations:

1. With uncooked Bombyx Batryticatus (*Sheng*

Jiang Can) and Buthus Martensi (*Quan Xie*) as in *Qian Zheng San* (Lead to Righteousness Powder [246])

2. With stir-fried Rhizoma Gastrodiae Elatae (*Chao Tian Ma*), uncooked Rhizoma Arisaematis (*Sheng Tian Nan Xing*), and Buthus Martensi (*Quan Xie*) as in *Bai Fu Yin* (Typhonium Drink [10])

3. With Fructus Tribuli Terrestris (*Bai Ji Li*) and uncooked Zaocys Dhummades (*Sheng Wu Shao She*). Reduce these three substances to powder and apply locally.

4. With uncooked Rhizoma Pinelliae Ternatae (*Sheng Ban Xia*). Reduce these two substances to powder and apply locally.

Dosage: 3-5g and up to 15g with prudence in severe cases

_____ Processed *(Zhi)*[1] _____

Names: *Zhi Bai Fu Zi, Bai Fu Zi, Yun Bai Fu Zi*

Flavors & nature: Slightly acrid and sweet; warm; slightly toxic

Functions: Scatters cold, transforms phlegm dampness

Indications: Headache due to either 1) cold dampness with headache aggravated by cold or 2) accumulation of phlegm dampness with vertigo, vomiting phlegmy fluids, a sensation of a heavy head...

Rhizoma Typhonii continued . . .

Typical combinations:

1. With Radix Angelicae Dahuricae (*Bai Zhi*), Radix Et Rhizoma Ligustici Chinensis (*Gao Ben*), and Rhizoma Arisaematis (*Tian Nan Xing*)

2. With Rhizoma Pinelliae Ternatae (*Ban Xia*), processed Rhizoma Arisaematis (*Zhi Tian Nan Xing*), and uncooked Rhizoma Atractylodis Macrocephalae (*Sheng Bai Zhu*)

Dosage: 3-5g and up to 15g in severe cases

Note: 1. Typhonium is boiled with tofu (*Dou Fu*), Radix Glycyrrhizae (*Gan Cao*), and Semen Phaseoli Hispidae (*Hei Dou*) until the rhizome is soaked to its center. Then it is dried slowly according to the method *hong*.

Addendum: There are two varieties of *Bai Fu Zi*: *Yu Bai Fu Zi* and *Guan Bai Fu Zi*. *Yu Bai Fu Zi* is toxic and drying, disperses phlegm wind, levels internal wind, settles tremors, and treats wind stroke (*zhong feng*) due to accumulation of phlegm, hemiplegia, tetany, etc. *Guan Bai Fu Zi* is very toxic and very drying, scatters cold dampness, stops pain, eliminates phlegm wind, treats *bi* of the wind cold dampness type, headaches, hemiplegia, deviated mouth and eyes due to phlegm wind, etc. *Yu Bai Fu Zi* is used more in clinical practice.

Radix Cynanchi Stautonii (Bai Qian)

—————— Uncooked (Sheng) ——————

Names: *Sheng Bai Qian, Sou Bai Qian, Bai Qian*

Flavors & nature: Acrid and sweet; slightly warm

Functions: Resolves the exterior, rectifies the lung qi, transforms phlegm, stops cough

Indications:

1. Cough[1] due to either A) wind cold with fever, chills, difficult to expectorate phlegm, a floating (*fu*) pulse or B) wind heat with thick, yellow phlegm which is difficult to expectorate, fever, chills...

2. Hemoptysis due to incessant cough damaging the network vessels of the lungs

Typical combinations:

1. A) With uncooked Radix Asteris Tatarici (*Sheng Zi Wan*), uncooked Herba Schizonepetae Tenuifoliae (*Sheng Jing Jie*), and steamed Radix Stemonae (*Zheng Bai Bu*) as in *Zhi Sou San* (Stop Cough Powder [437])
B) With uncooked Radix Peucedani (*Sheng Qian Hu*), Bulbus Fritillariae Thunbergii (*Zhe Bei Mu*), uncooked Folium Eriobotryae Japonicae (*Sheng Pi Pa Ye*), and uncooked Radix Platycodi Grandiflori (*Sheng Jie Geng*)

2. With honey mix-fried Radix Platycodi Grandiflori (*Mi Zhi Jie Geng*), uncooked Radix Glycyrrhizae (*Sheng Gan Cao*), honey mix-fried Cortex Radicis Mori Albi (*Mi Zhi Sang Bai Pi*), and honey mix-fried Fructus Aristolochiae (*Mi Zhi Ma Dou Ling*)

Dosage: 5-10g

Radix Cynanchi Stautonii continued . . .

_____ Stir-fried [till] Scorched (Chao Jiao)_____

Names: *Chao Bai Qian, Jiao Bai Qian*

Flavors & nature: Sweet and slightly acrid; warm

Functions: Warms the lungs, scatters cold, transforms phlegm, stops cough

Indications: Cough due to either 1) accumulation of phlegm cold in the lungs with expectoration of white or clear mucus, chest oppression, shortness of breath or 2) accumulation of phlegm dampness in the lungs with expectoration of abundant, thick, sticky mucus, chest and epigastric oppression, loss of appetite...

Typical combinations:

1. With dry Rhizoma Zingiberis (*Gan Jiang*),

uncooked Radix Asteris Tatarici (*Sheng Zi Wan*), stir-fried Semen Pruni Armeniacae (*Chao Xing Ren*), honey mix-fried Herba Ephedrae (*Mi Zhi Ma Huang*), and processed Rhizoma Arisaematis (*Zhi Tian Nan Xing*)

2. With clear Rhizoma Pinelliae Ternatae (*Qing Ban Xia*), processed Rhizoma Arisaematis (*Zhi Tian Nan Xing*), uncooked Pericarpium Citri Reticulatae (*Sheng Chen Pi*), uncooked Sclerotium Poriae Cocos (*Sheng Fu Ling*), and uncooked Semen Raphani Sativi (*Sheng Lai Fu Zi*)

Dosage: 6-12g and up to 30g in severe cases

_____Honey Mix-fried (Mi Zhi)_____

Names: *Mi Zhi Bai Qian, Zhi Bai Qian*

Flavors & nature: Sweet and slightly acrid; moistening; warm

Functions: Moistens the lungs, downbears counterflow qi, transforms phlegm, stops cough

Indications: Cough due to either 1) lung qi vacuity with weak cough, white phlegm, shortness of breath, a pale complexion, fatigue or 2) lung yin vacuity with dry cough, scanty, dry phlegm which is difficult to expectorate, a dry mouth and throat...

Typical combinations:

1. With honey mix-fried Radix Astragali

Membranacei (*Mi Zhi Huang Qi*), Gecko (*Ge Jie*), Radix Panacis Ginseng (*Ren Shen*), honey mix-fried Flos Tussilaginis Farfarae (*Mi Zhi Kuan Dong Hua*), and honey mix-fried Radix Asteris Tatarici (*Mi Zhi Zi Wan*)

2. With honey mix-fried Bulbus Lilii (*Mi Zhi Bai He*), honey mix-fried Radix Adenophorae Strictae (*Mi Zhi Nan Sha Shen*), uncooked Tuber Ophiopogonis Japonicae (*Sheng Mai Men Dong*), uncooked Folium Eriobotryae Japonicae (*Sheng Pi Pa Ye*), and honey mix-fried Fructus Aristolochiae (*Mi Zhi Ma Dou Ling*)

Dosage: 6-12g and up to 30g in severe cases

Rhizoma Pinelliae Ternatae (Ban Xia)

_____ Uncooked (Sheng)[1] _____

Names: *Sheng Ban Xia, Ban Xia Pian, Ban Xia*

Flavors & nature: Acrid; warm; toxic

Functions: Softens the hard, scatters nodulations, disperses swelling, stops pain

Indications:

1. Skin inflammations, abscesses, mastitis

2. Subcutaneous nodulations, goiter, scrofula[2] due to phlegm stagnation in the channels

3. Plum pit qi (*mei he qi*)[2] due to qi and phlegm stagnation with hysteria, a sensation of a pit in the throat, dysphagia, chest oppression...

Typical combinations:

1. Apply locally as a plaster made from powdered uncooked Pinelliae (*Sheng Ban Xia*).

2. Apply locally as a plaster made from powdered uncooked Pinelliae (*Sheng Ban Xia*). Orally, with Bulbus Fritillariae Thunbergii (*Zhe Bei Mu*),

Thallus Algae (*Kun Bu*), Radix Scrophulariae Ningpoensis (*Xuan Shen*), and uncooked Concha Ostreae (*Sheng Mu Li*)

3. With uncooked Cortex Magnoliae Officinalis (*Sheng Hou Po*) and Folium Perillae Frutescentis (*Zi Su Ye*) as in *Ban Xia Hou Po Tang* (Pinellia & Magnolia Decoction [27])[2]

Dosage: Applied locally, use whatever amount necessary. There is no overdosage when used topically.

Notes: 1. Uncooked Pinellia is toxic and should be strictly reserved for external use. 2. For these indications, clear salt[-processed] Pinellia (*Qing Yan Ban Xia*) can be equally prescribed. *Qing Yan Ban Xia* refers to uncooked Pinellia (*Sheng Ban Xia*) or lime-processed Pinellia (*Fa Ban Xia*) prepared with salt. This preparation permits one to strengthen Pinellia's actions of softening the hard and scattering nodulations due to stagnant phlegm. For local application, use *Qing Yan Ban Xia* starting from uncooked Pinellia (*Sheng Ban Xia*). Orally, use *Qing Yan Ban Xia* starting with lime-processed Pinellia (*Fa Ban Xia*). Dosage: 3-10g

_____ Ginger[-processed] (Jiang)[1] _____

Names: *Jiang Ban Xia, Jiang Xia Pian, Jiang Xia*

Flavors & nature: Acrid; drying; warm; very slightly toxic

Functions: Warms the center, transforms phlegm, dries dampness, downbears counterflow qi, stops vomiting

Indications:

1. Vomiting, nausea due to A) evil cold in the stomach with vomiting of clear fluids or watery phlegm, B) severe evil cold in the stomach, C)

accumulation of phlegm dampness with fullness in the epigastrium, loss of appetite, loose stools or D) cold which has transformed into heat

2. Epigastric distention due to stomach qi stagnation with nausea, vomiting, borborygmus...

3. Cough due to phlegm cold

Typical combinations:

1. A) With uncooked Rhizoma Zingiberis (*Sheng Jiang*) as in *Xiao Ban Xia Tang* (Minor Pinellia Decoction [372])

Rhizoma Pinelliae Ternatae continued. . .

B) With Flos Caryophylli (*Ding Xiang*) and Herba Agastachis Seu Pogostemi (*Huo Xiang*) as in *Huo Xiang Ban Xia Tang* (Agastaches & Pinellia Decoction [163])

C) With uncooked Sclerotium Poriae Cocos (*Sheng Fu Ling*) and uncooked Rhizoma Zingiberis (*Sheng Jiang*) as in *Xiao Ban Xia Jia Fu Ling Tang* (Minor Pinellia Plus Poria Decoction [371])

D) With ginger[-processed] Rhizoma Coptidis Chinensis (*Jiang Huang Lian*), stir-fried Pericarpium Citri Reticulatae (*Chao Chen Pi*), and ginger[-processed] Caulis In Taeniis Bambusae (*Jiang Zhu Ru*) as in *Huang Lian Zhu Ru Ju Pi Ban Xia Tang* (Coptis, Bambusa, Orange Peel & Pinellia Decoction [154])

2. With Rhizoma Coptidis Chinensis (*Huang Lian*) and dry Rhizoma Zingiberis (*Gan Jiang*) as in *Ban Xia Xie Xin Tang* (Pinellia Drain the Heart Decoction [28])

3. With dry Rhizoma Zingiberis (*Gan Jiang*), stir-fried Radix Cynanchi Stautonii (*Chao Bai Qian*), and honey mix-fried Flos Inulae (*Mi Zhi Xuan Fu Hua*)

Dosage: 3-10g and up to 15g in severe cases

Note: 1. Ginger[-processed] Pinellia is prepared with the aid of fresh Ginger and Alumen (*Bai Fan*). Sometimes Radix Glycyrrhizae (*Gan Cao*), Mirabilitum (*Pi Xiao*), and Fructus Gleditschiae Chinensis (*Zao Jiao*) are added.

_____Clear or Water[-processed] (*Qing or Shui*)[1]_____

Names: *Qing Ban Xia, Qing Xia Pian*

Flavors & nature: Slightly acrid; warm; drying; very slightly toxic

Functions: Dries dampness, transforms phlegm

Indications:

1. Cough due to either A) phlegm dampness with abundant, thick mucus which is difficult to expectorate or B) phlegm heat with thick, yellow mucus which is difficult to expectorate...

2. Rheumatic complaints due to stagnation of phlegm dampness and dampness in the channels with joint pain, generalized pain...

3. Chest pain due to accumulation of phlegm heat in the chest with expectoration of thick, yellow mucus, cough, epigastric and chest distention...

Typical combinations:

1. A) With uncooked Pericarpium Citri Reticulatae (*Sheng Chen Pi*), uncooked Sclerotium Po-

riae Cocos (*Sheng Fu Ling*), and stir-fried Semen Pruni Armeniacae (*Chao Xing Ren*) as in *Liu An Jian* (Six Quiets Decoction [202])

B) With bile-[-processed] Rhizoma Arisaematis (*Dan Nan Xing*) and stir-fried Semen Trichosanthis Kirlowii (*Chao Gua Lou Ren*) as in *Qing Qi Hua Tan Wan* (Clear the Qi & Transform Phlegm Pills [254])

2. With Radix Et Rhizoma Notopterygii (*Qiang Huo*) and uncooked Rhizoma Atractylodis (*Sheng Cang Zhu*) as in *Qing Shi Hua Tan Tang* (Clear Dampness & Transform Phlegm Decoction [255])

3. With wine[-processed] Radix Scutellariae Baicalensis (*Jiu Huang Qin*) and stir-fried Semen Trichosanthis Kirlowii (*Chao Gua Lou Ren*) as in *Xiao Xian Xiong Tang* (Minor Fell [*i.e.*, Drain] the Chest Decoction [379])

Dosage: 3-10g and up to 15g in severe cases

Note: 1. *Qing Shui Ban Xia* is prepared with the aid of Alumen (*Bai Fan*). Sometimes one also uses Radix Glycyrrhizae (*Gan Cao*), Radix Codonopsis Pilosulae (*Dang Shen*), Bulbus Fritillariae Cirrhosae (*Chuan Bei*

Rhizoma Pinelliae Ternatae continued. . .

Mu), and salt (*Qing Yan*) are also used. In that case, the preparation is called *Su Ban Xia* (i.e., Jiangsu Pinellia).

Addendum: The difference between *Qing Ban Xia* and *Fa Ban Xia* is fine. *Qing Ban Xia* is advantageously drying, while *Fa Ban Xia* is stronger for supplementing the spleen. In clinical practice, both types are often prescribed indiscriminately.

Lime-processed *(Fa)*[1]

Names: *Fa Ban Xia, Jing Ban Xia, Fa Xia, Jing Xia, Huang Fa Xia*

Flavors & nature: Slightly acrid; warm; drying; very slightly toxic

Functions: Dries dampness, transforms phlegm, fortifies the spleen, harmonizes the stomach

Indications:

1. Phlegm dampness due to spleen vacuity with whitish, abundant phlegm, lack of appetite, loose stools, fatigue...

2. Vertigo due to phlegm dampness harassing the upper body with headache, a sensation of a heavy head, chest and diaphragmatic oppression, a thick [tongue] coating, a slippery (*hua*) or wiry (*xian*) pulse...

3. Insomnia due to phlegm dampness and disharmony of the stomach

Typical combinations:

1. With uncooked Rhizoma Atractylodis Macrocephalae (*Sheng Bai Zhu*) and uncooked Sclerotium Poriae Cocos (*Sheng Fu Ling*) as in *Er Chen Tang* (Two Aged [Ingredients] Decoction [95])

2. With stir-fried Rhizoma Gastrodiae Elatae (*Chao Tian Ma*) and uncooked Rhizoma Atractylodis Macrocephalae (*Sheng Bai Zhu*) as in *Ban Xia Bai Zhu Tian Ma Tang* (Pinellia, Atractylodes & Gastrodia Decoction [26])

3. With Semen Panici Miliacei (*Shu Mi*) as in *Ban Xia Shu Mi Tang* (Pinellia & Millet Decoction [27a])

Dosage: 3-10g and up to 15g in severe cases

Note: 1. *Fa Ban Xia* is prepared with the aid of lime (*Shi Hui*) and Radix Glycyrrhizae (*Gan Cao*). Sometimes Fructus Gleditschiae Chinensis (*Zao Jiao*), Mirabilitum (*Pi Xiao*), and Pericarpium Citri Reticulatae (*Chen Pi*) are added to the preparation.

Bamboo Juice [Processed] *(Zhu Li)*[1]

Name: *Zhu Li Ban Xia*

Flavors & nature: Slightly acrid; slightly warm tending toward neutral; drying; very slightly toxic

Functions: Dries dampness, transforms phlegm, downbears counterflow qi, clears heat

Indications:

1. Vomiting due to stomach heat and stagnation of phlegm heat in the stomach with nausea, acid regurgitation, a bitter taste in the mouth, thirst...

2. Cough due to lung heat with expectoration of yellow, thick, sticky phlegm...

3. Loss of consciousness due to phlegm misting the portals of the heart

4. Epilepsy due to phlegm wind misting the portals of the heart

Typical combinations:

1. With ginger[-processed] Caulis In Taeniis Bambusae (*Jiang Zhu Ru*), ginger[-processed]

Rhizoma Pinelliae Ternatae continued. . .

Rhizoma Coptidis Chinensis (*Jiang Huang Lian*), stir-fried Folium Eriobotryae Japonicae (*Chao Pi Pa Ye*), and stir-fried Pericarpium Citri Reticulatae (*Chao Chen Pi*)

2. With wine[-processed] Radix Scutellariae Baicalensis (*Jiu Huang Qin*), honey mix-fried Cortex Radicis Mori Albi (*Mi Zhi Sang Bai Pi*), Bulbus Fritillariae Thunbergii (*Zhe Bei Mu*), and stir-fried Semen Lepidii (*Chao Ting Li Zi*)

3. With uncooked Rhizoma Arisaematis (*Sheng Tian Nan Xing*) and stir-fried Pericarpium Citri Reticulatae (*Chao Chen Pi*) as in *Dao Tan Tang* (Abduct Phlegm Decoction [81])

4. With Rhizoma Acori Graminei (*Shi Chang Pu*), bile[-processed] Rhizoma Arisaematis (*Dan Nan Xing*), and Buthus Martensi (*Quan Xie*) as in *Ding Xian Wan* (Stabilize Epilepsy Pills [87])

Dosage: 3-10g and up to 15g in severe cases

Note: 1. *Zhu Li Ban Xia* is prepared starting from *Fa Ban Xia* with Succus Bambusae (*Zhu Li*).

Fermented (Qu)[1]

Name: *Ban Xia Qu*

Flavors & nature: Slightly acrid; warm; drying; very slightly toxic

Functions: Dries dampness, transforms phlegm, harmonizes the stomach, disperses food stagnation

Indications:

1. Vomiting due to food stagnation with loss of appetite, nausea, disgust at [the idea of] eating, abdominal distention, diarrhea...

2. Abdominal distention due to stagnation of dampness and food with lack of appetite, loose stools, nausea...

3. Regurgitation, eructation due to stagnation of dampness and food with loss of appetite, nausea, abdominal distention, slow digestion...

Typical combinations:

1. With stir-fried Massa Medica Fermentata (*Chao Shen Qu*), stir-fried Fructus Crataegi (*Chao Shan Zha*), and bran stir-fried Rhizoma Atractylodis Macrocephalae (*Fu Chao Bai Zhu*)

2. With bran stir-fried Rhizoma Atractylodis Macrocephalae (*Fu Chao Bai Zhu*), uncooked Radix Saussureae Seu Vladimiriae (*Sheng Mu Xiang*), and stir-fried Semen Raphani Sativi (*Chao Lai Fu Zi*)

3. With processed Fructus Evodiae Rutecarpae (*Zhi Wu Zhu Yu*), stir-fried Massa Medica Fermentata (*Chao Shen Qu*), and bran stir-fried Rhizoma Atractylodis Macrocephalae (*Fu Chao Bai Zhu*)

Dosage: 3-10g and up to 15g in severe cases

Note: 1. *Ban Xia Qu* is a fermented product of uncooked Pinellia (*Sheng Ban Xia*), ginger juice, and wheat bran.

Rhizoma Arisaematis *(Tian Nan Xing)*

Uncooked *(Sheng)*

Names: *Sheng Tian Nan Xing, Sheng Nan Xing*

Flavors & nature: Bitter and acrid; warm; very drying; toxic

Functions: Dispels wind, stops convulsions, expels phlegm wind, scatters nodulations

Indications:

1. Tetany due to wind toxins with trismus, opisthotonos, muscular spasm...

2. Wind stroke (*zhong feng*) due to phlegm wind in the network vessels with hemiplegia, aphasia, deviated mouth and eyes...

3. Convulsions, spasms due to phlegm wind in the network vessels with paresthesia of the hands and feet...

4. Goiter, scrofula, subcutaneous nodules due to accumulation of phlegm

Typical combinations:

1. With uncooked Rhizoma Typhonii (*Sheng Bai Fu Zi*) and stir-fried Rhizoma Gastrodiae Elatae (*Chao Tian Ma*) as in *Yu Zhen San* (True Jade Powder [420])

2. With bamboo juice [processed] Rhizoma Pinelliae Ternatae (*Zhu Li Ban Xia*), uncooked Rhizoma Typhonii (*Sheng Bai Fu Zi*), stir-fried Rhizoma Gastrodiae Elatae (*Chao Tian Ma*), and Lumbricus (*Di Long*)

3. With Buthus Martensi (*Quan Xie*), stone-baked Scolopendra Subspinipes (*Bei Wu Gong*), and uncooked Bombyx Batryticatus (*Sheng Jiang Can*)

4. With uncooked Rhizoma Pinelliae Ternatae (*Sheng Ban Xia*). Reduce these two plants to powder, add a little vinegar, and make into a paste. Apply locally.

Dosage: 3-6g in decoction and up to 12g in severe cases and in a prudent manner; 0.3-1.2g in powder

Processed *(Zhi)*[1]

Names: *Zhi Tian Nan Xing, Zhi Nan Xing, Tian Nan Xing*

Flavors & nature: Bitter and acrid; warm

Functions: Dries dampness, transforms phlegm

Indications:

1. Cough due to either A) phlegm dampness with whitish, thick, difficult to expectorate expectorations, chest and epigastric oppression or B) phlegm cold with clear, fine, abundant rheum, shortness of breath, chest oppression...

2. Vertigo due to phlegm dampness harassing the head with a sensation of a heavy head, numbness, nausea, vomiting, insomnia...

3. Rheumatic complaints due to phlegm dampness stagnating in the network vessels

Typical combinations:

1. A) With uncooked Pericarpium Citri Reticulatae (*Sheng Chen Pi*) and ginger[-processed] Rhizoma Pinelliae Ternatae (*Jiang Ban Xia*) as in *Yu Fen Wan* (Jade Powder Pills [413])
B) With Cortex Cinnamomi (*Rou Gui*) and uncooked Rhizoma Zingiberis (*Sheng Jiang*) as in *Jiang Gui Wan* (Ginger & Cinnamon Pills [172])

2. With stir-fried Rhizoma Gastrodiae Elatae (*Chao Tian Ma*) and lime-processed Rhizoma

Rhizoma Arisaematis continued . . .

Pinelliae Ternatae (*Fa Ban Xia*) as in *Yu Hu Wan* (Jade Vase Pills [415])

3. With uncooked Rhizoma Atractylodis (*Sheng Cang Zhu*) and Radix Et Rhizoma Notopterygii (*Qiang Huo*) as in *Qing Shi Hua Tan Tang* (Clear Dampness & Transform Phlegm Decoction [255])

Dosage: 5-10g and up to 15g in severe cases

Note: 1. This refers to *Tian Nan Xing* prepared with Alumen (*Bai Fan*) and uncooked Rhizoma Zingiberis (*Sheng Jiang*).

_____ Bile[-processed] (*Dan*)[1] _____

Names: *Dan Nan Xing, Chen Dan Xing*

Flavors & nature: Bitter; cool

Functions: Clears heat, transforms phlegm, extinguishes wind, soothes tetany

Indications:

1. Cough due to phlegm heat accumulated in the lungs with thick, sticky, yellow, difficult to expectorate phlegm...

2. Infantile convulsions due to heat and phlegm wind with spasms in the hands and feet...

3. Epilepsy due to phlegm heat misting the portals of the heart with loss of consciousness, foaming mouth...

4. Loss of consciousness due to phlegm heat misting the portals of the heart with convulsions...

Typical combinations:

1. With wine[-processed] Radix Scutellariae Baicalensis (*Jiu Huang Qin*) and stir-fried Semen Trichosanthis Kirlowii (*Chao Gua Lou Ren*) as in *Qing Qi Hua Tan Wan* (Clear the Qi & Transform Phlegm Pills [254])

2. With Buthus Martensi (*Quan Xie*) and stir-fried Rhizoma Gastrodiae Elatae (*Chao Tian Ma*) as in *Qian Jin San* (Thousand [Ounces of] Gold Powder [243])

3. With Rhizoma Acori Graminei (*Shi Chang Pu*), Buthus Martensi (*Quan Xie*), and Succus Bambusae (*Zhu Li*) as in *Ding Xian Wan* (Stabilize Epilepsy Pills [87])

4. With Calculus Bovis (*Niu Huang*), Rhizoma Acori Graminei (*Shi Chang Pu*), and Borneol (*Bing Pian*)

Dosage: 3-10g. Do not exceed this dosage.

Note: 1. *Dan Nan Xing* is prepared with the aid of Alumen (*Bai Fan*) and pig bile (*Zhu Dan*). *Dan* means bile.

Flos Inulae (*Xuan Fu Hua*)

_____ Uncooked (*Sheng*) _____

Names: *Xuan Fu Hua, Quan Fu Hua, Jin Fei Hua*

Flavors & nature: Acrid, bitter, and salty; slightly warm

Functions: Transforms phlegm, disinhibits urination, downbears counterflow qi, stops vomiting

Indications:

1. Vomiting due to either A) phlegm rheum in the stomach with vomiting of clear fluids or watery

Flos Inulae continued . . .

rheum or B) stagnation of phlegm dampness and middle burner deficiency with nausea, eructation, chest and epigastric distention...

2. Chest and lateral costal oppression and fullness due to evil cold stagnating in the liver channel following a stagnation of qi and blood with pain and distention...

3. Ascites due to accumulation of dampness caused by spleen yang vacuity with oliguria, epigastric distention and swelling...

Typical combinations:

1. A) With uncooked Sclerotium Poriae Cocos (*Sheng Fu Ling*) and ginger[-processed] Rhizoma Pinelliae Ternatae (*Jiang Ban Xia*)
B) With uncooked Haematitum (*Sheng Dai Zhe Shi*) and Radix Panacis Ginseng (*Ren Shen*) as in *Xuan Fu Dai Zhe Tang* (Inula & Hematite Decoction [388])

2. With Bulbus Allii Fistulosi (*Cong Bai*) as in *Xuan Fu Hua Tang* (Inula Decoction [389])

3. With vinegar[-processed] Radix Euphorbiae Kansui (*Cu Gan Sui*), vinegar[-processed] Radix Euphorbiae Pekinensis (*Cu Jing Da Ji*), and uncooked Semen Arecae Catechu (*Sheng Bing Lang*)

Dosage: 5-10g and up to 20g in severe cases

Honey Mix-fried (*Mi Zhi*)

Names: *Mi Zhi Xuan Fu Hua, Zhi Xuan Fu Hua, Mi Zhi Quan Fu Hua, Mi Zhi Jin Fei Hua*

Flavors & nature: Sweet and salty; slightly warm

Functions: Eliminates phlegm, calms dyspnea, stops cough

Indications: Cough, asthma due to 1) phlegm cold with abundant expectorations, chest oppression, 2) phlegm heat, expectoration of thick, yellow mucus with chest oppression, or 3) wind cold with fever, chills...

Typical combinations:

1. With honey mix-fried Herba Ephedrae (*Mi Zhi Ma Huang*), stir-fried Fructus Perillae Frutescentis (*Chao Zi Su Zi*), stir-fried Semen Pruni Armeniacae (*Chao Xing Ren*), and ginger[-processed] Cortex Magnoliae Officinalis (*Jiang Hou Po*)

2. With honey mix-fried Cortex Radicis Mori Albi (*Mi Zhi Sang Bai Pi*), uncooked Radix Peucedani (*Sheng Qian Hu*), uncooked Radix Platycodi Grandiflori (*Sheng Jie Geng*), and Bulbus Fritillariae Thunbergii (*Zhe Bei Mu*)

3. With uncooked Herba Ephedrae (*Sheng Ma Huang*), uncooked Herba Schizonepetae Tenuifoliae (*Sheng Jing Jie*), ginger[-processed] Rhizoma Pinelliae Ternatae (*Jiang Ban Xia*), and uncooked Radix Peucedani (*Sheng Qian Hu*) as in *Jin Fei Cao San* (Inula Powder [179])

Dosage: 6-15g and up to 20g in severe cases

Addendum: Although flowers usually have an ascending property, Flos Inulae, on the contrary, downbears the qi, [thus having] a descending property.

13
Phlegm Heat Clearing & Transforming Medicinals

Semen Benincasae Hispidae (Dong Gua Ren)

Uncooked (Sheng)

Names: *Sheng Dong Gua Ren, Sheng Dong Gua Zi, Dong Gua Ren, Dong Gua Zi*

Flavors & nature: Slightly sweet; cold

Functions: Clears heat, transforms phlegm, evacuates pus, disinhibits urination

Indications:

1. Cough due to lung heat and accumulation of phlegm heat with chest oppression...

2. Lung abscess due to stagnation of heat in the lungs with expectoration of purulent, malodorous phlegm, chest pain...

3. Appendicitis due to stagnation of heat and blood stasis in the intestines with abdominal pain aggravated by pressure...

4. Dysuria due to accumulation of heat in the bladder with urodynia

Typical combinations:

1. With uncooked Radix Peucedani (*Sheng Qian Hu*) and uncooked Semen Coicis Lachryma-jobi (*Sheng Yi Yi Ren*) as in *Qian Bei Xing Gua Tang* (Peucedanum, Fritillaria, Armeniaca & Benincasa Decoction [239])

2. With Rhizoma Phragmitis Communis (*Lu Gen*) and uncooked Semen Coicis Lachryma-jobi (*Sheng Yi Yi Ren*) as in *Wei Jing Tang* (Phragmites Decoction [338])

3. With uncooked Radix Et Rhizoma Rhei (*Sheng Da Huang*) and uncooked Cortex Radicis Moutan (*Sheng Mu Dan Pi*) as in *Da Huang Mu Dan Pi Tang* (Rhubarb & Moutan Decoction [64])

4. With uncooked Rhizoma Alismatis (*Sheng Ze Xie*), Sclerotium Polypori Umbellati (*Zhu Ling*), and uncooked Fructus Gardeniae Jasminoidis (*Sheng Shan Zhi Zi*)

Dosage: 6-15g

Stir-fried [till] Scorched (Chao Jiao)

Names: *Chao Dong Gua Ren, Chao Dong Gua Zi*

Flavors & nature: Slightly sweet; slightly cold

Functions: Eliminates dampness, transforms phlegm, stimulates the appetite

Indications:

1. Cough due to stagnation of phlegm cold or phlegm heat (or not very intense heat) with expectoration of whitish mucus, shortness of breath, chest oppression...

Semen Benincasae Hispidae continued . . .

2. Abnormal vaginal discharge, urinary strangury with dribbling and dripping due to accumulation of damp heat in the lower burner

3. Loss of appetite[1] due to food stagnation caused by spleen and stomach vacuity with eructations, nausea, vomiting, a bland mouth, loss of taste, epigastric and abdominal distention...

Typical combinations:

1. With stir-fried Semen Pruni Armeniacae (*Chao Xing Ren*), stir-fried Radix Cynanchi Stautonii (*Chao Bai Qian*), and uncooked Radix Asteris Tatarici (*Sheng Zi Wan*)

2. With uncooked Cortex Phellodendri (*Sheng Huang Bai*), stir-fried Rhizoma Dioscoreae Hypoglaucae (*Chao Bei Xie*), uncooked Semen Coicis Lachryma-jobi (*Sheng Yi Yi Ren*), and Rhizoma Acori Graminei (*Shi Chang Pu*)

3. With bran stir-fried Rhizoma Atractylodis Macrocephalae (*Fu Chao Bai Zhu*), stir-fried Fructus Germinatus Hordei Vulgaris (*Chao Mai Ya*), and stir-fried Fructus Crataegi (*Chao Shan Zha*)

Dosage: 6-15g

Note: 1. For this indication, bran stir-fried Semen Benincasae (*Fu Chao Dong Gua Ren*) can be prescribed.

_____ **Honey Mix-fried** *(Mi Zhi)* _____

Names: *Mi Zhi Dong Gua Ren, Mi Zhi Dong Gua Zi, Zhi Dong Gua Ren, Zhi Dong Gua Zi*

Flavors & nature: Sweet; slightly cold

Functions: Moistens the lungs, eliminates phlegm

Indications: Cough due to 1) lung qi vacuity with whitish phlegm which is difficult to expectorate, weak cough, fatigue, spontaneous perspiration, shortness of breath or 2) lung yin vacuity with scanty, dry, difficult to expectorate phlegm, dry cough, dry throat, a sensation of heat in the chest, night sweats...

Typical combinations:

1. With honey mix-fried Radix Astragali Membranacei (*Mi Zhi Huang Qi*), Radix Panacis Ginseng (*Ren Shen*), uncooked Radix Dioscoreae Oppositae (*Sheng Shan Yao*), and Bulbus Fritillariae Cirrhosae (*Chuan Bei Mu*)

2. With uncooked Tuber Ophiopogonis Japonicae (*Sheng Mai Men Dong*), honey mix-fried Bulbus Lilii (*Mi Zhi Bai He*), honey mix-fried Radix Adenophorae Strictae (*Mi Zhi Nan Sha Shen*), and Bulbus Fritillariae Cirrhosae (*Chuan Bei Mu*)

Dosage: 10-15g

Fructus Trichosanthis Kirlowii *(Gua Lou)*[1]

_____ **Uncooked** *(Sheng)* _____

Names: *Quan Gua Lou, Yuan Gua Lou, Gua Lou Shi, Gua Lou*

Flavors & nature: Sweet and bitter; cold

Functions: Clears heat, moistens the lungs, dispels phlegm, treats mastitis

Indications:

1. Cough due to accumulation of phlegm heat in the lungs with chest oppression and pain, abundant, yellow mucus...

Fructus Trichosanthis Kirlowii continued . . .

2. Mastitis due to heat toxins and blood stasis with fever, chills...

Typical combinations:

1. With ginger[-processed] Rhizoma Coptidis Chinensis (*Jiang Huang Lian*) and clear Rhizoma Pinelliae Ternatae (*Qing Ban Xia*) as in *Xiao Xian Xiong Tang* (Minor Fell [*i.e.,* Drain] the Chest Decoction [379])

2. With uncooked Flos Lonicerae Japonicae (*Sheng Jin Yin Hua*), uncooked Fructus Forsythiae Suspensae (*Sheng Lian Qiao*), Herba Cum Radice Taraxaci Mongolici (*Pu Gong Ying*), and uncooked Radix Rubrus Paeoniae Lactiflorae (*Sheng Chi Shao Yao*)

Dosage: 10-15g and up to 30g in severe cases

Note: 1. *Gua Lou Pi* is the skin of Trichosanthis. *Gua Lou Ren* is the seed of the fruit of Trichosanthis. *Gua Lou* is the entire fruit of Trichosanthis. *Gua Lou Gen* (a.k.a. *Tian Hua Fen*) is the root of Trichosanthis.

_____ **Stir-fried [till] Scorched** (*Chao Jiao*) _____

Names: *Chao Quan Gua Lou, Chao Gua Lou Shi*

Flavors & nature: Bitter and sweet; cold tending to neutral

Functions: Loosens the chest, moves the qi, dispels phlegm

Indications:

1. Chest pain (*xiong bi*)[1] due to accumulation of phlegm dampness in the lungs and chest yang deficiency with chest oppression and pain, cough with whitish mucus, dyspnea, asthmatic breathing...

2. Heart pain (*xiong bi*)[1] due to heart blood stasis with chest pain radiating to the back or left arm, a purple tongue, a choppy (*se*) pulse...

Typical combinations:

1. With Bulbus Allii Macrostemi (*Xie Bai*), clear

Rhizoma Pinelliae Ternatae (*Qing Ban Xia*), and white alcohol (*Bai Jiu*) as in *Gua Lou Xie Bai Ban Xia Tang* (Trichosanthes, Allium Macrostemi, & Pinelliae Decoction [120])

2. With uncooked Pollen Typhae (*Sheng Pu Huang*), Flos Carthami Tinctorii (*Hong Hua*), stir-fried Resina Olibani (*Chao Ru Xiang*), Radix Pseudoginseng (*San Qi*), wine[-processed] Radix Salviae Miltiorrhizae (*Jiu Dan Shen*), and Bulbus Allii Macrostemi (*Xie Bai*)

Dosage: 10-15g and up to 30g in severe cases

Note: 1. Stir-fried Pericarpium Trichosanthis Kirlowii (*Chao Gua Lou Pi*) and *Chao Quan Gua Lou* have the same indications. However, the former is more powerful than the latter.

Pericarpium Trichosanthis Kirlowii (Gua Lou Pi)

Uncooked (Sheng)

Names: *Gua Lou Pi, Gua Lou Ke, Sheng Lou Pi*

Flavors & nature: Sweet and bitter; cold

Functions: Clears heat, transforms phlegm, diffuses the lungs

Indications:

1. Cough due to A) lung heat and stagnation of phlegm heat in the lungs with chest oppression, expectoration of yellowish, sticky phlegm, B) lung fire and stagnation of phlegm fire in the lungs with cough which follows pain in the chest, phlegm streaked with blood, or C) incessant cough damaging the lungs with vexation...

2. Sore, swollen throat due to lung heat with hoarseness...

Typical combinations:

1. A) With Bulbus Fritillariae Thunbergii (*Zhe Bei Mu*), uncooked Radix Platycodi Grandiflori (*Sheng Jie Geng*), and Herba Houttuyniae Cordatae (*Yu Xing Cao*)
B) With wine[-processed] Radix Scutellariae Baicalensis (*Jiu Huang Qin*), uncooked Fructus Gardeniae Jasminoidis (*Sheng Shan Zhi Zi*), and carbonized Radix Rubiae Cordifoliae (*Qian Cao Gen Tan*)
C) With uncooked Radix Glycyrrhizae (*Sheng Gan Cao*) and uncooked Honey (*Sheng Feng Mi*) as in *Gua Lou Jian* (Trichosanthes Decoction [119])

2. With uncooked Radix Glycyrrhizae (*Sheng Gan Cao*) as in *Fa Sheng San* (Emit the Voice Powder [102])

Dosage: 10-15g and up to 30g in severe cases

Addendum: Honey mix-fried Pericarpium Trichosanthis (*Mi Zhi Gua Lou Pi*) is sometimes prescribed in case of a dry cough due to lung yin vacuity with yellowish but scanty phlegm, difficult to expectorate.

Stir-fried [till] Scorched (Chao Jiao)

Names: *Chao Gua Lou Pi, Chao Lou Pi*

Flavors & nature: Sweet and bitter; cold tending to neutral

Functions: Loosens the chest, moves the qi, dispels phlegm

Indications:

1. Chest pain (*xiong bi*) due to accumulation of phlegm dampness in the lungs and chest yang deficiency with chest oppression and pain, cough with whitish mucus, dyspnea, asthmatic breathing...

2. With heart pain (*xiong bi*) due to heart blood stasis with chest pain radiating to the back or left arm, a purple tongue, a choppy (*se*) pulse...

Typical combinations:

1. With Bulbus Allii Macrostemi (*Xie Bai*), clear Rhizoma Pinelliae Ternatae (*Qing Ban Xia*), uncooked Cortex Magnoliae Officinalis (*Sheng Hou Po*), stir-fried Semen Sinapis Albae (*Chao Bai Jie Zi*), and uncooked Radix Asteris Tatarici (*Sheng Zi Wan*)

2. With Bulbus Allii Macrostemi (*Xie Bai*), Radix Pseudoginseng (*San Qi*), uncooked Pollen Typhae (*Sheng Pu Huang*), Flos Carthami Tinctorii (*Hong Hua*), stir-fried Resina Olibani (*Chao Ru Xiang*), and wine[-processed] Radix Salviae Miltiorrhizae (*Jiu Dan Shen*)

Dosage: 10-15g and up to 30g in severe cases

Semen Trichosanthis Kirlowii (*Gua Lou Ren*)

Uncooked (*Sheng*)

Names: *Gua Lou Zi, Gua Lou Ren*

Flavors & nature: Sweet and slightly bitter; cold

Functions: Clears the lungs, moistens the large intestine, frees the stool

Indications:

1. Constipation due to A) lung heat transmitted to the large intestine and which dries the fluids of the latter with dry, hard stools, cough, shortness of breath; B) dryness of the large intestine; or C) blood vacuity

2. Chronic appendicitis with constipation due to accumulation of heat and blood stasis in the intestines with hard stools, pain in the lower abdomen...

Typical combinations:

1. A) With uncooked Semen Pruni Armeniacae (*Sheng Xing Ren*), uncooked Rhizoma Anemarrhenae (*Sheng Zhi Mu*), and uncooked Honey (*Sheng Feng Mi*)
B) With Radix Scrophulariae Ningpoensis (*Xuan Shen*), Tuber Asparagi Cochinensis (*Tian Men Dong*), uncooked Radix Rehmanniae (*Sheng Di Huang*), and uncooked Tuber Ophiopogonis Japonicae (*Sheng Mai Men Dong*)
C) With uncooked Radix Polygoni Multiflori (*Sheng He Shou Wu*), uncooked Radix Angelicae Sinensis (*Sheng Dang Gui*), and stir-fried Semen Pruni Persicae (*Chao Tao Ren*)

2. With uncooked Cortex Radicis Moutan (*Sheng Mu Dan Pi*), uncooked Radix Et Rhizoma Rhei (*Sheng Da Huang*), and uncooked Semen Benincasae Hispidae (*Sheng Dong Gua Ren*)

Dosage: 12-30g

Stir-fried [till] Scorched (*Chao Jiao*)

Names: *Chao Gua Lou Ren, Chao Gua Lou Zi*

Flavors & nature: Sweet and slightly bitter; cold tending to neutral

Functions: Rectifies the lungs, dispels phlegm

Indications: Cough, asthma, due to 1) accumulation of phlegm heat in the lungs with dyspnea, yellow, thick, sticky mucus; 2) accumulation of phlegm dampness in the lungs with white, abundant mucus; 3) lung yin vacuity but accompanied by weakness of the spleen[1] with loose stools, lack of appetite, scanty phlegm, a dry cough, dry throat; or 4) phlegm dryness

Typical combinations:

1. With honey mix-fried Cortex Radicis Mori Albi (*Mi Zhi Sang Bai Pi*), bile[-processed] Rhizoma Arisaematis (*Dan Nan Xing*), and uncooked Semen Pruni Armeniacae (*Sheng Xing Ren*)

2. With clear Rhizoma Pinelliae Ternatae (*Qing Ban Xia*), stir-fried Semen Sinapis Albae (*Chao Bai Jie Zi*), uncooked Radix Asteris Tatarici (*Sheng Zi Wan*), and stir-fried Flos Tussilaginis Farfarae (*Chao Kuan Dong Hua*)

3. With uncooked Tuber Ophiopogonis Japonicae (*Sheng Mai Men Dong*), honey mix-fried Radix Adenophorae Strictae (*Mi Zhi Nan Sha Shen*), uncooked Radix Dioscoreae Oppositae (*Sheng Shan Yao*), and stir-fried Semen Dolichoris Lablab (*Chao Bai Bian Dou*)

4. With Bulbus Fritillariae Cirrhosae (*Chuan Bei Mu*), honey mix-fried Radix Platycodi Grandiflori (*Mi Zhi Jie Geng*), honey mix-fried Flos Tussilaginis Farfarae (*Mi Zhi Kuan Dong Hua*), and honey mix-fried Radix Adenophorae Strictae (*Mi Zhi Nan Sha Shen*)

Dosage: 10-30g

Semen Trichosanthis Kirlowii continued . . .

Note: 1. In this case, defatted Semen Trichosanthis (*Gua Lou Ren Shuang*) is often prescribed. This refers to *Gua Lou Ren* which has been rid of its fatty body.

Thus, *Gua Lou Ren Shuang* is always beneficial for the lungs without being moistening to the large intestine or spleen. This preparation is systematically used when the spleen and stomach's function of transportation and transformation is deficient.

Pumice *(Hai Fu Shi)*

Uncooked *(Sheng)*

Names: *Fu Hai Shi, Hai Fu Shi, Sheng Hai Shi, Sheng Fu Shi*

Flavors & nature: Salty; cold

Functions: Clears the lungs, transforms phlegm, opens strangury

Indications:

1. Cough due to lung heat and accumulation of phlegm heat in the lungs with chest oppression, shortness of breath, expectoration of thick, yellowish phlegm which is difficult to expectorate...

2. Hemoptysis due to fire damaging the network vessels of the lungs with cough, phlegm streaked with blood, chest pain and oppression, vexation...

3. Strangury with hematuria (*xue lin*) or with lithiasis (*shi lin*) due to damp heat in the bladder with urodynia, dysuria, urgent but scanty urination, reddish urine with blood clots or gravel...

4. Thirst due to lung or stomach heat damaging fluids

Typical combinations:

1. With wine[-processed] Radix Scutellariae Baicalensis (*Jiu Huang Qin*), bile[-processed] Rhizoma Arisaematis (*Dan Nan Xing*), Bulbus Fritillariae Thunbergii (*Zhe Bei Mu*), and uncooked Radix Peucedani (*Sheng Qian Hu*)

2. With Pulvis Indigonis (*Qing Dai*), uncooked Fructus Gardeniae Jasminoidis (*Sheng Shan Zhi Zi*), and stir-fried Semen Trichosanthis Kirlowii (*Chao Gua Lou Ren*) as in *Ke Xue Fang* (Coughing Blood Formula [194])

3. With Spora Lygodii (*Hai Jin Sha*), Folium Pyrrosiae (*Shi Wei*), uncooked Pollen Typhae (*Sheng Pu Huang*), and carbonized Herba Cephalanoploris Segeti (*Xiao Ji Tan*)

4. With Radix Trichosanthis Kirlowii (*Tian Hua Fen*), Rhizoma Phragmitis Communis (*Lu Gen*), and uncooked Rhizoma Polygonati Odorati (*Sheng Yu Zhu*)

Dosage: 5-15g and up to 30g in severe cases

Calcined *(Duan)*

Names: *Duan Fu Hai Shi, Duan Hai Fu Shi, Duan Hai Shi, Duan Fu Shi*

Flavors & nature: Salty; neutral

Functions: Softens nodulations, scatters nodulations

Indications:

1. Subcutaneous nodules, scrofula, goiter due to phlegm stagnating in the network vessels of the neck and throat...

2. Bone pain and swelling due to stagnation of

Pumice continued . . .

phlegm dampness and blood stasis in the joints with loss of mobility...

Typical combinations:

1. With Radix Scrophulariae Ningpoensis (*Xuan Shen*), Herba Sargassii (*Hai Zao*), and Thallus Algae (*Kun Bu*)

2. With uncooked Rhizoma Atractylodis (*Sheng Cang Zhu*), Lumbricus (*Di Long*), wine[-processed] Radix Clematidis Chinensis (*Jiu Wei Ling Xian*), Flos Carthami Tinctorii (*Hong Hua*), and stir-fried Semen Sinapis Albae (*Chao Bai Jie Zi*)

Dosage: 5-15g and up to 30g in severe cases

Concha Cyclinae *(Hai Ge Ke)*

_____ Uncooked *(Sheng)* _____

Names: *Sheng Ge Ke, Ge Ke, Hai Ge Ke*

Flavors & nature: Bitter and salty; cold

Functions: Clears the lungs, transforms phlegm, softens the hard, scatters nodulations, disinhibits urination

Indications:

1. Cough, asthma due to either A) heat and phlegm heat in the lungs with chest oppression, expectoration of thick, sticky, yellow phlegm or B) liver fire steaming the lungs with cough causing pain in the lungs and lateral costal region, blood-streaked phlegm or hemoptysis, irritability...

2. Subcutaneous nodules, scrofula due to stagnation of phlegm in the network vessels of the neck and throat...

3. Goiter due to stagnation of qi and phlegm

4. Edema due to accumulation of internal damp

heat with edema of the limbs and body, oliguria, fever...

Typical combinations:

1. A) With stir-fried Semen Trichosanthis Kirlowii (*Chao Gua Lou Ren*) as in *Hai Ge Wan* (Concha Cyclinae Pills [131])
B) With Pulvis Indigonis (*Qing Dai*) as in *Dai Ge San* (Indigo & Clam Shell Powder [71])

2. With uncooked Concha Ostreae (*Sheng Mu Li*), Herba Sargassii (*Hai Zao*), and Bulbus Fritillariae Thunbergii (*Zhe Bei Mu*) as in *Hua Jian Wan* (Transform the Hard Pills [148])

3. With Herba Sargassii (*Hai Zao*) and Herba Zosterae Marinae (*Hai Dai*) as in *Si Hai Shu Yu Wan* (Four Seas Soothe Depression Pills [309])

4. With Caulis Akebiae Mutong (*Mu Tong*) and uncooked Rhizoma Alismatis (*Sheng Ze Xie*) as in *Hai Ge Tang* (Concha Cyclinae Decoction [130])

Dosage: 10-15g

_____ Calcined *(Duan)* _____

Names: *Duan Ge Ke, Duan Hai Ge Ke*

Flavors & nature: Slightly bitter and slightly salty; neutral

Functions: Stops abnormal vaginal discharge, transforms turbidity, stops stomach acidity, stops pain, promotes the healing of sores

Concha Cyclinae continued . . .

Indications:

1. Abnormal vaginal discharge due to either A) damp heat in the lower burner with yellowish, thick, malodorous discharge or B) damp heat in the lower burner with reddish discharge...

2. Stomach acidity and pain due to disharmony of the liver and stomach with vomiting or acid regurgitation...

3. Skin ulcers, eczema, aphthae which are chronic and will not heal over...

Typical combinations:

1. A) With uncooked Cortex Phellodendri (*Sheng Huang Bai*), uncooked Cortex Ailanthi Altissimi (*Sheng Chun Gen Pi*), uncooked Rhizoma Alismatis (*Sheng Ze Xie*), and Rhizoma Smilacis Glabrae (*Tu Fu Ling*)
B) With uncooked Cortex Phellodendri (*Sheng Huang Bai*), uncooked Radix Rubrus Paeoniae Lactiflorae (*Sheng Chi Shao Yao*), and carbonized Radix Rubiae Cordifoliae (*Qian Cao Gen Tan*)

2. With calcined Concha Arcae (*Duan Wu Leng Zi*), uncooked Radix Glycyrrhizae (*Sheng Gan Cao*), uncooked Os Sepiae Seu Sepiellae (*Sheng Hai Piao Xiao*), and stir-fried Pericarpium Citri Reticulatae (*Chao Chen Pi*)

3. With uncooked Cortex Phellodendri (*Sheng Huang Bai*), calcined Gypsum Fibrosum (*Duan Shi Gao*), and Calomelas (*Qing Fen*). Reduce these four substances to powder and apply locally.

Dosage: 10-20g

Radix Platycodi Grandiflori *(Jie Geng)*

Uncooked *(Sheng)*

Names: *Jie Geng, Bai Jie Geng, Ku Jie Geng*

Flavors & nature: Bitter and acrid; neutral

Functions: Diffuses the lungs, transforms phlegm

Indications:

1. Cough, asthma due to A) wind heat blocking the lungs with yellow mucus, pain and itching of the throat, fever, chills; B) wind cold blocking the lungs with whitish mucus, itching of the throat, headache, fever, chills; C) severe wind cold; or D) slightly severe wind cold

2. Sore throat A) of all types; B) due to wind heat; or C) due to heat toxins

Typical combinations:

1. A) With uncooked Folium Mori Albi (*Sheng Sang Ye*) as in *Sang Ju Yin* (Morus & Chrysanthemum Drink [276])
B) With uncooked Herba Schizonepetae Tenuifoliae (*Sheng Jing Jie*) and uncooked Radix Ledebouriellae Sesloidis (*Sheng Fang Feng*) as in *Jing Fang Bai Du San* (Schizonepeta & Ledebouriella Vanquish Toxins Powder [183])
C) With Herba Ephedrae (*Ma Huang*) and Semen Pruni Armeniacae (*Xing Ren*) as in *Wu Ao Tang* (Five [Ingredients] Unbinding Decoction [343])
D) With uncooked Radix Cynanchi Stautonii (*Sheng Bai Qian*) and steamed Radix Stemonae (*Zheng Bai Bu*)

2. A) With uncooked Radix Glycyrrhizae (*Sheng Gan Cao*) as in *Jie Geng Tang* (Platycodon Decoction [176])
B) With Fructificatio Lasiosphaerae (*Ma Bo*), Periostracum Cicadae (*Chan Tui*), and Rhizoma Belamcandae (*She Gan*) as in *Jia Jian Jing Fang Bai Du San* (Additions & Subtractions Schizo-

Radix Platycodi Grandiflori continued . . .

nepeta & Ledebouriella Vanquish Toxins Powder [168])
C) With Radix Isatidis Seu Baphicacanthi (*Ban Lan Gen*), Radix Sophorae Subprostratae (*Shan Dou Gen*), uncooked Flos Lonicerae Japonicae (*Sheng Jin Yin Hua*), and uncooked Fructus Forsythiae Suspensae (*Sheng Lian Qiao*)

Dosage: 5-15g and up to 30g in severe cases

Stir-fried (Chao)

Name: *Chao Jie Geng*

Flavors & nature: Bitter and slightly acrid; slightly warm

Functions: Rectifies the lungs, eliminates phlegm

Indications:

1. Cough, asthma due to either A) accumulation of phlegm cold in the lungs with thin, clear phlegm or B) accumulation of phlegm dampness in the lungs caused by spleen vacuity with whitish, abundant, and difficult to expectorate mucus, chest oppression, shortness of breath...

2. Chest pain (*xiong bi*) due to stagnation of phlegm in the lungs

Typical combinations:

1. A) with dry Rhizoma Zingiberis (*Gan Jiang*), honey mix-fried Herba Cum Radice Asari (*Mi Zhi Xi Xin*), uncooked Sclerotium Poriae Cocos (*Sheng Fu Ling*), uncooked Radix Asteris Tatarici (*Sheng Zi Wan*), and stir-fried Flos Tussilaginis Farfarae (*Chao Kuan Dong Hua*)
B) With lime-processed Rhizoma Pinelliae Ternatae (*Fa Ban Xia*), uncooked Pericarpium Citri Reticulatae (*Sheng Chen Pi*), uncooked Cortex Magnoliae Officinalis (*Sheng Hou Po*), stir-fried Semen Pruni Armeniacae (*Chao Xing Ren*), and uncooked Sclerotium Poriae Cocos (*Sheng Fu Ling*)

2. With honey mix-fried Fructus Citri Seu Ponciri (*Mi Zhi Zhi Ke*) and stir-fried Pericarpium Trichosanthis Kirlowii (*Chao Gua Lou Pi*)

Dosage: 5-15g

Honey Mix-fried (Mi Zhi)

Names: *Mi Zhi Jie Geng, Zhi Jie Geng*

Flavors & nature: Bitter, sweet, and slightly acrid; neutral; moistening

Functions: Moistens the lungs, eliminates phlegm, outthrusts pus

Indications:

1. Lung abscesses[1] due to either A) blood stasis and heat stagnating in the lungs with expectoration of purulent, bloody phlegm, chest pain and oppression or B) the same plus yin vacuity

2. Aphonia or dry cough due to either A) lung yin vacuity with little or no phlegm which is difficult to expectorate or B) lung/kidney yin vacuity

Typical combinations:

1. A) With Semen Coicis Lachryma-jobi (*Yi Yi Ren*), uncooked Semen Benincasae Hispidae (*Sheng Dong Gua Ren*), Rhizoma Phragmitis Communis (*Lu Gen*), scalded Semen Pruni Persicae (*Dan Tao Ren*), and Herba Houttuyniae Cordatae (*Yu Xing Cao*)
B) With the same as above plus Tuber Ophiopogonis Japonicae (*Mai Men Dong*) and Radix Trichosanthis Kirlowii (*Tian Hua Fen*)

2. A) With honey mix-fried Bulbus Lilii (*Mi Zhi Bai He*), Radix Scrophulariae Ningpoensis (*Xuan Shen*), uncooked Tuber Ophiopogonis Japonicae

Radix Platycodi Grandiflori continued . . .

(*Sheng Mai Men Dong*), and Bulbus Fritillariae Cirrhosae (*Chuan Bei Mu*)
B) With the same as above plus prepared Radix Rehmanniae (*Shu Di Huang*) and uncooked Radix Rehmanniae (*Sheng Di Huang*)

Dosage: 5-15g and up to 30g for lung abscesses

Note: 1. If heat is severe, uncooked Platycodon can be prescribed (*Sheng Jie Geng*). However, if dryness is important, honey mix-fried Platycodon is better indicated.

Radix Peucedani *(Qian Hu)*

————————— Uncooked *(Sheng)* —————————

Names: *Qian Hu, Sou Qian Hu, Fen Qian Hu*

Flavors & nature: Acrid and bitter; slightly cold

Functions: Dispels wind, transforms phlegm, downbears counterflow qi

Indications:

1. Cough due to A) wind heat attacking the lungs with itchy throat, nasal congestion, rhinorrhea, fever, slight aversion to wind and cold; B) wind cold attacking the lungs with thin, clear mucus, headache, nasal congestion, clear rhinorrhea, chills, fever; or C) lung heat with thick, sticky, yellow phlegm, chest oppression...

2. Measles, due to wind heat with skin eruptions which emit badly

Typical combinations:

1. A) With uncooked Radix Platycodi Grandiflori (*Sheng Jie Geng*), uncooked Folium Mori Albi (*Sheng Sang Ye*), and uncooked Fructus Arctii Lappae (*Sheng Niu Bang Zi*) as in *Gan Mao Re Ke Fang* (Common Cold Hot Cough Formula [110])
B) With uncooked Semen Pruni Armeniacae (*Sheng Xing Ren*) and Folium Perillae Frutescentis (*Zi Su Ye*) as in *Xing Su San* (Armeniaca & Perilla Powder [384])
C) With Bulbus Fritillariae Thunbergii (*Zhe Bei Mu*), honey mix-fried Cortex Radicis Mori Albi (*Mi Zhi Sang Bai Pi*), and uncooked Semen Pruni Armeniacae (*Sheng Xing Ren*) as in *Qian Hu San* (Peucedanum Powder [242])

2. With uncooked Rhizoma Cimicifugae (*Sheng Sheng Ma*), uncooked Radix Puerariae (*Sheng Ge Gen*), and uncooked Radix Ledebouriellae Sesloidis (*Sheng Fang Feng*) as in *Xuan Du Jie Biao Tang* (Diffuse Toxins & Resolve the Exterior Decoction [387])

Dosage: 5-10g and up to 20g in severe cases

————————— Stir-fried [till] Scorched *(Chao Jiao)* —————————

Name: *Chao Qian Hu*

Flavors & nature: Bitter and slightly acrid; tending to neutral

Functions: Downbears counterflow qi, dispels phlegm, stops cough

Indications: Cough due to 1) counterflow lung qi caused by stagnation of phlegm and qi in the

lungs, 2) the same as above plus evil cold in the lungs, or 3) the same as 1 above plus evil heat in the lungs

Typical combinations:

1. With stir-fried Fructus Perillae Frutescentis (*Chao Zi Su Zi*), uncooked Semen Pruni Armeniacae (*Sheng Xing Ren*), uncooked Cortex Magnoliae Officinalis (*Sheng Hou Po*), uncooked Peri-

Radix Peucedani continued . . .

carpium Citri Reticulatae (*Sheng Chen Pi*), and clear Rhizoma Pinelliae Ternatae (*Qing Ban Xia*)

2. Same as above plus stir-fried Ramulus Cinnamomi (*Chao Gui Zhi*) and uncooked Radix Asteris Tatarici (*Sheng Zi Wan*)

3. Same as 1 above plus wine[-processed] Radix Scutellariae Baicalensis (*Jiu Huang Qin*) and honey mix-fried Cortex Radicis Mori Albi (*Mi Zhi Sang Bai Pi*)

Dosage: 5-10g and up to 20g in severe cases

_____Honey Mix-fried *(Mi Zhi)*_____

Names: *Mi Zhi Qian Hu, Zhi Qian Hu*

Flavors & nature: Bitter, sweet, and slightly acrid; slightly cold

Functions: Moistens the lungs, eliminates phlegm, downbears counterflow qi

Indications: Dry cough due to warm dryness damaging the lungs with yellow phlegm, a dry throat, shortness of breath, chest oppression...

Typical combinations: With honey mix-fried Radix Adenophorae Strictae (*Mi Zhi Nan Sha Shen*), stir-fried Semen Trichosanthis Kirlowii (*Chao Gua Lou Ren*), uncooked Tuber Ophiopogonis Japonicae (*Sheng Mai Men Dong*), honey mix-fried Flos Tussilaginis Farfarae (*Mi Zhi Kuan Dong Hua*), honey mix-fried Cortex Radicis Mori Albi (*Mi Zhi Sang Bai Pi*), and Bulbus Fritillariae Cirrhosae (*Chuan Bei Mu*)

Dosage: 6-12g and up to 20g in severe cases

Addendum: Radix Peucedani (*Qian Hu*) and Radix Cynanchi Stautonii (*Bai Qian*) have a similar action. They are often combined in prescriptions and form a pair called *Er Qian*, the two *Qian*.

Semen Lepidii *(Ting Li Zi)*

_____ Uncooked *(Sheng)*_____

Names: *Ting Li Zi, Sheng Ting Li, Gan Ting Li*

Flavors & nature: Acrid and bitter; very cold

Functions: Drains the lungs, disinhibits urination, expels water, disperses swelling

Indications:

1. Hydrothorax or pleural effusion due to accumulation of fluids in the chest with chest pain and distention

2. Ascites due to accumulation of fluids in the abdomen with abdominal distention, oliguria, dysuria, constipation...

3. Generalized edema due to accumulation of dampness with oliguria, dysuria...

Typical combinations:

1. With vinegar[-processed] Radix Euphorbiae Kansui (*Cu Gan Sui*), prepared Radix Et Rhizoma Rhei (*Shu Da Huang*), and Mirabilitum (*Mang Xiao*) as in *Da Xian Xiong Wan* (Great Fell [*i.e.*, Drain] the Chest Pills [69])

2. With prepared Radix Et Rhizoma Rhei (*Shu Da Huang*), Radix Stephaniae Tetrandrae (*Fang Ji*), and Semen Zanthoxyli Bungeani (*Jiao Mu*) as in *Ji Jiao Li Huang Wan* (Stephania, Zanthoxylum, Lepidium & Rhubarb Pills [166])

Semen Lepidii continued . . .

3. With Cortex Sclerotii Poriae Cocos (*Fu Ling Pi*), uncooked Cortex Radicis Mori Albi (*Sheng Sang Bai Pi*), and uncooked Rhizoma Atractylodis Macrocephalae (*Sheng Bai Zhu*) as in *Ting Li Zi San* (Lepidium Powder [328])

Dosage: 3-10g and up to 15g in severe cases

Addendum: Since the action of Lepidium is drastic, in clinical practice it is counseled to use it with Fructus Zizyphi Jujubae (*Da Zao*), which helps protect the stomach.

_____Stir-fried [till] Scorched *(Chao Jiao)*_____

Names: *Chao Ting Li, Chao Gan Ting Li*

Flavors & nature: Bitter and slightly acrid; cold

Functions: Rectifies the lungs, drains the lungs, calms dyspnea

Indications:

1. Lung abscesses due to stagnation of heat in the lungs with expectoration of pus, asthmatic breathing...

2. Asthma, cough[1] due to accumulation of phlegm heat in the lungs

Typical combinations:

1. With Fructus Zizyphi Jujubae (*Da Zao*) as in *Ting Li Zi Da Zao Xie Fei Tang* (Lepidium & Red Dates Drain the Lungs Decoction [327a])

2. With uncooked Pericarpium Trichosanthis Kirlowii (*Sheng Gua Lou Pi*), honey mix-fried Cortex Radicis Mori Albi (*Mi Zhi Sang Bai Pi*), Bulbus Fritillariae Thunbergii (*Zhe Bei Mu*), and wine[-processed] Radix Scutellariae Baicalensis (*Jiu Huang Qin*)

Dosage: 6-12g

Note: 1. In case of cough due to lung qi vacuity or lung yin vacuity, honey mix-fried Lepidium (*Mi Zhi Ting Li Zi*) is sometimes used.

Addendum: There are two types of *Ting Li Zi. Tian Ting Li* or sweet Lepidium's draining action is moderate. It drains the lungs without damaging the stomach. *Ku Ting Li* or bitter Lepidium's draining action is more powerful. It drains the lungs but damages the stomach. In order to avoid this side effect, *Ku Ting Li* is combined with Red Dates in order to protect the middle burner while still benefitting from the performance of its action.

Caulis In Taeniis Bambusae *(Zhu Ru)*

_____Uncooked *(Sheng)*_____

Names: *Gan Zhu Ru, Dan Zhu Ru, Zhu Er Qing, Zhu Ru*

Flavors & nature: Sweet; slightly cold

Functions: Clears the lungs, transforms phlegm

Indications:

1. Cough due to accumulation of phlegm heat in the lungs with fever, dry mouth, agitation, chest oppression, yellow mucus...

2. Hemoptysis due to heat with cough, blood-streaked phlegm...

3. Apoplexy due to wind stroke (*zhong feng*) set in motion by wind phlegm with loss of consciousness, stertorous breathing...

Caulis In Taeniis Bambusae continued . . .

Typical combinations:

1. With Bulbus Fritillariae Thunbergii (*Zhe Bei Mu*), stir-fried Semen Lepidii (*Chao Ting Li Zi*), wine[-processed] Radix Scutellariae Baicalensis (*Jiu Huang Qin*), and Rhizoma Phragmitis Communis (*Lu Gen*)

2. With carbonized Fructus Gardeniae Jasminoidis (*Zhi Zi Tan*), uncooked Rhizoma Imperatae Cylin-dricae (*Sheng Bai Mao Gen*), wine mix-fried Radix Scutellariae Baicalensis (*Jiu Zhi Huang Qin*), and Rhizoma Bletillae Striatae (*Bai Ji*)

3. With bile[-processed] Rhizoma Arisaematis (*Dan Nan Xing*), Rhizoma Acori Graminei (*Shi Chang Pu*), and clear Rhizoma Pinelliae Ternatae (*Qing Ban Xia*) as in *Di Tan Tang* (Scour Phlegm Decoction [85])

Dosage: 5-10g and up to 60g in severe cases

Ginger Mix-fried (*Jiang Zhi*)

Names: *Jiang Zhi Zhu Ru, Jiang Zhu Ru*

Flavors & nature: Sweet and acrid; cool tending to neutral

Functions: Harmonizes the stomach, clears the stomach, stops vomiting

Indications:

1. Nausea, vomiting due to A) stomach qi vacuity following qi counterflow accompanied by heat with eructation, regurgitation; B) heat in the stomach with regurgitation, thirst; or C) accumulation of damp heat in the stomach with chest, epigastric, and abdominal oppression and distention, a thick yellow, slimy tongue coating...

2. Nausea or vomiting during pregnancy due to disharmony of the stomach with chest and epigastric oppression and distention, vomiting in the morning or after meals, loss of appetite...

3. Insomnia, heart palpitations due to disharmony between the gallbladder and stomach accompanied by accumulation of phlegm heat with vertigo, chest distention, anxiety, a bitter taste in the mouth...

Typical combinations:

1. A) With Radix Panacis Ginseng (*Ren Shen*), stir-fried Pericarpium Citri Reticulatae (*Chao Chen Pi*), and uncooked Rhizoma Zingiberis (*Sheng Jiang*) as in *Ju Pi Zhu Ru Tang* (Orange Peel & Caulis Bambusae Decoction [191])
B) With uncooked Gypsum Fibrosum (*Sheng Shi Gao*), Folium Lophatheri Gracilis (*Dan Zhu Ye*), and Rhizoma Phragmitis Communis (*Lu Gen*)
C) With ginger[-processed] Rhizoma Coptidis Chinensis (*Jiang Huang Lian*) and ginger[-processed] Rhizoma Pinelliae Ternatae (*Jiang Ban Xia*)

2. With ginger[-processed] Radix Scutellariae Baicalensis (*Jiang Huang Qin*), bran stir-fried Rhizoma Atractylodis Macrocephalae (*Fu Chao Bai Zhu*), and Caulis Perillae Frutescentis (*Zi Su Geng*)

3. With uncooked Fructus Immaturus Citri Seu Ponciri (*Sheng Zhi Shi*), stir-fried Pericarpium Citri Reticulatae (*Chao Chen Pi*), and clear Rhizoma Pinelliae Ternatae (*Qing Ban Xia*) as in *Wen Dan Tang* (Warm the Gallbladder Decoction [340])

Dosage: 5-10g and up to 60g in severe cases

14
Cough-stopping, Dyspnea-calming Medicinals

Radix Stemonae (Bai Bu)

Uncooked (Sheng)

Name: *Sheng Bai Bu*

Flavors & nature: Sweet and bitter; slightly warm

Functions: Kills parasites, destroys lice

Indications:

1. Pinworms

2. Lice. It eliminates the entirety of lice and fleas.

3. Mycoses

4. Genital itching due to damp heat in the lower burner

Typical combinations:

1. Anal injection of 10-20ml of a decoction of

Stemonae for 5 days. (Decoction: 30g to 1/2 liter of water). Make an ointment with powdered uncooked Stemona and uncooked Semen Arecae Catechu (*Sheng Bing Lang*) and apply to the anus.

2. Soak 100g of Stemona in 500ml of alcohol for 2-3 days. Apply locally.

3. With Cortex Radicis Dictamni (*Bai Xian Pi*), uncooked Cortex Phellodendri (*Sheng Huang Bai*), and Realgar (*Xiong Huang*) as in *Bai Bu Gao* (Stemona Paste [6])

4. Wash locally with a decoction of Stemona, Radix Sophorae Flavescentis (*Ku Shen*), and Fructus Cnidii Monnieri (*She Chuang Zi*).

Dosage: 6-12g in decoction

Steamed (Zheng)

Name: *Zheng Bai Bu*

Flavors & nature: Sweet and bitter; warm

Functions: Warms the lungs, stops cough

Indications: Cough due to 1) wind cold blocking the lungs with whitish mucus or 2) phlegm cold with paroxysmal cough, difficult expectoration...

Typical combinations:

1. With uncooked Herba Ephedrae (*Sheng Ma*

Huang), uncooked Semen Pruni Armeniacae (*Sheng Xing Ren*), and uncooked Radix Glycyrrhizae (*Sheng Gan Cao*) as in *Bai Bu Wan* (Stemona Pills [9])

2. With uncooked Radix Asteris Tatarici (*Sheng Zi Wan*) and stir-fried Radix Cynanchi Stautonii (*Chao Bai Qian*) as in *Zhi Sou San* (Stop Coughing Powder [437])

Dosage: 6-12g and up to 30g in severe cases

_____Honey Mix-fried *(Mi Zhi)* _____

Names: *Mi Zhi Bai Bu, Zhi Bai Bu*

Flavors & nature: Sweet and slightly bitter; slightly moistening; slightly warm

Functions: Moistens the lungs, stops cough

Indications:

1. Cough due to lung yin vacuity, dry cough, little or no phlegm, phlegm streaked with blood, evening fever, night sweats...

2. Pertussis, paroxysmal cough in infants due to lung dryness (often due to yin vacuity accompanied by qi vacuity) with paroxysmal, spasmodic cough like a cock's crow

Typical combinations:

1. With uncooked Tuber Ophiopogonis Japonicae (*Sheng Mai Men Dong*), honey mix-fried Radix Adenophorae Strictae (*Mi Zhi Nan Sha Shen*), and honey mix-fried Bulbus Lilii (*Mi Zhi Bai He*) as in *Bai Bu Tang* (Stemona Decoction [8])

2. With honey mix-fried Radix Cynanchi Stautonii (*Mi Zhi Bai Qian*), honey mix-fried Radix Asteris Tatarici (*Mi Zhi Zi Wan*), honey mix-fried Radix Adenophorae Strictae (*Mi Zhi Nan Sha Shen*), and honey mix-fried Radix Astragali Membranacei (*Mi Zhi Huang Qi*) as in *Bai Bu Jian* (Stemona Decoction [7])

Dosage: 8-15g and up to 30g in severe cases

Flos Tussilaginis Farfarae *(Kuan Dong Hua)*

_____ Uncooked *(Sheng)* _____

Names: *Sheng Kuan Dong Hua, Sheng Dong Hua*

Flavors & nature: Acrid; warm

Functions: Scatters cold, stops cough

Indications: Cough, asthma due to 1) wind cold and accumulation of phlegm rheum with stertorous breathing, thin, clear mucus, fever, chills; 2) external cold penetrating the lungs with incessant cough; or 3) external heat penetrating the lungs

Typical combinations:

1. With Rhizoma Belamcandae (*She Gan*), uncooked Radix Asteris Tatarici (*Sheng Zi Wan*), and uncooked Herba Ephedrae (*Sheng Ma Huang*) as in *She Gan Ma Huang Tang* (Belamcanda & Ephedra Decoction [287])

2. With honey mix-fried Herba Cum Radice Asari (*Mi Zhi Xi Xin*), uncooked Radix Asteris Tatarici (*Sheng Zi Wan*), and uncooked Semen Pruni Armeniacae (*Sheng Xing Ren*) as in *Zi Wan San* (Aster Powder [1; 448])

3. With honey mix-fried Cortex Radicis Mori Albi (*Mi Zhi Sang Bai Pi*), uncooked Semen Pruni Armeniacae (*Sheng Xing Ren*), and uncooked Rhizoma Anemarrhenae (*Sheng Zhi Mu*) as in *Kuan Dong Hua Tang* (Tussilago Decoction [195a])

Dosage: 5-10g and up to 20g in severe cases

Flos Tussilaginis Farfarae continued . . .

_____Stir-fried [till] Scorched (Chao Jiao)_____

Names: _Chao Kuan Dong Hua, Chao Dong Hua_

Flavors & nature: Slightly acrid; warm; drying

Functions: Warms the lungs, stops cough

Indications: Cough due to 1) phlegm cold or 2) phlegm dampness

Typical combinations:

1. With processed Rhizoma Typhonii (_Zhi Bai Fu Zi_), honey mix-fried Flos Inulae (_Mi Zhi Xuan Fu Hua_), stir-fried Radix Cynanchi Stautonii (_Chao Bai Qian_), dry Rhizoma Zingiberis (_Gan Jiang_), and wine-steamed Fructus Schizandrae Chinensis (_Jiu Zheng Wu Wei Zi_)

2. With clear Rhizoma Pinelliae Ternatae (_Qing Ban Xia_), uncooked Pericarpium Citri Reticulatae (_Sheng Chen Pi_), and uncooked Sclerotium Poriae Cocos (_Sheng Fu Ling_)

Dosage: 5-10g and up to 20g in severe cases

_____ Honey Mix-fried (Mi Zhi)_____

Names: _Mi Zhi Kuan Dong Hua, Zhi Kuan Dong Hua_

Flavors & nature: Slightly acrid and slightly sweet; warm; moistening

Functions: Moistens the lungs, stops cough

Indications:

1. Cough due to either A) lung qi vacuity with whitish mucus, weak cough, fatigue, shortness of breath, a pale complexion, spontaneous sweating or B) lung yin vacuity with scanty mucus, dry mouth and throat, dry cough, possible night sweats, evening fever...

2. Hemoptysis due to lung yin vacuity with chronic dry cough, phlegm streaked with blood, a dry mouth and throat, heat in the chest, evening fever, night sweats...

Typical combinations:

1. A) With uncooked Radix Astragali Membranacei (_Sheng Huang Qi_), Radix Panacis Ginseng (_Ren Shen_), uncooked Radix Asteris Tatarici (_Sheng Zi Wan_), and uncooked Fructus Schizandrae Chinensis (_Sheng Wu Wei Zi_)
B) With uncooked Tuber Ophiopogonis Japonicae (_Sheng Mai Men Dong_), uncooked Rhizoma Anemarrhenae (_Sheng Zhi Mu_), honey mix-fried Bulbus Lilii (_Mi Zhi Bai He_), honey mix-fried Radix Adenophorae Strictae (_Mi Zhi Nan Sha Shen_), and Bulbus Fritillariae Cirrhosae (_Chuan Bei Mu_)

2. With honey mix-fried Bulbus Lilii (_Mi Zhi Bai He_), uncooked Tuber Ophiopogonis Japonicae (_Sheng Mai Men Dong_), Pollen Typhae stir-fried Gelatinum Corii Asini (_Pu Huang Chao E Jiao_), uncooked Rhizoma Anemarrhenae (_Sheng Zhi Mu_), uncooked Pumice (_Sheng Hai Fu Shi_), and honey mix-fried Fructus Aristolochiae (_Mi Zhi Ma Dou Ling_)

Dosage: 8-15g and up to 25g in severe cases

Fructus Aristolochiae (Ma Dou Ling)

Uncooked (Sheng)

Names: *Ma Dou Ling, Sheng Ma Dou Ling*

Flavors & nature: Bitter and slightly acrid; cold

Functions: Clears the lungs, stops cough, calms dyspnea, treats hemorrhoids

Indications:

1. Asthma due to lung heat with yellow mucus, chest oppression...

2. Cough due to lung heat with sore throat, yellow mucus...

3. Bleeding hemorrhoids due to accumulation of heat in the large intestine with pain, swelling, and distention of the anus...

Typical combinations:

1. With honey mix-fried Cortex Radicis Mori Albi (*Mi Zhi Sang Bai Pi*) and stir-fried Semen Lepidii (*Chao Ting Li Zi*) as in *Ma Dou Ling Tang* (Aristolochia Decoction [212])

2. With uncooked Radix Platycodi Grandiflori (*Sheng Jie Geng*), wine[-processed] Radix Scutellariae Baicalensis (*Jiu Huang Qin*), Rhizoma Phragmitis Communis (*Lu Gen*), and Fructificatio Lasiosphaerae (*Ma Bo*)

3. Apply locally as a paste made from Aristolochia

Dosage: 3-10g and up to 15g in severe cases

Honey Mix-fried (Mi Zhi)

Names: *Mi Zhi Ma Dou Ling, Zhi Ma Dou Ling*

Flavors & nature: Bitter, slightly acrid, and slightly sweet; cold

Functions: Clears heat, moistens the lungs

Indications:

1. Dry cough due to lung yin vacuity accompanied by phlegm heat with scanty expectoration, dry throat, evening fever, night sweats...

2. Hemoptysis due to lung heat (vacuous or replete)...

3. Dyspnea, cough following measles due to heat dragging on with dry throat, insomnia, vexation...

Typical combinations:

1. With honey mix-fried Radix Adenophorae Strictae (*Mi Zhi Nan Sha Shen*), uncooked Tuber Ophiopogonis Japonicae (*Sheng Mai Men Dong*), honey mix-fried Radix Stemonae (*Mi Zhi Bai Bu*), honey mix-fried Bulbus Lilii (*Mi Zhi Bai He*), and Bulbus Fritillariae Cirrhosae (*Chuan Bei Mu*)

2. With Pollen Typhae stir-fried Gelatinum Corii Asini (*Pu Huang Chao E Jiao*) as in *Bu Fei E Jiao Tang* (Supplement the Lungs Donkey Skin Glue Decoction [32])

3. With Cortex Radicis Lycii (*Di Gu Pi*), honey mix-fried Folium Eriobotryae Japonicae (*Mi Zhi Pi Pa Ye*), honey mix-fried Radix Adenophorae Strictae (*Mi Zhi Nan Sha Shen*), uncooked Pumice (*Sheng Hai Fu Shi*), and uncooked Fructus Gardeniae Jasminoidis (*Sheng Shan Zhi Zi*)

Dosage: 6-12g and up to 20g in severe cases

Folium Eriobotryae Japonicae (Pi Pa Ye)

Uncooked (Sheng)

Names: *Pi Pa Ye, Sheng Pi Pa Ye*

Flavors & nature: Slightly bitter; slightly cold

Functions: Clears the lungs, downbears counterflow qi, stops cough

Indications:

1. Cough, dyspnea due to A) wind heat attacking the lungs, B) lung heat, or C) accumulation of phlegm heat in the lungs

2. Diphtheria due to heat toxins in the lungs with fever, chills, barking cough...

Typical combinations:

1. A) With uncooked Folium Mori Albi (*Sheng Sang Ye*), uncooked Radix Platycodi Grandiflori (*Sheng Jie Geng*), and uncooked Radix Peucedani (*Sheng Qian Hu*)

B) With uncooked Gypsum Fibrosum (*Sheng Shi Gao*), uncooked Rhizoma Anemarrhenae (*Sheng Zhi Mu*), wine[-processed] Radix Scutellariae Baicalensis (*Jiu Huang Qin*), and Rhizoma Phragmitis Communis (*Lu Gen*)

C) With uncooked Pericarpium Trichosanthis Kirlowii (*Sheng Gua Lou Pi*), Bulbus Fritillariae Thunbergii (*Zhe Bei Mu*), and stir-fried Semen Lepidii (*Chao Ting Li Zi*)

2. With uncooked Flos Lonicerae Japonicae (*Sheng Jin Yin Hua*), uncooked Folium Mori Albi (*Sheng Sang Ye*), Herba Menthae Haplocalycis (*Bo He*), and uncooked Radix Glycyrrhizae (*Sheng Gan Cao*) as in *Chu Wen Hua Du Tang* (Eliminate Warm [Disease] & Transform Toxins Decoction [49a])

Dosage: 6-12g and up to 60g in severe cases

Stir-fried [till] Scorched (Chao Jiao)

Name: *Chao Pi Pa Ye*

Flavors & nature: Slightly bitter; neutral

Functions: Harmonizes the stomach, stops vomiting

Indications: Nausea, vomiting[1] due to 1) stomach disharmony; 2) lung heat disturbing the stomach;[2] 3) stomach heat;[3] or 4) damp heat

Typical combinations:

1. With ginger[-processed] Rhizoma Pinelliae Ternatae (*Jiang Ban Xia*) and uncooked Rhizoma Zingiberis (*Sheng Jiang*)

2. With ginger[-processed] Caulis In Taeniis Bambusae (*Jiang Zhu Ru*) and Rhizoma Phragmitis Communis (*Lu Gen*)

3. With ginger[-processed] Rhizoma Coptidis Chinensis (*Jiang Huang Lian*), uncooked Rhizoma Imperatae Cylindricae (*Sheng Bai Mao Gen*), and uncooked Haematitum (*Sheng Dai Zhe Shi*)

4. With Radix Gentianae Scabrae (*Long Dan Cao*) and ginger[-processed] Rhizoma Coptidis Chinensis (*Jiang Huang Lian*)

Dosage: 6-12g and up to 60g in severe cases

Notes: 1. Ginger[-processed] Eriobotryae (*Jiang Zhi Pi Pa Ye*) can also be used. 2. If heat is important, uncooked Eriobotryae (*Sheng Pi Pa Ye*) can be prescribed. 3. If heat is important, uncooked Folium Eriobotryae may be prescribed.

Folium Eriobotryae Japonicae continued . . .

_____Honey Mix-fried *(Mi Zhi)*_____

Names: *Mi Zhi Pi Pa Ye, Zhi Pi Pa Ye*

Flavors & nature: Slightly bitter and slightly sweet; moistening; neutral

Functions: Moistens the lungs, stops cough

Indications: Cough due to either 1) lung dryness caused by attack of external heat or dryness with dry cough, little or no mucus, phlegm streaked with blood, a dry throat or 2) lung yin and qi vacuity with weak cough, shortness of breath, dry throat, fatigue, thirst...

Typical combinations:

1. With uncooked Tuber Ophiopogonis Japonicae (*Sheng Mai Men Dong*), Concha Cyclinae powder stir-fried Gelatinum Corii Asini (*Ge Fen Chao E Jiao*), and uncooked Semen Pruni Armeniacae (*Sheng Xing Ren*) as in *Qing Zao Jiu Fei Tang* (Clear Dryness & Rescue the Lungs Decoction [260])

2. With honey mix-fried Radix Astragali Membranacei (*Mi Zhi Huang Qi*), Radix Panacis Ginseng (*Ren Shen*), and uncooked Fructus Schizandrae Chinensis (*Sheng Wu Wei Zi*), honey mix-fried Radix Adenophorae Strictae (*Mi Zhi Nan Sha Shen*), and honey mix-fried Bulbus Lilii (*Mi Zhi Bai He*)

Dosage: 8-15g and up to 60g in severe cases

Cortex Radicis Mori Albi *(Sang Bai Pi)*

_____Uncooked *(Sheng)*_____

Names: *Sang Bai Pi, Sang Gen Pi, Sheng Sang Bai Pi*

Flavors & nature: Sweet; cold

Functions: Disinhibits urination; disperses swelling

Indications:

1. Edema due to A) accumulation of dampness with edema of the face, four limbs, chest and abdomen, dysuria; B) external wind (*feng shui*) with edema beginning in the eyelids and preponderant in the upper body, fever, chills; or C) damp heat with generalized edema, shiny skin, oliguria, fever, irritability, vexation...

2. Oliguria due to either A) damp heat or B) accumulation of dampness

Typical combinations:

1. A) With uncooked Cortex Rhizomatis Zingiberis (*Sheng Jiang Pi*), Cortex Sclerotii Poriae Cocos (*Fu Ling Pi*), and Pericarpium Arecae Catechu (*Da Fu Pi*) as in *Wu Pi San* (Five Peels Powder [351])
B) With uncooked Herba Ephedrae (*Sheng Ma Huang*), Herba Elsholtziae (*Xiang Ru*), Sclerotium Polypori Umbellati (*Zhu Ling*), and uncooked Rhizoma Alismatis (*Sheng Ze Xie*)
C) With salt[-processed] Semen Plantaginis (*Yan Che Qian Zi*), Talcum (*Hua Shi*), Radix Stephaniae Tetrandrae (*Fang Ji*), and Sclerotium Polypori Umbellati (*Zhu Ling*)

2. A) With uncooked Rhizoma Alismatis (*Sheng Ze Xie*), salt[-processed] Semen Plantaginis (*Yan Che Qian Zi*), and Sclerotium Polypori Umbellati (*Zhu Ling*)

Cortex Radicis Mori Albi continued . . .

B) With Cortex Sclerotii Poriae Cocos (*Fu Ling Pi*), Pericarpium Arecae Catechu (*Da Fu Pi*), and uncooked Cortex Rhizomatis Zingiberis (*Sheng Jiang Pi*)

Dosage: 5-15g and up to 30g in severe cases

_____**Honey Mix-fried** *(Mi Zhi)*_____

Names: *Mi Zhi Sang Bai Pi, Zhi Sang Bai Pi, Zhi Sang Gen Pi*

Flavors & nature: Sweet; cold; tends to be moistening

Functions: Moistens the lungs, clears heat, stops cough, calms dyspnea

Indications: Cough, asthma due to 1) lung heat;[1] lung heat with hemoptysis; 3) lung yin vacuity; or 4) stagnation of phlegm rheum in the lungs[1...]

Typical combinations:

1. With Cortex Radicis Lycii (*Di Gu Pi*) and uncooked Radix Glycyrrhizae (*Sheng Gan Cao*) as in *Xie Bai San* (Drain the White Powder [381])

2. With uncooked Rhizoma Imperatae Cylindricae (*Sheng Bai Mao Gen*) and carbonized Radix Rubiae Cordifoliae (*Qian Cao Gen Tan*)

3. With uncooked Tuber Ophiopogonis Japonicae (*Sheng Mai Men Dong*), honey mix-fried Tuber Asparagi Cochinensis (*Mi Zhi Tian Men Dong*), and honey mix-fried Radix Adenophorae Strictae (*Mi Zhi Nan Sha Shen*)

4. With honey mix-fried Herba Ephedrae (*Mi Zhi Ma Huang*), uncooked Semen Pruni Armeniacae (*Sheng Xing Ren*), and dry Rhizoma Zingiberis (*Gan Jiang*) as in *Sang Bai Pi Tang* (Cortex Mori Decoction [275])

Dosage: 8-20g and up to 30g in severe cases

Note: 1. For this indication, stir-fried [till] scorched Cortex Mori (*Chao Jiao Sang Bai Pi*) is often prescribed.

Semen Pruni Armeniacae *(Xing Ren)*

_____**Uncooked** *(Sheng)*[1]_____

Flavors & nature: Bitter; warm; slightly toxic

Functions: Diffuses lung qi, downbears counterflow qi, stops cough, moistens the intestines, frees the stools

Indications:

1. Cough, asthma due to A) wind cold with nasal congestion, chest oppression, thin, abundant phlegm; B) external cold which has transformed into heat with rapid breathing, fever, thirst; C) external dryness and coolness with fever, chills,

dry cough, dry mouth, throat, and nose, little or no mucus, or D) wind heat with fever, chills, sore throat, thirst, yellowish, thick mucus...

2. Constipation due to either A) large intestine dryness or blood vacuity or B) heat in the stomach and intestines

Typical combinations:

1. A) With uncooked Herba Ephedrae (*Sheng Ma Huang*) as in *San Ao Tang* (Three [Ingredients] Unbinding Decoction [271])

Semen Pruni Armeniacae continued . . .

B) With uncooked Gypsum Fibrosum (*Sheng Shi Gao*) as in *Ma Xing Shi Gan Tang* (Ephedra, Armeniaca, Gypsum & Licorice Decoction [216])

C) With Folium Perillae Frutescentis (*Zi Su Ye*) as in *Xing Su San* (Armeniaca & Perilla Powder [384])

D) With uncooked Folium Mori Albi (*Sheng Sang Ye*) as in *Sang Xing Tang* (Morus & Armeniaca Decoction [279])

2. A) With stir-fried Semen Cannabis Sativae (*Chao Huo Ma Ren*) and uncooked Radix Angelicae Sinensis (*Sheng Dang Gui*) as in *Run Chang Wan* (Moisten the Intestines Pills [269])

B) With uncooked Radix Et Rhizoma Rhei (*Sheng Da Huang*) as in *Ma Zi Ren Wan* (Cannabis Seed Pills [218])

Dosage: 5-10g. Overdosage is prohibited for babies and infants.

Note: 1. In fact, uncooked Armeniaca is rarely used. It is typically replaced by scalded Armeniaca (*Dan Xing Ren*) from which one has eliminated the superficial skin and the tip of the kernel in order to reduce its toxicity.

_____Stir-fried [till] Yellow *(Chao Huang)* _____

Names: *Chao Xing Ren, Chao Ku Xing Ren*

Flavors & nature: Bitter; warm; tends to be drying

Functions: Warms the lungs, scatters cold, stops cough

Indications: Cough due to either 1) phlegm cold accumulated in the lungs with shortness of breath, thin, clear mucus or 2) phlegm dampness accumulated in the lungs with white, abundant mucus...

Typical combinations:

1. With honey mix-fried Herba Cum Radice Asari (*Mi Zhi Xi Xin*), dry Rhizoma Zingiberis (*Gan Jiang*), wine-steamed Fructus Schizandrae Chinensis (*Jiu Zheng Wu Wei Zi*), stir-fried Flos Tussilaginis Farfarae (*Chao Kuan Dong Hua*), and uncooked Radix Asteris Tatarici (*Sheng Zi Wan*)

2. With lime-processed Rhizoma Pinelliae Ternatae (*Fa Ban Xia*), uncooked Sclerotium Poriae Cocos (*Sheng Fu Ling*), uncooked Pericarpium Citri Reticulatae (*Sheng Chen Pi*), uncooked Radix Asteris Tatarici (*Sheng Zi Wan*), uncooked Cortex Magnoliae Officinalis (*Sheng Hou Po*), and uncooked Fructus Perillae Frutescentis (*Sheng Zi Su Zi*)

Dosage: 5-10g and up to 20g in severe cases

_____Defatted *(Shuang)* _____

Names: *Xing Ren Shuang, Ku Xing Ren Shuang*

Flavors & nature: Bitter; warm

Functions: Downbears lung qi, stops cough

Indications: Cough due to either 1) spleen/lung qi vacuity with weak cough, whitish phlegm, fatigue, shortness of breath, spontaneous perspiration, a pale, wan complexion, loose stools, loss of appe-

tite or 2) spleen qi vacuity and lung yin vacuity with dry cough, little phlegm, dry mouth and throat, loose stools, fatigue...

Typical combinations:

1. With honey mix-fried Flos Tussilaginis Farfarae (*Mi Zhi Kuan Dong Hua*), honey mix-fried Radix Stemonae (*Mi Zhi Bai Bu*), honey mix-fried or uncooked Radix Astragali Membran-

Semen Pruni Armeniacae continued . . .

acei (*Mi Zhi* or *Sheng Huang Qi*), and honey mix-fried Radix Codonopsis Pilosulae (*Mi Zhi Dang Shen*)

2. With honey mix-fried Radix Adenophorae Strictae (*Mi Zhi Nan Sha Shen*), uncooked Tuber Ophiopogonis Japonicae (*Sheng Mai Men Dong*), honey mix-fried Bulbus Lilii (*Mi Zhi Bai He*), uncooked Radix Dioscoreae Oppositae (*Sheng Shan Yao*), and honey mix-fried Radix Astragali Membranacei (*Mi Zhi Huang Qi*)

Dosage: 3-8g

Addendum: There are two types of *Xing Ren*. *Ku Xing Ren* or bitter Armeniaca, also called *Bei Xing Ren*, northern Armeniaca, is most often prescribed in clinical practice. Its flavor is bitter and its nature is warm. Its property is descending and dispersing and it is toxic. It is favorably used for dyspnea or cough of the replete type (internal or external) and colds and flu accompanied by cough with very abundant mucus. *Tian Xing Ren*, sweet Armeniaca, or *Nan Xing Ren*, southern Armeniaca, is sweet in flavor, neutral in nature, and its property is moistening (lungs and large intestine). It is not toxic and can be favorably used for dyspnea and cough of the vacuity type and constipation of the dry type.

Fructus Perillae Frutescentis (*Zi Su Zi*)

────────── Uncooked (*Sheng*) ──────────

Names: *Sheng Su Zi, Sheng Zi Su Zi*

Flavors & nature: Acrid; warm

Functions: Eliminates phlegm, downbears qi, moistens the intestines, frees the stool

Indications:

1. Cough due to accumulation of phlegm dampness with chest oppression, abundant, thick, sticky phlegm, loss of appetite, possible nausea...

2. Constipation due to either A) qi stagnation with epigastric and abdominal distention or B) large intestine dryness with dry, hard stools...

Typical combinations:

1. With lime-processed Rhizoma Pinelliae Ternatae (*Fa Ban Xia*), uncooked Pericarpium Citri Reticulatae (*Sheng Chen Pi*), and uncooked Sclerotium Poriae Cocos (*Sheng Fu Ling*)

2. A) With stir-fried Semen Cannabis Sativae (*Chao Huo Ma Ren*), uncooked Fructus Citri Seu Ponciri (*Sheng Zhi Ke*), and ginger[-processed] Cortex Magnoliae Officinalis (*Jiang Hou Po*)
B) With uncooked Semen Biotae Orientalis (*Sheng Bai Zi Ren*), Semen Sesami Indici (*Hei Zhi Ma*), stir-fried Semen Cannabis Sativae (*Chao Huo Ma Ren*), and uncooked Radix Angelicae Sinensis (*Sheng Dang Gui*)

Dosage: 5-15g and up to 30g in severe cases

──────── Stir-fried [till] Scorched (*Chao Jiao*) ────────

Names: *Chao Su Zi, Chao Zi Su Zi, Zi Su Zi, Su Zi*

Flavors & nature: Slightly acrid; warm; drying

Functions: Warms the lungs, scatters cold, elimi-

nates phlegm, calms dyspnea

Indications: Cough, asthma due to either 1) phlegm cold accumulated in the lungs and spleen qi vacuity with thin, clear phlegm, chest and epi-

Fructus Perillae Frutescentis continued . . .

gastric oppression, loss of appetite or 2) phlegm accumulated in the lungs and kidney qi vacuity with abundant phlegm, dyspnea on exertion...

Typical combinations:

1. With stir-fried Semen Sinapis Albae (*Chao Bai Jie Zi*) and uncooked Semen Raphani Sativi

(*Sheng Lai Fu Zi*) as in *San Zi Yang Xin Tang* (Three Seeds Nourish the Aged Decoction [274])

2. With Cortex Cinnamomi (*Rou Gui*), uncooked Cortex Magnoliae Officinalis (*Sheng Hou Po*), and stir-fried Radix Peucedani (*Chao Qian Hu*) as in *Su Zi Jiang Qi Tang* (Perilla Seed Downbear Qi Decoction [316])

Dosage: 5-15g and up to 30g in severe cases

―――――――――――――――**Honey Mix-fried (Mi Zhi)**―――――――――――――――

Names: *Mi Zhi Su Zi, Zhi Su Zi*

Flavors & nature: Slightly acrid and slightly sweet; warm; moistening

Functions: Moistens the lungs, eliminates phlegm, downbears qi, calms dyspnea

Indications: Cough due to either 1) lung qi vacuity with shortness of breath, weak cough, fatigue, spontaneous perspiration or 2) lung yin vacuity with shortness of breath, dry cough, scant, sticky, difficult to expectorate phlegm, dry mouth and throat...

Typical combinations:

1. With uncooked Radix Astragali Membranacei (*Sheng Huang Qi*), uncooked Radix Dioscoreae Oppositae (*Sheng Shan Yao*), uncooked Radix Asteris Tatarici (*Sheng Zi Wan*), and honey mix-fried Flos Tussilaginis Farfarae (*Mi Zhi Kuan Dong Hua*)

2. With honey mix-fried Radix Adenophorae Strictae (*Mi Zhi Nan Sha Shen*), uncooked Tuber Ophiopogonis Japonicae (*Sheng Mai Men Dong*), Bulbus Fritillariae Cirrhosae (*Chuan Bei Mu*), honey mix-fried Radix Platycodi Grandiflori (*Mi Zhi Jie Geng*), and honey mix-fried Bulbus Lilii (*Mi Zhi Bai He*)

Dosage: 5-15g and up to 30g in severe cases

Radix Asteris Tatarici (*Zi Wan*)

―――――――――――――――**Uncooked (Sheng)**―――――――――――――――

Names: *Sheng Zi Wan, Zi Wan*

Flavors & nature: Acrid and bitter; warm

Functions: Scatters cold, eliminates phlegm

Indications: Cough due to either 1) wind cold with whitish mucus, fever, chills or 2) phlegm cold accumulated in the lungs with asthmatic breathing...[1]

Typical combinations:

1. With steamed Radix Stemonae (*Zheng Bai Bu*), uncooked Radix Cynanchi Stautonii (*Sheng Bai Qian*), and uncooked Herba Schizonepetae Tenuifoliae (*Sheng Jing Jie*) as in *Zhi Sou San* (Stop Cough Powder [437])

2. With honey mix-fried Herba Ephedrae (*Mi Zhi Ma Huang*), honey mix-fried Herba Cum Radice

Radix Asteris Tatarici continued . . .

Asari (*Mi Zhi Xi Xin*), and stir-fried Flos Tussilaginis Farfarae (*Chao Kuan Dong Hua*) as in *She Gan Ma Huang Tang* (Belamcanda & Ephedra Decoction [287])

Dosage: 5-12g and up to 30g in severe cases

Note: 1. For warming the lungs, stir-fried Perilla (*Chao Zi Su Zi*) can be used.

Honey Mix-fried (*Mi Zhi*)

Names: *Mi Zhi Zi Wan, Zhi Zi Wan*

Flavors & nature: Slightly acrid and slightly sweet; warm; moistening

Functions: Moistens the lungs, eliminates phlegm

Indications: Cough due to either 1) lung qi vacuity with shortness of breath, weak cough, fatigue, a pale, wan complexion, spontaneous perspiration or 2) lung yin vacuity with dry cough, dry mouth and throat, little or no phlegm, phlegm streaked with blood or hemoptysis...

Typical combinations:

1. With uncooked Radix Astragali Membranacei (*Sheng Huang Qi*), Radix Panacis Ginseng (*Ren Shen*), honey mix-fried Flos Tussilaginis Farfarae (*Mi Zhi Kuan Dong Hua*), and stir-fried Semen Pruni Armeniacae (*Chao Xing Ren*)

2. With uncooked Tuber Ophiopogonis Japonicae (*Sheng Mai Men Dong*), Concha Cyclinae powder stir-fried Gelatinum Corii Asini (*Ge Ke Fen E Jiao*), and Bulbus Fritillariae Cirrhosae (*Chuan Bei Mu*) as in *Zi Wan San* (Aster Powder [II; 449])

Dosage: 5-12g and up to 30g in severe cases

15
Spirit-quieting Medicinals

Semen Biotae Orientalis (Bai Zi Ren)

Uncooked (Sheng)

Names: *Bai Zi Ren, Sheng Bai Zi Ren, Sheng Bai Ren*

Flavors & nature: Sweet and slightly acrid; neutral

Functions: Moistens the intestines, frees the stool

Indications: Constipation due to 1) large intestine dryness, 2) blood vacuity, or 3) yin vacuity

Typical combinations:

1. With Semen Pini (*Song Zi Ren*), uncooked Semen Pruni Armeniacae (*Sheng Xing Ren*), and stir-fried Semen Pruni (*Chao Yu Li Ren*) as in *Wu Ren Wan* (Five Seeds Pills [353])

2. With uncooked Radix Angelicae Sinensis (*Sheng Dang Gui*), uncooked Radix Polygoni Multiflori (*Sheng He Shou Wu*), and Fructus Mori Albi (*Sang Shen*)

3. With uncooked Radix Rehmanniae (*Sheng Di Huang*), Radix Scrophulariae Ningpoensis (*Xuan Shen*), and Tuber Asparagi Cochinensis (*Tian Men Dong*)

Dosage: 5-10g and up to 20g in severe cases

Defatted (Shuang)[1]

Names: *Bai Zi Ren Shuang, Bai Zi Shuang, Bai Ren Shuang*

Flavors & nature: Sweet; neutral

Functions: Nourishes heart blood, quiets the spirit, enriches yin, stops perspiration

Indications:

1. Heart palpitations due to heart blood vacuity with insomnia, poor memory, agitation...

2. Insomnia, amnesia due to heart blood vacuity with agitation, abundant dreams, insomnia...

3. Night sweats due to A) yin vacuity, B) severe yin vacuity, or C) yin and qi vacuity

Typical combinations:

1. With uncooked Semen Zizyphi Spinosae (*Sheng Suan Zao Ren*) and uncooked Fructus Schizandrae Chinensis (*Sheng Wu Wei Zi*) as in *Yang Xin Tang* (Nourish the Heart Decoction [397])

2. With wine[-processed] Radix Angelicae Sinensis (*Jiu Dang Gui*), Rhizoma Acori Graminei (*Shi Chang Pu*), and Cinnabar[-processed] Sclerotium Pararadicis Poriae Cocos (*Zhu Sha Ban Fu Shen*) as in *Bai Zi Yang Xin Wan* (Biota Seed Nourish the Heart Pills [25])

Semen Biotae Orientalis continued . . .

3. A) With calcined Concha Ostreae (*Duan Mu Li*) and Radix Ephedrae (*Ma Huang Gen*) as in *Bai Zi Ren Wan* (Biota Seed Pills [24])
B) With the same as above plus uncooked Radix Rehmanniae (*Sheng Di Huang*), Cortex Radicis Lycii (*Di Gu Pi*), and uncooked Radix Albus Paeoniae Lactiflorae (*Sheng Bai Shao Yao*)

C) With the same as A) above plus stir-fried Rhizoma Atractylodis Macrocephalae (*Chao Bai Zhu*), and uncooked Radix Astragali Membranacei (*Sheng Huang Qi*)

Dosage: 5-15g and up to 30g in severe cases

Note: 1. This refers to Semen Biotae prepared by the method of defatting. See the chapter "Methods of Preparing the Chinese Materia Medica."

Magnetitum *(Ci Shi)*

Uncooked *(Sheng)*

Names: *Ci Shi, Ling Ci Shi, Huo Ci Shi, Sheng Ci Shi*

Flavors & nature: Acrid; cold

Functions: Quiets the liver, downbears yang, settles tetany, quiets the spirit

Indications:

1. Vertigo due to liver yang rising

2. Heart palpitations, insomnia due to heart yang rising caused by disharmony between the heart and kidneys

3. Epilepsy of the yang type with clenched jaws, salivation, piercing cries, urinary incontinence...

Typical combinations:

1. With uncooked Concha Ostreae (*Sheng Mu Li*), uncooked Os Draconis (*Sheng Long Gu*), and uncooked Radix Albus Paeoniae Lactiflorae (*Sheng Bai Shao Yao*)

2. With Cinnabar (*Zhu Sha*) as in *Ci Zhu Wan* (Magnetite & Cinnabar Pills [54])

3. With bile[-processed] Rhizoma Arisaematis (*Dan Nan Xing*), Rhizoma Acori Graminei (*Shi Chang Pu*), and uncooked Bombyx Batryticatus (*Sheng Jiang Can*)

Dosage: 15-30g

Vinegar Dip Calcined *(Cu Cui)*[1]

Names: *Duan Ci Shi, Cui Ci Shi*

Flavors & nature: Acrid and slightly sour; slightly cold

Functions: Nourishes the kidneys, promotes the absorption of qi, benefits hearing and vision, stops bleeding

Indications:

1. Dyspnea due to kidney qi vacuity not absorbing the qi

2. Deafness, tinnitus due to kidney yin vacuity

3. Diminished visual acuity due to liver/kidney yin vacuity

4. Hemorrhage due to traumatic injury with pain...

Magnetitum continued . . .

Typical combinations:

1. With Lignum Aquilariae Agallochae (*Chen Xiang*), salt[-processed] Fructus Psoraleae Coryli-foliae (*Yan Bu Gu Zhi*), prepared Radix Rehmanniae (*Shu Di Huang*), wine-steamed Fruc-tus Schizandrae Chinensis (*Jiu Zheng Wu Wei Zi*), and Gecko (*Ge Jie*)

2. With prepared Radix Rehmanniae (*Shu Di Huang*) and wine-steamed Fructus Corni Offi-cinalis (*Jiu Zheng Shan Yu*) as in *Ci Shi Liu Wei Wan* (Magnetite Six Flavors Pills [53])

3. With prepared Radix Rehmanniae (*Shu Di Huang*), uncooked Fructus Ligustri Lucidi (*Sheng Nu Zhen Zi*), Fructus Lycii Chinensis (*Gou Qi Zi*), and uncooked Semen Cuscutae (*Sheng Tu Si Zi*)

4. Apply powdered Magnetite locally.

Dosage: 15-30g

Note: 1. Vinegar dip calcined Magnetite is obtained by heating the *Ci Shi* till red hot and then plunging it while still hot into a vinegar solution. This operation is repeated several times.

Dens Draconis (*Long Chi*)

——————————— Uncooked (*Sheng*) ———————————

Names: *Long Chi, Qing Long Chi, Bai Long Chi, Sheng Long Chi*

Flavors & nature: Sweet and astringent; cool

Functions: Quiets the heart, settles tetany, resolves vexation

Indications:

1. Epilepsy, psychoses A) due to heart fire or B) in infants

2. Vexation due to evil heat disturbing the heart with fever, a dry red mouth and tongue, chest and diaphragmatic oppression

Typical combinations:

1. A) With Cinnabar[-processed] Sclerotium Para-radicis Poriae Cocos (*Zhu Sha Ban Fu Shen*), Frustra Ferri (*Tie Luo*), and Calcitum (*Han Shui Shi*)
B) With Ramulus Uncariae Cum Uncis (*Gou Teng*), Periostracum Cicadae (*Chan Tui*), and Cinnabar (*Zhu Sha*) as in *Long Chi San* (Dragon Tooth Powder [205])

2. With Rhizoma Picrorrhizae (*Hu Huang Lian*), Cortex Radicis Lycii (*Di Gu Pi*), stir-fried Fructus Gardeniae Jasminoidis (*Chao Zhi Zi*), clear Semen Praeparatum Sojae (*Qing Dan Dou Chi*), and Ra-dix Scrophulariae Ningpoensis (*Xuan Shen*)

Dosage: 10-20g

——————————— Calcined (*Duan*) ———————————

Name: *Duan Long Chi*

Flavors & nature: Sweet and astringent; neutral

Functions: Quiets the spirit and calms the heart

Indications: Insomnia with abundant dreams, heart palpitations due to 1) heart blood vacuity with palpitations, poor memory, 2) heart blood and yin vacuity with agitated sleep, night sweats, or 3) heart qi and blood vacuity with palpitations, shortness of breath...

Dens Draconis continued . . .

Typical combinations:

1. With defatted Semen Biotae Orientalis (*Bai Zi Ren Shuang*), uncooked Semen Zizyphi Spinosae (*Sheng Suan Zao Ren*), processed Radix Polygalae Tenuifoliae (*Zhi Yuan Zhi*), Cinnabar[-processed] Sclerotium Pararadicis Poriae Cocos (*Zhu Sha Ban Fu Shen*), and uncooked Fructus Schizandrae Chinensis (*Sheng Wu Wei Zi*)

2. With same as 1 above plus uncooked Radix Rehmanniae (*Sheng Di Huang*), Radix Scrophulariae Ningpoensis (*Xuan Shen*), and wine[-processed] Radix Angelicae Sinensis (*Jiu Dang Gui*)

3. With same as 1 above plus Radix Panacis Ginseng (*Ren Shen*) and stir-fried Radix Astragali Membranacei (*Chao Huang Qi*)

Dosage: 10-20g

Os Draconis *(Long Gu)*

Uncooked *(Sheng)*

Names: *Long Gu, Hua Long Gu, Bai Long Gu, Sheng Long Gu*

Flavors & nature: Sweet and astringent; slightly cold

Functions: Settles the liver, downbears yang, settles tetany, quiets the spirit

Indications:

1. Insomnia, heart palpitations[1] due to heart qi and blood vacuity with poor memory, a pale complexion, fatigue...

2. Convulsions, epilepsy, psychoses due to heart yang rising or phlegm fire harassing the spirit

3. Vertigo, headache, or tinnitus due to liver yang rising

Typical combinations:

1. With uncooked Semen Zizyphi Spinosae (*Sheng Suan Zao Ren*), processed Radix Polygalae Tenuifoliae (*Zhi Yuan Zhi*), Arillus Euphoriae Longanae (*Long Yan Rou*), Radix Panacis Ginseng (*Ren Shen*), and stir-fried Radix Astragali Membranacei (*Chao Huang Qi*)

2. With Cinnabar (*Zhu Sha*), pig blood[-processed] Radix Salviae Miltiorrhizae (*Zhu Xue Ban Dan Shen*), bile[-processed] Rhizoma Arisaematis (*Dan Nan Xing*), Rhizoma Acori Graminei (*Shi Chang Pu*), and uncooked Concha Margaritiferae (*Sheng Zhen Zhu Mu*)

3. With uncooked Haematitum (*Sheng Dai Zhe Shi*), uncooked Concha Ostreae (*Sheng Mu Li*), uncooked Radix Achyranthis Bidentatae (*Sheng Huai Niu Xi*), and uncooked Radix Albus Paeoniae Lactiflorae (*Sheng Bai Shao Yao*) as in *Zhen Gan Xi Feng Tang* (Settle the Liver & Extinguish Wind Decoction [428])

Dosage: 15-30g and up to 60g in severe cases

Note: 1. For this indication, Cinnabar[-processed] Dragon Bone (*Zhu Sha Ban Long Gu*) is sometimes used.

Os Draconis continued . . .

Name: *Duan Long Gu*

Flavors & nature: Sweet and astringent; neutral

Functions: Astringes, restrains that which is escaping

Indications:

1. Spontaneous perspiration, night sweats due to A) qi vacuity, B) yin vacuity, or C) yang desertion

2. Spermatorrhea with erotic dreams due to kidney qi not securing , weak low back and knees...

3. Chronic, incessant diarrhea due to spleen/-kidney vacuity

4. Metrorrhagia due to *chong* and *ren* not securing

5. Abnormal vaginal discharge due to *dai mai* vacuity

6. Sores which will not heal over

Typical combinations:

1. A) With Calcined Concha Ostreae (*Duan Mu Li*), stir-fried Rhizoma Atractylodis Macro-cephalae (*Chao Bai Zhu*), and uncooked Radix Astragali Membranacei (*Sheng Huang Qi*)
B) With uncooked Radix Albus Paeoniae Lacti-florae (*Sheng Bai Shao Yao*), defatted Semen Bio-tae Orientalis (*Bai Zi Ren Shuang*), and calcined Concha Ostreae (*Duan Mu Li*)
C) With processed Radix Lateralis Praeparatus Aconiti Carmichaeli (*Zhi Fu Zi*), Radix Panacis Ginseng (*Ren Shen*), uncooked Fructus Schizan-drae Chinensis (*Sheng Wu Wei Zi*), and calcined Concha Ostreae (*Duan Mu Li*)

2. With uncooked Semen Euryalis Ferocis (*Sheng Qian Shi*) and calcined Concha Ostreae (*Duan Mu Li*) as in *Jin Suo Gu Jing Wan* (Golden Lock Se-cure the Essence Pills [182])

3. With stir-fried Fructus Terminaliae Chebulae (*Chao He Zi*) and calcined Hallyositum Rubrum (*Duan Chi Shi Zhi*) as in *Long Gu San* (Dragon Bone Powder [207])

4. With carbonized Folium Et Petiolus Trachy-carpi (*Zong Lu Tan*) and carbonized Radix Rubiae Cordifoliae (*Qian Cao Gen Tan*)

5. With stir-fried Radix Dioscoreae Oppositae (*Chao Shan Yao*) and stir-fried Os Sepiae Seu Sepiellae (*Chao Hai Piao Xiao*) as in *Qing Dai Tang* (Clear Vaginal Discharge Decoction [250])

6. Apply powdered *Duan Long Gu* and calcined Alum (*Duan Bai Fan*) locally.

Dosage: 15-30g and up to 60g in severe cases

Concha Ostreae (*Mu Li*)

Names: *Mu Li, Sheng Mu Li*

Flavors & nature: Salty and astringent; slightly cold

Functions: Settles the liver, downbears yang, softens the hard, scatters nodulations

Indications:

1. Vertigo, headache, tinnitus, or congested eyes due to liver yang rising

Concha Ostreae continued . . .

2. Clonic convulsions due to liver yang producing wind in the body in a person with a warm disease which has damaged yin with dry mouth and throat, muscular spasms, a scarlet red tongue...

3. Goiter, subcutaneous nodules, scrofula due to stagnation of qi and phlegm

Typical combinations:

1. With uncooked Haematitum (*Sheng Dai Zhe Shi*) and uncooked Os Draconis (*Sheng Long Gu*) as in *Zhen Gan Xi Feng Tang* (Settle the Liver & Extinguish Wind Decoction [428])

2. With uncooked Plastrum Testudinis (*Sheng Gui Ban*), uncooked Radix Rehmanniae (*Sheng Di Huang*), and uncooked Radix Albus Paeoniae Lactiflorae (*Sheng Bai Shao Yao*) as in *Da Ding Feng Zhu* (Great Stabilize Wind Pearls [62a])

3. With Radix Scrophulariae Ningpoensis (*Xuan Shen*), Spica Prunellae Vulgaris (*Xia Ku Cao*), Bulbus Fritillariae Thunbergii (*Zhe Bei Mu*), Herba Sargassii (*Hai Zao*), and Thallus Algae (*Kun Bu*)

Dosage: 15-30g and up to 60g in severe cases

Calcined (Duan)

Name: *Duan Mu Li*

Flavors & nature: Salty and astringent; neutral

Functions: Astringes, restrains that which is escaping, stops stomach acidity, stops pain

Indications:

1. Spontaneous perspiration, night sweats due to qi and yin vacuity

2. Spermatorrhea with erotic dreams due to kidney qi not securing, weak low back and knees...

3. Abnormal vaginal discharge due to spleen/-kidney vacuity

4. Metrorrhagia due to *chong* and *ren* not securing

5. Stomach acidity and pain

Typical combinations:

1. With Radix Ephedrae (*Ma Huang Gen*) and uncooked Radix Astragali Membranacei (*Sheng Huang Qi*) as in *Mu Li San* (Oyster Shell Powder [224])

2. With uncooked Semen Euryalis Ferocis (*Sheng Qian Shi*) and Semen Nelumbinis Nuciferae (*Lian Zi*) as in *Jin Suo Gu Jing Wan* (Golden Lock Secure the Essence Pills [182])

3. With stir-fried Radix Dioscoreae Oppositae (*Chao Shan Yao*), stir-fried Rhizoma Atractylodis Macrocephalae (*Chao Bai Zhu*), Semen Nelumbinis Nuciferae (*Lian Zi*), and uncooked Semen Euryalis Ferocis (*Sheng Qian Shi*)

4. With carbonized Folium Et Petiolus Trachycarpi (*Zong Lun Tan*) and stir-fried Os Sepiae Seu Sepiellae (*Chao Hai Piao Xiao*) as in *Gu Chong Tang* (Secure the *Chong* Decoction [117])

5. With calcined Concha Arcae (*Duan Wa Leng Zi*), uncooked Radix Glycyrrhizae (*Sheng Gan Cao*), and uncooked Radix Saussureae Seu Vladimiriae (*Sheng Mu Xiang*)

Dosage: 15-30g and up to 60g in severe cases

Semen Zizyphi Spinosae (Suan Zao Ren)

Uncooked (Sheng)

Names: *Suan Zao Ren, Sheng Zao Ren*

Flavors & nature: Sweet and sour; neutral

Functions: Nourishes the heart and liver, quiets the spirit

Indications:

1. Insomnia due to either A) heart yin or blood vacuity with abundant dreams, agitation, poor memory, palpitations or B) heart and liver yin vacuity with dream-disturbed sleep, nightmares, irritability, palpitations...

2. Heart palpitations due to heart yin or blood vacuity with anxiety when there are palpitations, vexation, insomnia...

3. Vertigo, tinnitus due to liver/kidney yin vacuity with insomnia, dream-disturbed sleep...

Typical combinations:

1. A) With Semen Biotae Orientalis (*Bai Zi Ren*), processed Radix Polygalae Tenuifoliae (*Zhi Yuan Zhi*), and Cinnabar[-processed] Tuber Ophiopogonis Japonicae (*Zhu Sha Ban Mai Men Dong*) as in *Tian Wang Bu Xin Dan* (Heavenly Emperor Supplement the Heart Elixir [326])
B) With Cinnabar[-processed] Sclerotium Pararadicis Poriae Cocos (*Zhu Sha Ban Fu Shen*) as in *Suan Zao Ren Tang* (Zizyphus Spinosa Decoction [317])

2. With defatted Semen Biotae Orientalis (*Bai Zi Ren Shuang*), Arillus Euphoriae Longanae (*Long Yan Rou*), Cinnabar[-processed] Tuber Ophiopogonis Japonicae (*Zhu Sha Ban Mai Men Dong*), and uncooked Os Draconis (*Sheng Long Gu*)

3. With Fructus Lycii Chinensis (*Gou Qi Zi*), wine-steamed Fructus Ligustri Lucidi (*Jiu Zheng Nu Zhen Zi*), wine-steamed Fructus Corni Officinalis (*Jiu Zheng Shan Zhu Yu*), and uncooked Radix Albus Paeoniae Lactiflorae (*Sheng Bai Shao Yao*)

Dosage: 10-15g and up to 30g in severe cases; 1.5-2g in powder

Stir-fried [till] Yellow (Chao Huang)

Names: *Chao Suan Zao Ren, Chao Zao Ren*

Flavors & nature: Sweet and sour; neutral tending to neutral

Functions: Restrains yin, stops sweating

Indications:

1. Spontaneous perspiration due to qi vacuity with sweating on slight effort, a pale, wan complexion, fatigue...

2. Night sweats due to vacuity heat caused by yin vacuity with heat in the five hearts, evening fever...

Typical combinations:

1. With uncooked Radix Astragali Membranacei (*Sheng Huang Qi*), stir-fried Rhizoma Atractylodis Macrocephalae (*Chao Bai Zhu*), Radix Panacis Ginseng (*Ren Shen*), and uncooked Fructus Schizandrae Chinensis (*Sheng Wu Wei Zi*)

Semen Zizyphi Spinosae continued . . .

2. With uncooked Radix Albus Paeoniae Lactiflorae (*Sheng Bai Shao Yao*), Fructus Levis Tritici Aestivi (*Fu Xiao Mai*), uncooked Radix Rehmanniae (*Sheng Di Huang*), Cortex Radicis Lycii (*Di Gu Pi*), and defatted Semen Biotae Orientalis (*Bai Zi Ren Shuang*)

Dosage: 10-15g and up to 30g in severe cases; 1.5-2g in powder

Radix Polygalae Tenuifoliae *(Yuan Zhi)*

Licorice-processed *(Gan Cao Zhi)*[1]

Names: *Zhi Yuan Zhi, Yuan Zhi*

Flavors & nature: Bitter and slightly sweet; warm

Functions: Quiets the spirit, calms the heart, strengthens the intellect

Indications:

1. Insomnia[2] due to heart blood vacuity

2. Heart palpitations[2] due to heart qi vacuity

3. Spermatorrhea due to heart and kidneys not interacting with agitation, erotic dreams, restless sleep...

4. Mental agitation, anxiety[2] due to heart and kidneys not interacting

5. Poor memory, mental confusion due to heart qi vacuity

Typical combinations:

1. With uncooked Semen Zizyphi Spinosae (*Sheng Suan Zao Ren*) as in *Yuan Zhi Tang* (Polygala Decoction [422])

2. With uncooked Dens Draconis (*Sheng Long Chi*), Cinnabar[-processed] Sclerotium Pararadicis Poriae Cocos (*Zhu Sha Ban Fu Shen*), and Radix Panacis Ginseng (*Ren Shen*) as in *An Shen Ding Zhi Wan* (Quiet the Spirit & Stabilize the Will Pills [1])

3. With Cinnabar[-processed] Sclerotium Pararadicis Poriae Cocos (*Zhu Sha Ban Fu Shen*), Rhizoma Acori Graminei (*Shi Chang Pu*), calcined Os Draconis (*Duan Long Gu*), and salt[-processed] Ootheca Mantidis (*Yan Sang Piao Xiao*) as in *Sang Piao Xiao San* (Mantis Egg-case Powder [278])

4. With Cinnabar[-processed] Sclerotium Pararadicis Poriae Cocos (*Zhu Sha Ban Fu Shen*), Rhizoma Acori Graminei (*Shi Chang Pu*), prepared Radix Rehmanniae (*Shu Di Huang*), and uncooked Semen Zizyphi Spinosae (*Sheng Suan Zao Ren*)

5. With Radix Panacis Ginseng (*Ren Shen*) and Rhizoma Acori Graminei (*Shi Chang Pu*) as in *Bu Wang San* (No Forgetting Powder [36])

Dosage: 5-10g. Do not exceed 15g if there is stomach weakness, such as ulcers, gastritis, etc.

Notes: 1. Polygala is boiled in a decoction of Radix Glycyrrhizae (*Gan Cao*). 2. For these indications, Cinnabar[-processed] Polygala (*Zhu Sha Ban Yuan Zhi*) is sometimes prescribed to reinforce its function of quieting the spirit. This refers to *Zhi Yuan Zhi* prepared with Cinnabar (*Zhu Sha*).

Radix Polygalae Tenuifoliae continued . . .

Honey Mix-fried (Mi Zhi)

Names: *Mi Zhi Yuan Zhi, Zhi Yuan Zhi*

Flavors & nature: Acrid, bitter, and slightly sweet; tends to be moistening; warm

Functions: Eliminates phlegm, stops cough

Indications: Cough[1] due to accumulation of phlegm in the lungs

Typical combinations: With uncooked Semen Pruni Armeniacae (*Sheng Xing Ren*), Bulbus Fritillariae Thunbergii (*Zhe Bei Mu*), and uncooked Radix Asteris Tatarici (*Sheng Zi Wan*)

Dosage: 5-10g. Do not exceed 15g if there is stomach weakness.[2]

Notes: 1. Honey mix-fried Polygala is less powerful and is seldom used for this indication. However, it is prescribed for loss of consciousness due to accumulation of phlegm misting the portals of the heart. In any case, it is equally less powerful for treating this condition and is only used as an auxiliary medicinal. 2. Uncooked Polygala irritates the stomach mucosa, which is followed by nausea and vomiting. It is for this reason that Polygala is prepared in licorice or honey and it is contraindicated in cases of gastritis and gastric ulcers.

Fluoritum (Zi Shi Ying)

Uncooked (Sheng)

Names: *Zi Shi Ying, Chi Shi Ying, Sheng Zi Shi Yin*

Flavors & nature: Sweet; warm

Functions: Quiets the heart, settles tetany

Indications:

1. Clonic convulsions, epilepsy, spasms due to a disquieted heart spirit

2. Heart palpitations due to heart vacuity with insomnia, poor memory...

Typical combinations:

1. With uncooked Os Draconis (*Sheng Long Gu*) and uncooked Concha Ostreae (*Sheng Mu Li*) as in *Yin Feng Tang* (Conduct Wind Decoction [411])

2. With uncooked Semen Zizyphi Spinosae (*Sheng Suan Zao Ren*), processed Radix Polygalae Tenuifoliae (*Zhi Yuan Zhi*), Cinnabar-processed] Sclerotium Pararadicis Poriae Cocos (*Zhu Sha Ban Fu Shen*), defatted Semen Biotae Orientalis (*Bai Zi Ren Shuang*), and uncooked Rhizoma Coptidis Chinensis (*Sheng Huang Lian*)

Dosage: 10-15g

Vinegar Dip Calcined (Cu Cui)[1]

Names: *Cui Zi Shi Ying, Cu Cui Zi Shi Ying, Duan Zi Shi Ying*

Flavors & nature: Sweet, slightly sour, and slightly astringent; warm

Functions: Warms the lungs, downbears counterflow qi, scatters cold, warms the uterus

Indications:

1. Cough due to evil cold lodging in the lungs

Fluoritum continued . . .

with shortness of breath, thin, whitish mucus...

2. Infertility due to cold in the uterus with a long menstrual cycle, pain and a sensation of cold in the lower abdomen...

Typical combinations:

1. With uncooked Radix Asteris Tatarici (*Sheng Zi Wan*), uncooked Flos Tussilaginis Farfarae (*Sheng Kuan Dong Hua*), and uncooked Semen Pruni Armeniacae (*Sheng Xing Ren*)

2. With processed Radix Lateralis Praeparatus Aconiti Carmichaeli (*Zhi Fu Zi*), processed Fructus Evodiae Rutecarpae (*Zhi Wu Zhu Yu*), wine[-processed] Radix Angelicae Sinensis (*Jiu Dang Gui*), and wine[-processed] Radix Ligustici Walli-chii (*Jiu Chuan Xiong*)

Dosage: 10-15g

Note: 1. Vinegar dip calcined Fluoritum is obtained by heating Fluoritum till red hot and then plunging it while still hot into a vinegar solution. This operation is repeated several times.

16
Liver-settling, Wind-extinguishing Medicinals

Haematitium (Dai Zhe Shi)

_____Uncooked *(Sheng)*_____

Names: *Dai Zhe, Zhe Shi, Dai Zhe Shi, Sheng Zhe Shi*

Flavors & nature: Bitter and sweet; cold

Functions: Settles the liver, downbears yang, downbears counterflow qi

Indications:

1. Vertigo due to liver yang rising with headache and distention, tinnitus, congested eyes...

2. Vomiting due to disharmony of the stomach with nausea, eructation, regurgitation...

3. Dyspnea, asthma due to either A) qi stagnation in the lungs with cough, asthmatic breathing, chest oppression or B) lung/kidney vacuity with dyspnea on exertion, fatigue, spontaneous perspiration, weakness of the low back and knees...

Typical combinations:

1. With Concha Ostreae (*Sheng Mu Li*),

uncooked Os Draconis (*Sheng Long Gu*), and uncooked Radix Achyranthis Bidentatae (*Sheng Huai Niu Xi*) as in *Zhen Gan Xi Feng Tang* (Settle the Liver & Extinguish Wind Decoction [428])

2. With uncooked Flos Inulae (*Sheng Xuan Fu Hua*), ginger[-processed] Rhizoma Pinelliae Ternatae (*Jiang Ban Xia*), and uncooked Rhizoma Zingiberis (*Sheng Jiang*) as in *Xuan Fu Dai Zhe Tang* (Inula & Hematite Decoction [388])

3. A) With uncooked Semen Pruni Armeniacae (*Sheng Xing Ren*), uncooked Fructus Perillae Frutescentis (*Sheng Zi Su Zi*), stir-fried Semen Gingkonis Bilobae (*Chao Bai Guo*), and honey mix-fried Cortex Radicis Mori Albi (*Mi Zhi Sang Bai Pi*)
B) With Radix Panacis Ginseng (*Ren Shen*), Gecko (*Ge Jie*), calcined Magnetitum (*Cui Ci Shi*), Lignum Aquilariae Agallochae (*Chen Xiang*), and uncooked Radix Astragali Membranacei (*Sheng Huang Qi*)

Dosage: 20-30g

_____Vinegar Dip Calcined *(Cu Cui)*¹_____

Names: *Cui Dai Zhe Shi, Cu Cui Dai Zhe Shi, Duan Dai Zhe Shi, Cui Dai Zhe, Cui Zhe Shi*

Flavors & nature: Bitter, sweet, and slightly sour; slightly cold

Haematitum continued . . .

Functions: Astringes, stops bleeding

Indications:

1. Hemoptysis due to heat damaging the network vessels of the lungs

2. Hematemesis due to disharmony of the stomach injuring the network vessels of the stomach with vomiting of dark blood possibly mixed with food...

3. Epistaxis due to heat in the liver and lungs

4. Metrorrhagia, menorrhagia due to *chong* and *ren* not securing

Typical combinations:

1. With carbonized Radix Rubiae Cordifoliae

(*Qian Cao Gen Tan*), uncooked Cacumen Biotae Orientalis (*Sheng Ce Bai Ye*), and Cortex Radicis Lycii (*Di Gu Pi*)

2. With Radix Pseudoginseng (*San Qi*) and Rhizoma Bletillae Striatae (*Bai Ji*)

3. With uncooked Rhizoma Imperatae Cylindricae (*Sheng Bai Mao Gen*) and uncooked Fructus Gardeniae Jasminoidis (*Sheng Shan Zhi Zi*)

4. With stir-fried Os Sepiae Seu Sepiellae (*Chao Hai Piao Xiao*) and carbonized Folium Et Petiolus Trachycarpi (*Zong Lu Tan*)

Dosage: 20-30g

Note: 1. This refers to the method of dip calcining in vinegar. See the chaper titled "Methods of Preparing the Chinese Materia Medica."

Bombyx Batryticus (*Jiang Can*)

Uncooked (*Sheng*)

Names: *Sheng Jiang Can, Sheng Jiang Chong, Sheng Tian Chong*

Flavors & nature: Acrid and salty; neutral

Functions: Dispels wind, settles tetany, stops pain

Indications:

1. Convulsions, epilepsy due to either A) internal wind or B) internal wind and spleen vacuity with chronic convulsions, chronic diarrhea...

2. Pruritus, rubeola due to either A) external wind or B) external wind and heat toxins

3. Headache due to wind heat with headache and distention, tearing...

4. Sore, swollen throat due to wind heat

5. Aphonia due to wind heat

6. Deviated mouth and eyes, hemiplegia due to wind stroke (*zhong feng*)

Typical combinations:

1. A) With Buthus Martensi (*Quan Xie*) and stone-baked Scolopendra Subspinipes (*Bei Wu Gong*) B) With earth stir-fried Rhizoma Atractylodis Macrocephalae (*Tu Chao Bai Zhu*), Radix Panacis Ginseng (*Ren Shen*), stir-fried Rhizoma Gastrodiae Elatae (*Chao Tian Ma*), uncooked Rhizoma Typhonii (*Sheng Bai Fu Zi*), and Buthus Martensi (*Quan Xie*)

2. A) With Periostracum Cicadae (*Chan Tui*), Herba Menthae Haplocalycis (*Bo He*), Fructus Kochiae Scopariae (*Di Fu Zi*), and Fructus Tribuli Terrestris (*Bai Ji Li*)

Bombyx Batryticatus continued . . .

B) With the same as above plus uncooked Flos Lonicerae Japonicae (*Sheng Jin Yin Hua*) and uncooked Cortex Radicis Moutan (*Sheng Mu Dan Pi*)

3. With uncooked Folium Mori Albi (*Sheng Sang Ye*) and uncooked Herba Schizonepetae Tenuifoliae (*Sheng Jing Jie*) as in *Bai Jiang Can San* (White Silkworm Powder [17]) or uncooked Radix Ligustici Wallichii (*Sheng Chuan Xiong*) and uncooked Flos Chrysanthemi Morifolii (*Sheng Ju Hua*) as in *Ju Hua Cha Tiao San* (Chrysanthemum & Tea Regulating Powder [188])

4. With uncooked Radix Platycodi Grandiflori (*Sheng Jie Geng*), uncooked Radix Glycyrrhizae (*Sheng Gan Cao*), Herba Menthae Haplocalycis (*Bo He*), and Periostracum Cicadae (*Chan Tui*)

5. With uncooked Radix Glycyrrhizae (*Sheng Gan Cao*) and uncooked Pericarpium Trichosanthis Kirlowii (*Sheng Gua Lou Pi*) as in *Fa Sheng San* (Emit the Voice Powder [102])

6. With uncooked Rhizoma Typhonii (*Sheng Bai Fu Zi*) and Buthus Martensi (*Quan Xie*) as in *Qian Zheng San* (Lead to Righteousness Powder [246])

Dosage: 5-10g and up to 20g in severe cases

_____ **Bran Stir-fried** *(Fu Chao)*[1] _____

Names: *Chao Jiang Can, Chao Tian Chong, Chao Jiang Chong, Jiang Can*

Flavors & nature: Acrid and salty; slightly warm

Functions: Resolves toxins, scatters nodulations, eliminates phlegm (wind)

Indications:

1. Subcutaneous nodules, scrofula due to accumulation of phlegm

2. Aphasia due to wind stroke (*zhong feng*) with impossibility of expressing the slightest sound, stertorous breathing...

3. Asthmatic breathing, dyspnea due to accumulation of phlegm with stertorous breathing...

Typical combinations:

1. With Bulbus Fritillariae Thunbergii (*Zhe Bei*

Mu) and Spica Prunellae Vulgaris (*Xia Ku Cao*)

2. With Secretio Moschi Moschiferi (*She Xiang*) and Radix Et Rhizoma Notopterygii (*Qiang Huo*) as in *Tong Guan San* (Open the Gate Powder [329])

3. With uncooked Semen Pruni Armeniacae (*Sheng Xing Ren*), uncooked Radix Asteris Tatarici (*Sheng Zi Wan*), and stir-fried Semen Gingkonis Bilobae (*Chao Bai Guo*)

Dosage: 5-10g and up to 20g in severe cases

Note: 1. In order to obtain bran stir-fried Bombyx, the silkworms are fried till yellow in ginger juice and wheat bran. This preparation permits one to reinforce its phlegm-dispersing action thanks to ginger and to eliminate its irritating effect on the stomach mucosa thanks to the wheat bran.

Concha Haliotidis (Shi Jue Ming)

Uncooked (Sheng)

Names: *Shi Jue Ming, Jiu Kong Jue Ming, Sheng Shi Jue Ming*

Flavors & nature: Salty; slightly cold

Functions: Settles the liver, downbears yang

Indications:

1. Vertigo, headache, congested eyes due to liver yang rising

2. Convulsions, spasms, epilepsy due to internal wind

Typical combinations:

1. With uncooked Radix Albus Paeoniae Lactiflorae (*Sheng Bai Shao Yao*), uncooked Radix Achyranthis Bidentatae (*Sheng Huai Niu Xi*), stir-fried Rhizoma Gastrodiae Elatae (*Chao Tian Ma*), and Ramulus Uncariae Cum Uncis (*Gou Teng*)

2. With uncooked Bombyx Batryticatus (*Sheng Jiang Can*), bile[-processed] Rhizoma Arisaematis (*Dan Nan Xing*), and Buthus Martensi (*Quan Xie*)

Dosage: 15-30g

Calcined (Duan)

Name: *Duan Shi Jue Ming*

Flavors & nature: Salty and slightly astringent; neutral

Functions: Clears the liver and vacuity heat, brightens the eyes, eliminates film

Indications:

1. Bone steaming fever due to vacuity heat caused by yin vacuity with red cheeks, evening fever, night sweats, fatigue...

2. Red, painful, swollen eyes due to wind heat penetrating the liver channel

3. Glaucoma, optic atrophy due to heat penetrating the liver channel

Typical combinations:

1. With Cortex Radicis Lycii (*Di Gu Pi*), uncooked Carapax Amydae Sinensis (*Sheng Bie Jia*), uncooked Radix Rehmanniae (*Sheng Di Huang*), and salt[-processed] Rhizoma Anemarrhenae (*Yan Zhi Mu*)

2. With Herba Menthae Haplocalycis (*Bo He*), uncooked Flos Chrysanthemi Morifolii (*Sheng Ju Hua*), uncooked Folium Mori Albi (*Sheng Sang Ye*), and uncooked Fructus Viticis (*Sheng Man Jing Zi*)

3. With Scapus Et Inflorescentia Eriocaulonis Buergeriani (*Gu Jing Cao*) and Herba Equiseti Hiemalis (*Mu Zei*) as in *Shi Jue Ming San* (Concha Haliotidis Powder [300])

Rhizoma Gastrodiae Elatae *(Tian Ma)*

Uncooked *(Sheng)*

Names: *Tian Ma, Ming Tian Ma*

Flavors & nature: Sweet and slightly acrid; neutral

Functions: Dispels wind, stops pain

Indications:

1. Headache due to A) external wind with vertigo, B) liver blood vacuity, or C) liver yang rising

2. Rheumatic complaints, numbness of the extremities due to wind cold dampness

3. Hemiplegia due to wind stroke (*zhong feng*)

Typical combinations:

1. A) With uncooked Radix Ligustici Wallichii (*Sheng Chuan Xiong*), Radix Angelicae Dahuricae (*Bai Zhi*), and uncooked Bombyx Batryticatus (*Sheng Jiang Can*)

B) With uncooked Radix Albus Paeoniae Lactiflorae (*Sheng Bai Shao Yao*) and wine[-processed] Radix Angelicae Sinensis (*Jiu Dang Gui*)
C) With Ramulus Uncariae Cum Uncis (*Gou Teng*), uncooked Flos Chrysanthemi Morifolii (*Sheng Ju Hua*), and uncooked Radix Achyranthis Bidentatae (*Sheng Huai Niu Xi*)

2. With wine[-processed] Radix Gentianae Macrophyllae (*Jiu Qin Jiao*), Radix Et Rhizoma Notopterygii (*Qiang Huo*), and wine[-processed] Ramulus Mori Albi (*Jiu Sang Zhi*) as in *Qin Jiao Tian Ma Tang* (Gentiana Macrophylla & Gastrodia Decoction [248])

3. With Buthus Martensi (*Quan Xie*), uncooked Rhizoma Arisaematis (*Tian Nan Xing*), Lumbricus (*Di Long*), and uncooked Radix Ligustici Wallichii (*Sheng Chuan Xiong*) as in *Tian Ma Wan* (Gastrodia Pills [324])

Dosage: 3-10g and up to 30g in severe cases or if Gastrodia is used alone

Stir-fried [till] Yellow *(Chao Huang)*

Names: *Chao Tian Ma, Wei Tian Ma*

Flavors & nature: Sweet; slightly warm

Functions: Settles the liver, extinguishes wind, settles tetany

Indications:

1. Vertigo due to A) liver yang rising with headache, insomnia; B) liver wind with severe vertigo even when the eyes are shut; or C) phlegm dampness with a sensation of a heavy head...

2. Convulsions, spasms due to A) internal wind, B) warm disease, or C) tetanus

Typical combinations:

1. A) With Ramulus Uncariae Cum Uncis (*Gou Teng*), uncooked Concha Haliotidis (*Sheng Shi Jue Ming*), and uncooked Radix Achyranthis Bidentatae (*Sheng Huai Niu Xi*)
B) With Cornu Antelopis (*Ling Yang Jiao*), uncooked Flos Chrysanthemi Morifolii (*Sheng Ju Hua*), and Ramulus Uncariae Cum Uncis (*Gou Teng*)
C) With bran stir-fried Rhizoma Atractylodis Macrocephalae (*Fu Chao Bai Zhu*) and lime-processed Rhizoma Pinelliae Ternatae (*Fa Ban*

Rhizoma Gastrodiae Elatae continued . . .

Xia) as in *Ban Xia Bai Zhu Tian Ma Tang* (Pinellia, Atractylodes & Gastrodia Decoction [26])

2. A) With Buthus Martensi (*Quan Xie*) and stone-baked Scolopendra Subspinipes (*Bei Wu Gong*)
B) With Ramulus Uncariae Cum Uncis (*Gou Teng*), Cornu Antelopis (*Ling Yang Jiao*), and uncooked Fructus Gardeniae Jasminoidis (*Sheng Shan Zhi Zi*)
C) With uncooked Rhizoma Arisaematis (*Sheng Tian Nan Xing*), uncooked Radix Ledebouriellae Sesloidis (*Sheng Fang Feng*), and uncooked Rhizoma Typhonii (*Sheng Bai Fu Zi*)

Dosage: 3-10g and 30g if used alone

Concha Margaritiferae *(Zhen Zhu Mu)*

Uncooked *(Sheng)*

Names: *Zhen Zhu Mu, Sheng Zhen Zhu Mu*

Flavors & nature: Salty; cold

Functions: Settles the liver, downbears yang, brightens the eyes

Indications:

1. Headache, vertigo, tinnitus, deafness due to liver yang rising

2. Red, swollen eyes, hemeralopia, glaucoma due to either A) liver blood and yin vacuity or B) heat penetrating the liver channel

3. Heart palpitations, insomnia due to liver yang rising which disturbs the heart spirit with agitation and irritability...

Typical combinations:

1. With uncooked Radix Achyranthis Bidentatae (*Sheng Huai Niu Xi*), uncooked Radix Albus Paeoniae Lactiflorae (*Sheng Bai Shao Yao*), stir-fried Rhizoma Gastrodiae Elatae (*Chao Tian Ma*), and Ramulus Uncariae Cum Uncis (*Gou Teng*)

2. A) With uncooked Rhizoma Atractylodis (*Sheng Cang Zhu*), Feces Vespertilionis Murini (*Ye Ming Sha*), Fructus Lycii Chinensis (*Gou Qi Zi*), and uncooked Fructus Ligustri Lucidi (*Sheng Nu Zhen Zi*)
B) With Herba Equiseti Hiemalis (*Mu Zei*), Scapus Et Inflorescentia Eriocaulonis Buergeriani (*Gu Jing Cao*), Spica Prunellae Vulgaris (*Xia Ku Cao*), and uncooked Semen Cassiae Torae (*Sheng Jue Ming Zi*)

3. With processed Radix Polygalae Tenuifoliae (*Zhi Yuan Zhi*), uncooked Semen Zizyphi Spinosae (*Sheng Suan Zao Ren*), Cinnabar[-processed] Sclerotium Pararadicis Poriae Cocos (*Zhu Sha Ban Fu Shen*), and calcined Dens Draconis (*Duan Long Chi*)

Dosage: 15-30g

Concha Margaritiferae continued . . .

Calcined (Duan)

Name: *Duan Zhen Zhu Mu*

Flavors & nature: Salty and astringent; slightly cold

Functions: Dries dampness, stops bleeding

Indications:

1. Oozing sores with pruritus due to dampness

2. Metrorrhagia, epistaxis, hematemesis due to spleen qi not restraining the blood

Typical combinations:

1. Apply locally powdered calcined Concha Ostreae (*Duan Mu Li*), calcined Concha Margaritiferae (*Duan Zhen Zhu Mu*), and calcined Alumen (*Duan Bai Fan*).

2. With uncooked Rhizoma Imperatae Cylindricae (*Sheng Bai Mao Gen*), carbonized Radix Rubiae Cordifoliae (*Qian Cao Gen Tan*), Crinis Carbonisatus (*Xue Yu Tan*), rice stir-fried Radix Codonopsis Pilosulae (*Mi Chao Dang Shen*), and stir-fried Radix Astragali Membranacei (*Chao Huang Qi*)

Dosage: 15-30g

17
Qi-supplementing Medicinals

Semen Dolichoris Lablab *(Bai Bian Dou)*

Uncooked *(Sheng)*

Names: *Sheng Bian Dou, Bai Bian Dou, Nan Bian Dou*

Flavors & nature: Sweet; neutral

Functions: Clears summerheat, transforms dampness

Indications:

1. Vomiting, diarrhea due to summerheat and dampness with fever, aversion to cold, headache with a sensation of distention and heavy head, a sensation of oppression and fullness in the chest...

2. Strong thirst due to injury of fluids by summerheat with accumulation of heat in the spleen and stomach

Typical combinations:

1. With Herba Elsholtziae *(Xiang Ru)* and ginger[-processed] Cortex Magnoliae Officinalis *(Jiang Hou Po)* as in *Xiang Ru San* (Elsholtzia Powder [368])

2. With Radix Trichosanthis Kirlowii *(Tian Hua Fen)*

Dosage: 10-20g and up to 50g in severe cases

Addendum: Uncooked Dolichoris is used to combat intoxication from fish toxins, alcohol, and certain toxic Chinese plants.

Stir-fried *(Chao)*[1]

Name: *Chao Bian Dou*

Flavors & nature: Sweet; slightly warm

Functions: Fortifies the spleen, supplements the qi, stops diarrhea, stops vaginal discharge

Indications:

1. Diarrhea due to spleen and stomach qi vacuity with fatigue, loss of appetite...

2. Abnormal vaginal discharge due to spleen qi vacuity with whitish, abundant, fluid discharge...

Typical combinations:

1. With earth stir-fried Rhizoma Atractylodis Macrocephalae *(Tu Chao Bai Zhu)*, earth stir-fried Radix Dioscoreae Oppositae *(Tu Chao Shan Yao)*, and Radix Panacis Ginseng *(Ren Shen)* as in *Shen Ling Bai Zhu San* (Ginseng, Poria & Atractylodes Powder [288])

2. With Semen Euryalis Ferocis *(Qian Shi)*, Stamen Nelumbinis Nuciferae *(Lian Xu)*, and bran stir-fried Rhizoma Atractylodis Macrocephalae *(Fu Chao Bai Zhu)*

Dosage: 10-20g and up to 50g in severe cases

Semen Dolichoris Lablab continued . . .

Note: 1. If one wants to reinforce the astringing aspect or warming action of Dolichoris, one can use stir-fried [till] yellow Dolichoris (*Chao Huang Bai Bian Dou*) or earth stir-fried Dolichoris (*Tu Chao Bai Bian Dou*).

Rhizoma Atractylodis Macrocephalae (Bai Zhu)

Uncooked (Sheng)

Names: *Sheng Bai Zhu, Bai Zhu*

Flavors & nature: Sweet and bitter; warm

Functions: Fortifies the spleen, dries dampness, disinhibits urination, disperses swelling

Indications:

1. Edema due to accumulation of dampness internally with edematous face and limbs, oliguria...

2. Phlegm rheum due to spleen weakness with edema, dizziness, palpitations, shortness of breath, cough...

3. Rheumatic complaints (*bi*) due to wind dampness with pain in the entire body, a sensation of discomfort, loss of movement of the joints, a sensation of joint pain...

Typical combinations:

1. With Sclerotium Polypori Umbellati (*Zhu Ling*), uncooked Rhizoma Alismatis (*Sheng Ze Xie*), and uncooked Sclerotium Poriae Cocos (*Sheng Fu Ling*) as in *Wu Ling San* (Five [Ingredients] *Ling* Powder [348])

2. With stir-fried Ramulus Cinnamomi (*Chao Gui Zhi*), uncooked Sclerotium Poriae Cocos (*Sheng Fu Ling*), and mix-fried Radix Glycyrrhizae (*Zhi Gan Cao*) as in *Ling Gui Zhu Gan Tang* (Poria, Cinnamon, Atractylodes & Licorice Decoction [201])

3. With processed Radix Lateralis Praeparatus Aconiti Carmichaeli (*Zhi Fu Zi*) and uncooked Rhizoma Zingiberis (*Sheng Jiang*) as in *Bai Zhu Fu Zi Tang* (Atractylodes & Aconite Decoction [22])

Dosage: 10-15g and up to 30g in severe cases

Bran Stir-fried (Fu Chao)

Names: *Chao Bai Zhu, Chao Dong Zhu, Chao Yu Zhu*

Flavors & nature: Sweet and bitter, warm

Functions: Fortifies the spleen, supplements the qi

Indications:

1. Epigastric and abdominal distention and fullness due to spleen qi vacuity with loss of appetite, borborygmus, loose stools...

2. Food stagnation, loss of appetite due to spleen vacuity

3. Middle burner qi fall due to spleen qi vacuity with a sensation of weight in the stomach, possible stomach ptosis, anal prolapse, uterine prolapse...

4. Spontaneous perspiration due to qi vacuity with fatigue, aversion to wind, a tendency to catch cold...

Rhizoma Atractylodis Macrocephalae continued . . .

5. Restless fetus and threatened abortion due to qi and blood vacuity

Typical combinations:

1. With bran stir-fried Fructus Immaturus Citri Seu Ponciri (*Fu Chao Zhi Shi*) as in *Zhi Zhu Wan* (Immature Citrus & Atractylodes Pills [439])

2. With stir-fried Fructus Germinatus Hordei Vulgaris (*Chao Mai Ya*), stir-fried Fructus Crataegi (*Chao Shan Zha*), and stir-fried Pericarpium Citri Reticulatae (*Chao Chen Pi*) as in *Jian Pi Wan* (Fortify the Spleen Pills [171])

3. With stir-fried Radix Astragali Membranacei (*Chao Huang Qi*), Radix Panacis Ginseng (*Ren Shen*), honey mix-fried Rhizoma Cimicifugae (*Mi Zhi Sheng Ma*), and stir-fried Radix Bupleuri (*Chao Chai Hu*) as in *Bu Zhong Yi Qi Tang* (Supplement the Center & Boost the Qi Decoction [38])

4. With uncooked Radix Astragali Membranacei (*Sheng Huang Qi*) and uncooked Radix Ledebouriellae Sesloidis (*Sheng Fang Feng*) as in *Yu Ping Feng San* (Jade Windscreen Powder [417])

5. With uncooked Radix Angelicae Sinensis (*Sheng Dang Gui*) and stir-fried Radix Scutellariae Baicalensis (*Chao Huang Qin*) as in *Dang Gui San* (*Dang Gui* Powder [I; 76])

Dosage: 10-15g and up to 30g in severe cases; up to 120g in cases of severe epigastric and abdominal distention. (It is often used alone in this case.)

_____ **Earth Stir-fried** *(Tu Chao)*_____

Names: *Chao Bai Zhu, Tu Chao Bai Zhu, Bai Zhu Tan[1], Jiao Bai Zhu[1]*

Flavors & nature: Sweet, bitter, and slightly astringent; warm

Functions: Fortifies the spleen, stops diarrhea

Indications:

1. Diarrhea[1] due to either A) spleen qi vacuity with fatigue, loss of appetite or B) spleen yang vacuity with accumulation internally of cold with aversion to cold, cold limbs, absence of thirst...

2. Diarrhea accompanied by abdominal pain[1] due to disharmony of the liver and spleen with diarrhea preceded by borborygmus and followed by abdominal pain, a wiry (*xian*) pulse...

Typical combinations:

1. A) With Radix Panacis Ginseng (*Ren Shen*), stir-fried Semen Nelumbinis Nuciferae (*Chao Lian Zi*), roasted Semen Myristicae Fragrantis (*Wei Rou Dou Kou*), and roasted Fructus Terminaliae Chebulae (*Wei He Zi*) as in *Shen Zhu San* (Ginseng & Atractylodes Powder [292])
B) With dry Rhizoma Zingiberis (*Gan Jiang*), Radix Panacis Ginseng (*Ren Shen*), and mix-fried Radix Glycyrrhizae (*Zhi Gan Cao*) as in *Li Zhong Wan* (Rectify the Center Pills [196])

2. With stir-fried Radix Albus Paeoniae Lactiflorae (*Chao Bai Shao Yao*), carbonized Radix Ledebouriellae Sesloidis (*Fang Feng Tan*), and stir-fried Pericarpium Citri Reticulatae (*Chao Chen Pi*) as in *Tong Xie Yao Fang* (Painful Diarrhea Essential Formula [333])

Dosage: 10-15g and up to 30g in severe cases

Note: 1. Earth stir-fried Atractylodes can be equally replaced by carbonized Atractylodes (*Bai Zhu Tan*) or stir-fried [till] scorched Atractylodes (*Chao Jiao Bai Zhu*).

Radix Codonopsis Pilosulae *(Dang Shen)*

Uncooked *(Sheng)*

Names: *Sheng Dang Shen, Dang Shen, Xi Lu Shen, Tai Shen*

Flavors & nature: Sweet; neutral

Functions: Supplements the qi, engenders fluids

Indications:

1. Simultaneous injury of qi and fluids, notably of the lungs with dry mouth and tongue, thirst, fatigue or dry, weak cough, feeble voice...

2. Qi and blood vacuity with fatigue, a pale, wan complexion, emaciation, general weakness, insomnia...

Typical combinations:

1. With Radix Glehniae Littoralis (*Bei Sha Shen*)

as in *Shang Dang Shen Tang* (Superior Codonopsis Decoction [283])

2. With prepared Radix Rehmanniae (*Shu Di Huang*) as in *Liang Yi Tang* (Two Principles Decoction [199])[1]

Dosage: 10-15g and up to 30-60g in severe cases

Note: 1. *Liang yi* refers to the two fundamental principles of the *Yi Jing (Classic of Change)*, *i.e.*, yang as represented in this formula by Codonopsis and yin as represented by Rehmannia.

Addendum: Similar to Radix Panacis Ginseng (*Ren Shen*), Codonopsis can be used in external injury due to colds or flu when combined with remedies which resolve the exterior and when the defensive and righteous qi are deficient.

Rice Stir-fried *(Mi Chao)*[1]

Names: *Mi Chao Dang Shen, Chao Dang Shen, Chao Lu Shen, Chao Tai Shen*

Flavors & nature: Sweet; neutral tending to warm

Functions: Fortifies the spleen, stops diarrhea

Indications: Diarrhea due to either 1) spleen and stomach qi vacuity with loss of appetite, fatigue or 2) spleen yang vacuity with loss of appetite, aversion to cold, cold limbs, undigested food in the stool...

Typical combinations:

1. With earth stir-fried Rhizoma Atractylodis

Macrocephalae (*Tu Chao Bai Zhu*), earth stir-fried Radix Dioscoreae Oppositae (*Tu Chao Shan Yao*), and earth stir-fried Semen Dolichoris Lablab (*Tu Chao Bai Bian Dou*)

2. With earth stir-fried Rhizoma Atractylodis Macrocephalae (*Tu Chao Bai Zhu*), dry Rhizoma Zingiberis (*Gan Jiang*), and mix-fried Radix Glycyrrhizae (*Zhi Gan Cao*) as in *Li Zhong Wan* (Rectify the Center Pills [196])

Dosage: 10-15g and up to 30-60g in severe cases

Note: 1. The *mi* in *Mi Chao Dang Shen* does not correspond to the *mi* in *feng mi*, *i.e.*, honey, but rather to the *mi* in *geng mi*, rice.

Radix Codonopsis Pilosulae continued . . .

_____**Honey Mix-fried (Mi Zhi)**_____

Names: *Mi Zhi Dang Shen, Zhi Dang Shen*

Flavors & nature: Sweet; neutral tending to warm; slightly moistening

Functions: Supplements the center, boosts the qi

Indications:

1. Cough, asthma due to lung qi vacuity with fatigue, weak voice...

2. Fall of qi due to spleen qi vacuity with stomach ptosis, prolapsed uterus, prolapsed anus, chronic diarrhea...

3. Fatigue due to spleen qi vacuity with lack of appetite, loose stools, lack of strength in the four extremities...

Typical combinations:

1. With honey mix-fried Radix Astragali Membranacei (*Mi Zhi Huang Qi*), uncooked Fructus Schizandrae Chinensis (*Sheng Wu Wei Zi*), and honey mix-fried Radix Asteris Tatarici (*Mi Zhi Zi Wan*) as in *Bu Fei Tang* (Supplement the Lungs Decoction [33])

2. With stir-fried Radix Astragali Membranacei (*Chao Huang Qi*), bran stir-fried Rhizoma Atractylodis Macrocephalae (*Fu Chao Bai Zhu*), and honey mix-fried Rhizoma Cimicifugae (*Mi Zhi Sheng Ma*) as in *Shen Qi Bai Zhu Tang* (Codonopsis, Astragalus & Atractylodes Decoction [289])

3. With bran stir-fried Rhizoma Atractylodis Macrocephalae (*Fu Chao Bai Zhu*), uncooked Sclerotium Poriae Cocos (*Sheng Fu Ling*), and mix-fried Radix Glycyrrhizae (*Zhi Gan Cao*) as in *Si Jun Zi Tang* (Four Gentlemen Decoction [310])

Dosage: 10-15g and up to 30-60g in severe cases[1]

Note: 1. When Codonopsis is used as a substitute for Radix Panacis Ginseng (*Ren Shen*), its dosage should be 40-50g per day. In any case, Codonopsis does not treat qi desertion.

Radix Glycyrrhizae (Gan Cao)

_____**Uncooked (Sheng)**_____

Names: *Sheng Gan Cao, Gan Cao*

Flavors & nature: Sweet; neutral

Functions: Clears heat, resolves toxins, moistens the lungs, soothes the throat, stops cough

Indications:

1. Skin inflammation due to heat toxins with pain, redness, and swelling...

2. Sore, swollen throat due to A) heat toxins, B) wind heat, or C) vacuity fire caused by yin vacuity

3. Cough[1] due to either A) lung heat and/or phlegm heat with thick, yellow mucus which is difficult to expectorate or B) lung heat damaging the network vessels with hemoptysis

4. Stomach acidity and pain

5. Intoxication. Licorice treats food intoxication

Radix Glycyrrhizae continued . . .

and intoxication by a number of medicinal substances, such as Aconite, Arisaema, Typhonium, etc.

Typical combinations:

1. With uncooked Flos Lonicerae Japonicae (*Sheng Jin Yin Hua*), Flos Chrysanthemi Indici (*Ye Ju Hua*), and Herba Cum Radice Taraxaci Mongolici (*Pu Gong Ying*)

2. A) With uncooked Radix Platycodi Grandiflori (*Sheng Jie Geng*) as in *Jie Geng Tang* (Platycodon Decoction [176])
B) With Herba Menthae Haplocalycis (*Bo He*) and uncooked Fructus Arctii (*Sheng Niu Bang Zi*)
C) With Radix Scrophulariae Ningpoensis (*Xuan Shen*) and uncooked Tuber Ophiopogonis Japonicae (*Sheng Mai Men Dong*) as in *Xuan Mai Gan Jie Tang* (Scrophularia, Ophiopogon, Licorice & Platycodon Decoction [391])

3. A) With uncooked Radix Peucedani (*Sheng*

Qian Hu), Bulbus Fritillariae Thunbergii (*Zhe Bei Mu*), and Herba Houttuyniae Cordatae (*Yu Xing Cao*)
B) With Rhizoma Bletillae Striatae (*Bai Ji*), uncooked Rhizoma Imperatae Cylindricae (*Sheng Bai Mao Gen*), and honey mix-fried Cortex Radicis Mori Albi (*Mi Zhi Sang Bai Pi*)

4. With calcined Concha Arcae (*Duan Wa Leng Zi*) and stir-fried Fructus Meliae Toosendan (*Chao Chuan Lian Zi*)

5. With uncooked Semen Phaseoli Munginis (*Lu Dou*)

Dosage: 3-6g and 10-30g if Licorice is used as the principal ingredient in the prescription[2]; 50-100g in severe cases

Notes: 1. In case of cough with phlegm cold, one can use mix-fried Licorice (*Zhi Gan Cao*) with Ramulus Cinnamomi (*Gui Zhi*) and Rhizoma Atractylodis Macrocephalae (*Bai Zhu*) as in *Ling Gui Zhu Gan Tang* (Poria, Cinnamon, Atractylodes & Licorice Decoction). 2. In case of prolonged use, do not prescribe more than 10g per day so as not to risk edema, since Licorice promotes the retention of sodium.

_____**Honey Mix-fried** *(Mi Zhi)*_____

Names: *Mi Zhi Gan Cao, Zhi Gan Cao*

Flavors & nature: Sweet; slightly warm

Functions: Supplements the center, boosts the qi, relaxes tension, stops pain

Indications:

1. Spleen and stomach qi vacuity with fatigue, loss of appetite, loose stools or diarrhea, borborygmus, abdominal distention...

2. Heart palpitations due to qi and blood vacuity with a regularly interrupted (*dai*) or bound *(jie)* pulse...

3. Muscular spasms or contracture with abdominal or limb pain...

4. Epigastric distention and fullness due to stomach qi vacuity with a sensation of discomfort or epigastric mass, borborygmus, indigestion...

5. To harmonize other medicinal substances[1]

Typical combinations:

1. With Radix Panacis Ginseng (*Ren Shen*), bran stir-fried Rhizoma Atractylodis Macrocephalae (*Fu Chao Bai Zhu*), and uncooked Sclerotium Poriae Cocos (*Sheng Fu Ling*) as in *Si Jun Zi Tang* (Four Gentlemen Decoction [310])

Radix Glycyrrhizae continued . . .

2. With Radix Panacis Ginseng (*Ren Shen*), stir-fried Ramulus Cinnamomi (*Chao Gui Zhi*), uncooked Radix Rehmanniae (*Sheng Di Huang*), and uncooked Gelatinum Corii Asini (*Sheng E Jiao*) as in *Zhi Gan Cao Tang* (Mix-fried Licorice Decoction [432])

3. With wine[-processed] Radix Albus Paeoniae Lactiflorae (*Jiu Bai Shao Yao*) as in *Shao Yao Gan Cao Tang* (Peony & Licorice Decoction [284])

4. With ginger[-processed] Rhizoma Coptidis Chinensis (*Jiang Huang Lian*), dry Rhizoma Zingiberis (*Gan Jiang*), and lime-processed Rhizoma Pinelliae Ternatae (*Fa Ban Xia*) as in *Gan Cao Xie Xin Tang* (Licorice Drain the Heart Decoction [109])

Dosage: 6-10g and 15-30g if Licorice is used as the principal ingredient in the prescription[2]; 50-100g in severe cases

Notes: 1. Mix-fried Licorice balances the action of numerous remedies. For example: It lessens the heating action of dry Ginger, Aconite, etc., and conserves yin. It moderates the refrigerating action of Gypsum, Anemarrhena, etc., and protects the stomach. It softens the purgative action of Rhubarb, Mirabilitum, etc., and safeguards the righteous qi. It tempers the supplementing action of Codonopsis, Astragalus, *Dang Gui*, prepared Rehmannia, etc., and permits the prolonged usage of [such] supplements. And it conciliates those substances having opposed actions and natures, such as dry Ginger and Coptis.
2. In case of prolonged use, do not prescribe more than 10g per day so as not to risk edema. Licorice promotes the retention of sodium.

Rhizoma Polygonati (*Huang Jing*)

————————— Steamed (*Zheng*) —————————

Names: *Huang Jing, Zheng Huang Jing, Shu Huang Jing, Zhi Huang Jing*

Flavors & nature: Sweet; neutral; slightly moistening

Functions: Moistens the lungs, enriches yin, fulfills the essence, nourishes the kidneys

Indications:

1. Dry cough due to lung/kidney yin vacuity with little or no phlegm, a dry, sore throat...

2. Diabetes due to vacuity heat caused by kidney yin vacuity with strong thirst, abundant urination...

3. Thirst due to stomach/kidney yin vacuity

4. Kidney essence insufficiency with low back weakness, premature aging, diminished hearing, premature greying of the hair...

Typical combinations:

1. With honey mix-fried Bulbus Lilii (*Mai Zhi Bai He*), uncooked Tuber Ophiopogonis Japonicae (*Sheng Mai Men Dong*), honey mix-fried Radix Adenophorae Strictae (*Mi Zhi Nan Sha Shen*) and uncooked Rhizoma Anemarrhenae (*Sheng Zhi Mu*)

2. With uncooked Radix Dioscoreae Oppositae (*Sheng Shan Yao*), Radix Trichosanthis Kirlowii (*Tian Hua Fen*), honey mix-fried Radix Astragali Membranacei (*Mi Zhi Huang Qi*), and Radix Scrophulariae Ningpoensis (*Xuan Shen*)

3. With Radix Glehniae Littoralis (*Bei Sha Shen*), uncooked Rhizoma Polygonati Odorati (*Sheng Yu*

Rhizoma Polygonati continued . . .

Zhu), uncooked Tuber Ophiopogonis Japonicae (*Sheng Mai Men Dong*), and prepared Radix Rehmanniae (*Shu Di Huang*)

4. With Fructus Lycii Chinensis (*Gou Qi Zi*) as in *Gou Qi Wan* (Lycium Pills [116])

Dosage: 10-20g and up to 30g in severe cases

Addendum: Uncooked Polygonatum (*Sheng Huang Jing*) is very irritating to the throat and therefore should always be prepared. Steamed Polygonatum is very rich and heavy to digest. Therefore, this preparation is contraindicated in spleen vacuity with dampness, phlegm, loose stools, abdominal distention, etc.

_____Wine-steamed *(Jiu Zheng)*_____

Names: *Jiu Huang Jing, Jiu Zhen Huang Jing*

Flavors & nature: Sweet; warm

Functions: Supplements the spleen, supplements the qi, supplements the kidneys

Indications:

1. Spleen qi vacuity with lack of appetite, borborygmus, loose stools, fatigue, shortness of breath...

2. Qi and blood vacuity with wan complexion, fatigue, loss of appetite, emaciation, insomnia...

3. Impotence, spermatorrhea due to kidney yang vacuity with low back and knee soreness, tinnitus...

Typical combinations:

1. With stir-fried Radix Astragali Membranacei (*Chao Huang Qi*), bran stir-fried Radix

Dioscoreae Oppositae (*Fu Chao Shan Yao*), rice stir-fried Radix Codonopsis Pilosulae (*Mi Chao Dang Shen*), and bran stir-fried Rhizoma Atractylodis Macrocephalae (*Fu Chao Bai Zhu*)

2. With wine[-processed] Radix Angelicae Sinensis (*Jiu Dang Gui*), prepared Radix Rehmanniae (*Shu Di Huang*), stir-fried Radix Astragali Membranacei (*Chao Huang Qi*), and honey mix-fried Radix Codonopsis Pilosulae (*Mi Zhi Dang Shen*)

3. With Hippocampus (*Hai Ma*), Cornu Parvum Cervi (*Lu Rong*), and Herba Cynomorii Songarici (*Suo Yang*)

Dosage: 10-20g and up to 30g in severe cases

Addendum: Wine-steamed Polygonatum possesses a less greasy nature and is thus more easily assimilated. However, it is counseled to avoid prescribing this remedy in case of dampness or abundant phlegm dampness.

Radix Astragali Membranacei *(Huang Qi)*

_____Uncooked *(Sheng)*_____

Names: *Huang Qi, Sheng Huang Qi, Mian Huang Qi, Sheng Jian Qi*

Flavors & nature: Sweet; slightly warm

Functions: Secures the exterior, stops perspiration, disinhibits urination, disperses swelling, outthrusts pus and toxins

Radix Astragali Membranacei continued . . .

Indications:

1. Spontaneous perspiration due to exterior (*biao*) and defensive qi (*wei qi*) vacuity with sweating on slight exertion or night sweats...

2. Frequent colds, predisposition to infections of the respiratory system due to righteous qi (*zheng qi*) and defensive qi (*wei qi*) vacuity

3. Edema of the wind type with edema beginning in the eyelids and then extending to the entire face and limbs, fever, aversion to wind and cold...

4. Rheumatic complaints due to qi and blood vacuity and disharmony between the defensive and constructive qi. This vacuity provides the opportunity for attack of the channels and network vessels by evil wind.

5. Hemiplegia due to wind stroke (*zhong feng*) with qi stagnation and blood stasis in the network vessels

6. Skin infection which heals poorly due to qi and blood vacuity with inflammation with redness, difficult evacuation of pus, chronic abscesses which do not ripen...

Typical combinations:

1. With calcined Concha Ostreae (*Duan Mu Li*), Semen Levis Tritici Aestivi (*Fu Xiao Mai*), and Radix Ephedrae (*Ma Huang Gen*) as in *Mu Li San* Oyster Shell Powder [224])

2. With bran stir-fried Rhizoma Atractylodis Macrocephalae (*Fu Chao Bai Zhu*) and uncooked Radix Ledebouriellae Sesloidis (*Sheng Fang Feng*) as in *Yu Ping Feng San* (Jade Windscreen Powder [417])

3. With uncooked Rhizoma Atractylodis Macrocephalae (*Sheng Bai Zhu*) and Radix Stephaniae Tetrandrae (*Han Fang Ji*) as in *Fang Ji Huang Qi Tang* (Stephania & Astragalus Decoction [104])

4. With uncooked Ramulus Cinnamomi (*Sheng Gui Zhi*) and wine[-processed] Radix Albus Paeoniae Lactiflorae (*Jiu Bai Shao Yao*) as in *Huang Qi Gui Zhi Wu Wu Tang* (Astragalus & Cinnamon Twig Five Materials Decoction [156])

5. With wine[-processed] Radix Angelicae Sinensis (*Jiu Dang Gui*), wine[-processed] Radix Ligustici Wallichii (*Jiu Chuan Xiong*), and Lumbricus (*Di Long*) as in *Bu Yang Huan Wu Tang* (Supplement Yang & Slacken (*i.e.*, Relax) the Five [Viscera] Decoction [37])

6. With uncooked Squama Manitis Pentadactylis (*Sheng Chuan Shan Jia*), Fructus Gleditschiae Chinensis (*Zao Jiao*), and wine[-processed] Radix Angelicae Sinensis (*Jiu Dang Gui*) as in *Tuo Nong San* (Outthrust Pus Powder [334])

Dosage: 10-15g and up to 30-120g in severe cases

Stir-fried (*Chao*)[1]

Names: *Chao Huang Qi, Chao Mian Qi*

Flavors & nature: Sweet; warm

Functions: Supplements the spleen qi, upbears yang, tends to warm yang

Indications:

1. Diarrhea due to spleen qi vacuity with diarrhea or loose stools, fatigue...

2. Fatigue[2] due to severe spleen qi vacuity with generalized weakness, fatigued, forceless limbs...

3. Uterine or rectal prolapse, gastric ptosis[2] due to middle burner qi fall with fatigue, shortness of breath...

4. Fever[2] due to either A) qi vacuity with intermittent fever aggravated by exertion, spontaneous perspiration, thirst for warm drinks, shortness of breath, fatigue or B) blood vacuity with low grade

Radix Astragali Membranacei continued . . .

fever postpartum, sweating, a sensation of heat in the muscles, a vacuity (*xu*), forceless (*wu li*) pulse...

5. Metrorrhagia[2] due to spleen qi vacuity unable to hold the blood within its vessels

Typical combinations:

1. With roasted Radix Puerariae (*Wei Ge Gen*), earth stir-fried Rhizoma Atractylodis Macrocephalae (*Tu Chao Bai Zhu*), and earth stir-fried Radix Dioscoreae Oppositae (*Tu Chao Shan Yao*)

2. With Radix Panacis Ginseng (*Ren Shen*) as in *Shen Qi Tang* (Ginseng & Astragalus Decoction [290])

3. With Radix Panacis Ginseng (*Ren Shen*), bran stir-fried Rhizoma Atractylodis Macrocephalae (*Fu Chao Bai Zhu*), honey mix-fried Rhizoma Cimicifugae (*Mi Zhi Sheng Ma*), and stir-fried Radix Bupleuri (*Chao Chai Hu*) as in *Bu Zhong Yi Qi Tang* (Supplement the Center & Boost the Qi Decoction [38])

4. A) With Radix Panacis Ginseng (*Ren Shen*) and bran stir-fried Rhizoma Atractylodis Macrocephalae (*Fu Chao Bai Zhu*) as in *Bu Zhong Yi Qi Tang* (Supplement the Center & Boost the Qi Decoction [38])
B) With wine[-processed] Radix Angelicae Sinensis (*Jiu Dang Gui*) as in *Dang Gui Bu Xue Tang* (*Dang Gui* Supplement the Blood Decoction [73])

5. With carbonized Radix Angelicae Sinensis (*Dang Gui Tan*), honey mix-fried Radix Codonopsis Pilosulae (*Mi Zhi Dang Shen*), and Herba Agrimoniae Pilosae (*Xian He Cao*) as in *Zhi Xue Gui Pi Tang* (Stop Bleeding Return the Spleen Decoction [438])

Dosage: 10-15g and up to 30-120g in severe cases

Notes: 1. This refers to either stir-fried [till] yellow Astragalus (*Chao Huang Huang Qi*) or bran stir-fried Astragalus (*Fu Chao Huang Qi*). 2. For these indications, it is possible to equally use honey mix-fried Astragalus (*Mi Zhi Huang Qi*) safely even if the spleen is suffering severely from an excess of dampness.

Honey Mix-fried (*Mi Zhi*)

Names: *Mi Zhi Huang Qi, Zhi Huang Qi, Zhi Mian Qi, Zhi Jiang Qi*

Flavors & nature: Sweet; slightly warm; slightly moistening

Functions: Supplements the lung qi, tends to moisten dryness, supplements vacuity

Indications:

1. Shortness of breath due to lung qi vacuity with dyspnea, cough, chronic asthma, a pale complexion, a pale tongue, a forceless (*wu li*), weak (*ruo*) pulse...

2. Constipation due to qi vacuity with constipation without dry stools, the expulsion of stools without

force, exhausted defecation following breathlessness and perspiration...

3. Spasmodic abdominal pain due to vacuity cold of the middle burner with fatigue, a pale complexion...

4. Diabetes due to heat in the middle burner with strong thirst, strong hunger, abundant urination

Typical combinations:

1. With uncooked Fructus Schizandrae Chinensis (*Sheng Wu Wei Zi*) and Radix Asteris Tatarici (*Sheng Zi Wan*) as in *Bu Fei Tang* (Supplement the Lungs Decoction [33])

Radix Astragali Membranacei continued . . .

2. With stir-fried Semen Cannabis Sativae (*Chao Huo Ma Ren*), uncooked Honey (*Sheng Feng Mi*), and uncooked Pericarpium Citri Reticulatae (*Sheng Chen Pi*) as in *Huang Qi Tang* (Astragalus Decoction [158])

3. With mix-fried Radix Glycyrrhizae (*Zhi Gan Cao*) and wine[-processed] Radix Albus Paeoniae Lactiflorae (*Jiu Bai Shao Yao*) as in *Huang Qi*

Jian Zhong Tang (Astragalus Fortify the Center Decoction [157])

4. With uncooked Radix Dioscoreae Oppositae (*Sheng Shan Yao*), Radix Trichosanthis Kirlowii (*Tian Hua Fen*), uncooked Radix Rehmanniae (*Sheng Di Huang*), and Tuber Ophiopogonis Japonicae (*Mai Men Dong*)

Dosage: 10-15g and up to 30-120g in severe cases

Radix Panacis Ginseng *(Ren Shen)*

I. General Presentation

Flavors & nature: Sweet and slightly bitter; slightly warm

Tropism: Lungs, spleen

Functions: Strongly supplements the source or *yuan qi*, supplements the spleen and lungs, engenders fluids and stops sweating, quiets the spirit, strengthens the intellect, strengthens the righteous qi, disperses external evils

Indications:

1. Yang qi desertion, fatigue, loss of appetite,

vomiting, diarrhea...

2. Shortness of breath, asthmatic breathing, cough, dyspnea, spontaneous perspiration, thirst, a dry mouth...

3. Agitation, insomnia, palpitations, poor memory...

4. Blood vacuity, abundant dreams, impotence...

Dosage: 5-10g in a long-cooked decoction; 1-3g in powder; 15-30g for desertion

II. Differentiations

Ren Shen is a generic term which is not used in prescriptions. Chinese prescribers employ different names which delineate the type of Ginseng being used. This depends on the quality and properties which are modified based on their place of culture, method of culture, age, and method of preparation.

1. Place of culture

There are four principal origins of Ginseng:

A) Ginseng from northwest China, called *Ji Lin Ren Shen* or *Ji Lin Shen*, literally Ginseng from

Jilin. This grows in the mountains of Jilin Province and most notably in the region of Chang Bai Shan.

Ji Lin Shen is prestigious and considered to be the best quality and most powerful along with *Gao Li Shen*. It is also one of the most expensive. It harmoniously supplements the qi and yin. It is very often used for great deficiencies.

B) Ginseng from North Korea, called *Gao Li Shen*, literally Korean Ginseng (Gao Li was an ancient name of Korea), or *Chao Xian Shen*, again literally Korean Ginseng (*Chao Xian* being the

Radix Panacis Ginseng continued . . .

modern name of Korea). This grows in the mountains of North Korea.

Gao Li Shen is also very famous. However, it is less harmonious in its action and tends to be used specifically for supplementing the qi and yang. It is used very frequently in clinical practice.

C) Ginseng from Japan, called *Dong Yang Shen*, literally Ginseng of the eastern foreigners. It grows in Japan.

Dong Yang Shen supplements the qi (of the spleen and stomach). It is much less powerful than *Ji Lin Shen* or *Gao Li Shen*. It is not used for qi desertion or for engendering fluids. It is equivalent to Radix Codonopsis Pilosulae (*Dang Shen*) in terms of its quality. It is only used for minor troubles at present.

D) Ginseng from the United States of America or Canada, called *Xi Yang Shen*, literally Ginseng of the western foreigners. It grows in the United States and Canada, but it is also now cultivated in China.

Xi Yang Shen, although considered a type of Ginseng, has very different properties from the above. Its nature is cool. It nourishes lung yin, supplements the qi, clears vacuity heat, and engenders fluids. It supplements the qi less forcefully than the three preceding medicinals, but it is more powerful for enriching yin. In clinical practice, *Ren Shen* is used in the winter and to supplement the qi without signs of heat, while *Xi Yang Shen* is used in summer and to supplement the qi in the presence of heat signs.

Comparison of Therapeutic Efficacy

Qi : *Ji Lin Shen* > or = *Gao Li Shen* > *Dong Yang Shen* > *Xi Yang Shen*[1]

Yang: *Gao Li Shen* > or = *Ji Lin Shen* > *Dong Yang Shen*

Yin: *Xi Yang Shen* > *Ji Lin Shen*

2. Mode of Cultivation

There are three methods of cultivation of Ginseng:

A) Wild Ginseng, called *Ye Shan Shen* or *Shan Shen*, literally Wild Mountian Ginseng. It grows naturally in the mountains without human intervention. It is sometimes called *Ji Lin Ye Shen*, literally Wild Jilin Ginseng, since the most wild Ginseng originates in Jilin Province.

Ye Shan Shen is the most prestigious Ginseng, the most sought after, the most powerful, and the most expensive. It is slightly warm and not drying. It strongly supplements the *yuan qi* and nourishes yin. It is used for either acute, severe diseases or for chronic maladies with a great deficiency of yang and yin. It is favorably employed in qi desertion (as in *Du Shen Tang* [Solitary Ginseng Decoction]) or in yang desertion (as in *Jia Ren Shen Tang* [Added Ginseng Decoction]).

B) Transplanted Ginseng, called *Yi Shan Shen*, literally Removed Mountain Ginseng. This mode of culture may use either of two distinct methods: 1) one may dig up a young wild Ginseng and then transplant it in a garden or 2) one may dig up a young cultivated Ginseng and transplant it in the mountains. Thus *Yi Shan Shen* is half cultivated and half wild.

Yi Shan Shen has an analogous action to *Ye Shan Shen* but is less powerful. It is very often used for qi vacuity and yin vacuity patterns.

C) Cultivated Ginseng, called *Yuan Shen*, literally Garden Ginseng. This is cultivated in China in Jilin, Liaoning, and Heilongjiang Provinces. In addition, *Dong Yang Shen* (Japanese Ginseng) and *Xi Yang Shen* (American Ginseng) are always cultivated. *Gao Li Shen* is sometimes wild and

Radix Panacis Ginseng continued . . .

sometimes cultivated, while *Ji Lin Shen* is very often wild.

Yuan Shen is less powerful than the two preceding Ginsengs but also less expensive. Therefore, it is largely used in clinical practice for common problems.

Comparison of Therapeutic Efficacy

Ye Shan Shen > Yi Shan Shen > Yuan Shen

3. Age

The older a Ginseng is, the more powerful it is. *Yuan Shen* is cultivated at least 5-7 years. *Ye Shan Shen* or Wild Mountain Ginseng should be at least 10 years old and may attain 200 years of age. In that case, it is called *Lao Ren Shen*, Old Ginseng. In prior times, *Lao Ren Shen* was reserved for the Emperor or offered as a prestigious gift to meritorious ministers.

4. Methods of Preparation

There are four methods of preparation of Ginseng:

A) Uncooked, sun-dried Ginseng, called *Sheng Shai Shen*, literally uncooked, sun-dried Ginseng. This is a Ginseng which has been washed in water and then dried in the sun. Its color is grayish yellow. The neck, rootlets, and secondary roots are kept. For this reason it is also called *Quan Xu Sheng Shai Shen*, literally whole Ginseng with rootlets, crude and dried in the sun. In addition, if the superficial skin of the root is scraped, it then becomes whitish and is called *Bai Gan Shen*, literally white, dry Ginseng. If the neck (*lu*) and the rootlets (*xu*) are removed, the root is then called *Da Li Shen*, literally great force Ginseng. This is because one keeps the large principal root where the active principles of the Ginseng are concentrated and because one has taken away the neck which is emetic and the rootlets which are only weak supplements.

One can speak equally of *Sheng Shai Ye Shen*, literally uncooked, sun-dried wild Ginseng. Wild Mountain Ginseng is most often prepared in the mode which makes even more valuable its superior qualities. *Sheng Shai Shen* is prepared most often starting with *Ye Shan Shen*, sometimes from *Yi Shan Shen*, and rarely from *Yuan Shen*.

Sheng Shai Shen is the most powerful. It is slightly warm and is not drying. It harmoniously supplements qi, yin, and fluids and humors.

B) Ginseng cooked in steam is called *Hong Shen* or literally Red Ginseng because, in the process of cooking it in steam and then drying it, it becomes reddish brown. It is sometimes also called *Chao Xian Hong Shen*, Korean Red Ginseng, since Korean Ginseng is the most adaptable for producing Red Ginseng. *Chao Xian Hong Shen*, like *Hong Shen,* tends to be warm and supplements specifically the qi and yang. *Hong Shen* is most often produced beginning from *Yuan Shen* or cultivated Ginseng.

Hong Shen is less powerful than *Sheng Shai Shen* but is clearly warm and specifically supplements the qi and yang.

C) Sugar-prepared Ginseng, called *Bai Ren Shen*, literally White Ginseng. It is so-called because it is lightly cooked and then soaked in a sugar solution or is impregnated with sugar and thus becomes whitish.

Bai Shen is less powerful than *Sheng Shai Shen* or *Hong Shen*. However, it has the advantage in engendering fluids and humors and is used when there is a qi and yin vacuity or when qi vacuity follows a vacuity heat (as in *Bu Zhong Yi Qi Tang* [Supplement the Center & Boost the Qi]). *Bai Shen* does supplement the qi, however, more forcefully than *Xi Yang Shen*.

Radix Panacis Ginseng continued . . .

D) Ginseng Rootlets, called *Ren Shen Xu*, literally Ginseng thorns. This refers to the long, fine secondary rootlets of Ginseng which are gathered when *Hong Shen* and *Bai Shen* are prepared. Therefore, during this method of preparation, one obtains either *Hong Shen Xu*, Red Ginseng Rootlets, or *Bai Shen Xu*, white Ginseng rootlets.

Ren Shen Xu is much less powerful than the preceding three medicinals. *Hong Shen Xu* tends to mostly supplement the qi. *Bai Shen Xu* tends to mostly nourish fluids and humors. In the case of great deficiencies, it is counseled against at first prescribing a very powerful supplementation.

This can damage the organism. In such cases, it is advantageous to first treat with moderate supplementation using *Ren Shen Xu*.

Comparison of Therapeutic Efficacy

Qi: *Sheng Shai Shen > Hong Shen > Bai Shen > Hong Shen Xu*

Yang: *Hong Shen > or = Sheng Shai Shen > Hong Shen Xu*

Yin Fluids: *Sheng Shai Shen > or = Bai Shen > Bai Shen Xu*

Note: > meaning "greater than"

Radix Dioscoreae Oppositae *(Shan Yao)*

Uncooked *(Sheng)*

Names: *Sheng Shan Yao, Shan Yao, Huai Shan Yao*

Flavors & nature: Sweet; neutral

Functions: Moistens the lungs, quiets cough, engenders fluids, stops thirst

Indications:

1. Cough due to lung qi and yin vacuity with shortness of breath, fatigue, a pale complexion...

2. Thirst due to either A) kidney yin vacuity followed by vacuity fire with night sweats, evening fever or B) simultaneous damage of qi and yin with strong thirst, emaciation, fatigue...

3. Diabetes due to heat in the middle burner with excessive thirst...

Typical combinations:

1. With uncooked Tuber Ophiopogonis Japonicae (*Sheng Mai Men Dong*), stir-fried Semen Pruni

Armeniacae (*Chao Xing Ren*), uncooked Gelatinum Corii Asini (*Sheng E Jiao*), and Radix Panacis Ginseng (*Ren Shen*) as in *Shu Yu Wan* (Dioscorea Pills [304])

2. A) With Radix Trichosanthis Kirlowii (*Tian Hua Fen*) and uncooked Fructus Schizandrae Chinensis (*Sheng Wu Wei Zi*) as in *Yu Ye Tang* (Jade Humors Decoction [419])
B) With uncooked Tuber Ophiopogonis Japonicae (*Sheng Mai Men Dong*), Radix Trichosanthis Kirlowii (*Tian Hua Fen*), and honey mix-fried Radix Astragali Membranacei (*Mi Zhi Huang Qi*) as in *Shan Yao Xiao Ke Yin* (Dioscorea Wasting Thirst Drink [281])

3. With uncooked Radix Rehmanniae (*Sheng Di Huang*), Radix Trichosanthis Kirlowii (*Tian Hua Fen*), uncooked Tuber Ophiopogonis Japonicae (*Sheng Mai Men Dong*), and honey mix-fried Radix Astragali Membranacei (*Mi Zhi Huang Qi*)

Dosage: 10-30g and up to 60-100g in severe cases; up to 250g in case of thirst in a diabetic

Radix Dioscoreae Oppositae continued . . .

Stir-fried *(Chao)*

Names: *Chao Shan Yao, Chao Shu Yu*

Flavors & nature: Sweet; slightly warm

Functions: Fortifies the spleen, stops diarrhea, supplements the kidneys, secures the essence

Indications:

1. Diarrhea[1] due to spleen qi vacuity with loss of appetite, epigastric and abdominal distention...

2. Lack of appetite, anorexia[2] due to spleen and stomach vacuity with loose stools...

3. Spermatorrhea[2] due to kidney qi not securing with weak low back and knees...

4. Enuresis, urinary incontinence[2] due to kidney qi vacuity

5. Abnormal vaginal discharge[2] due to spleen qi vacuity with whitish, fluid, abundant discharge, little or not bad odor...

Typical combinations:

1. With earth stir-fried Rhizoma Atractylodis Macrocephalae (*Tu Chao Bai Zhu*) and Radix Panacis Ginseng (*Ren Shen*) as in *Shan Yu Wan* (Dioscorea Pills [282])

2. With bran stir-fried Rhizoma Atractylodis Macrocephalae (*Fu Chao Bai Zhu*), Radix Panacis Ginseng (*Ren Shen*), and uncooked Sclerotium Poriae Cocos (*Sheng Fu Ling*) as in *Shen Ling Bai Zhu San* (Ginseng, Poria & Atractylodes Powder [288])

3. With uncooked Semen Euryalis Ferocis (*Sheng Qian Shi*), Fructus Rosae Laevigatae (*Jin Ying Zi*), and wine-steamed Fructus Schizandrae Chinensis (*Jiu Zheng Wu Wei Zi*) as in *Mi Yuan Jian* (Secret Source Decoction [220])

4. With salt[-processed] Fructus Alpiniae Oxyphyllae (*Yan Yi Zhi Ren*) as in *Suo Quan Wan* (Shut the Spring Pills [319])

5. With bran stir-fried Rhizoma Atractylodis Macrocephalae (*Fu Chao Bai Zhu*), stir-fried [till] scorched Rhizoma Atractylodis (*Chao Jiao Cang Zhu*), and stir-fried Semen Plantaginis (*Chao Che Qian Zi*) as in *Wan Dai Tang* (End Abnormal Vaginal Discharge Decoction [335])

Dosage: 15-30g and up to 60-100g in severe cases

Notes: 1. For this indication, earth stir-fried Dioscorea (*Tu Chao Shan Yao*) is prescribed. 2. For these indications, bran stir-fried Dioscorea (*Fu Chao Shan Yao*) is prescribed.

18
Yang-supplementing Medicinals

Radix Morindae Officinalis (Ba Ji Tian)

Uncooked (Sheng)

Names: *Ba Ji Tian, Ba Ji Rou, Ba Ji*

Flavors & nature: Acrid and sweet; slightly warm

Functions: Strengthens the sinews and bones, dispels wind dampness

Indications:

1. Rheumatic complaints due to wind cold dampness and kidney yang vacuity with joint pain aggravated by cold, the night, and fatigue, rheumatic complaints localized especially in the hips, low back, knees, ankles...

2. Low back pain due to kidney yang vacuity and wind cold dampness with low back pain aggravated by cold, damp weather as well as fatigue...

3. Dyspnea due to the kidneys not absorbing the qi with asthmatic breathing, dyspnea on exertion, low back weakness...

Typical combinations:

1. With Radix Angelicae Pubescentis (*Du Huo*), Radix Et Rhizoma Notopterygii (*Qiang Huo*), uncooked Cortex Radicis Acanthopanacis (*Sheng Wu Jia Pi*), and uncooked Radix Dipsaci (*Sheng Xu Duan*)

2. With salt[-processed] Radix Achyranthis Bidentatae (*Yan Huai Niu Xi*), salt[-processed] Cortex Eucommiae Ulmoidis (*Yan Du Zhong*), and Radix Et Rhizoma Notopterygii (*Qiang Huo*) as in *Ba Ji Wan* (Morinda Pills [3])

3. With Lignum Aquilariae Agallochae (*Chen Xiang*), salt[-processed] Fructus Psoraleae Corylifoliae (*Yan Bu Gu Zhi*), and calcined Magnetitum (*Cui Ci Shi*)

Dosage: 8-15g and up to 30g in severe cases

Salt Mix-fried (Yan Zhi)

Names: *Yan Zhi Ba Ji, Yan Ba Ji Tian*

Flavors & nature: Sweet, salty and slightly acrid; warm

Functions: Supplements the kidneys, strengthens yang

Indications:

1. Daybreak diarrhea due to kidney yang vacuity with loose stools containing undigested food or barely malodorous diarrhea...

2. Impotence, premature ejaculation due to kidney yang vacuity with mental apathy, fatigue, low back weakness...

3. Female infertility, menstrual irregularity, dysmenorrhea due to cold in the uterus

Radix Morindae Officinalis continued . . .

4. Enuresis, urinary incontinence, nocturia due to kidney qi vacuity with excessive, clear urination...

5. Urinary strangury with dribbling and dripping due to kidney qi vacuity

Typical combinations:

1. With salt[-processed] Fructus Psoraleae Corylifoliae (*Yan Bu Gu Zhi*), stir-fried Fructus Alpiniae Oxyphyllae (*Chao Yi Zhi Ren*), and processed Fructus Evodiae Rutecarpae (*Zhi Wu Zhu Yu*)

2. With wine[-processed] Rhizoma Curculiginis Orchioidis (*Xian Mao*) and mix-fried Herba Epimedii (*Zhi Yin Yang Huo*)

3. Fluoritum (*Zi Shi Ying*), processed Fructus Evodiae Rutecarpae (*Zhi Wu Zhu Yu*), and processed Radix Lateralis Praeparatus Aconiti Carmichaeli (*Zhi Fu Zi*)

4. With salt[-processed] Fructus Alpiniae Oxyphyllae (*Yan Yi Zhi Ren*), salt[-processed] Ootheca Mantidis (*Yan Sang Piao Xiao*), and salt[-processed] Semen Cuscutae (*Yan Tu Si Zi*)

5. With salt[-processed] Rhizoma Dioscoreae Hypoglaucae (*Yan Bei Xie*), Rhizoma Acori Graminei (*Shi Chang Pu*), bran stir-fried Radix Dioscoreae Oppositae (*Fu Chao Shan Yao*), and wine[-processed] Herba Cistanchis (*Jiu Rou Cong Rong*)

Dosage: 8-15g and up to 30g in severe cases

Fructus Psoraleae Corylifoliae *(Bu Gu Zhi)*

Uncooked *(Sheng)*

Names: *Sheng Bu Gu Zhi, Sheng Po Gu Zhi*

Flavors & nature: Bitter and acrid; very warm

Functions: Harmonizes the blood, dispels wind, treats vitiligo

Indication: Vitiligo

Typical combinations: Allow 30g of previously crushed uncooked Psoralea to soak for 7 days in 100ml of 70% alcohol. Apply 3 times per day. The skin should be massaged until it becomes red.

Dosage: Use externally whatever quantity necessary

Salt mix-fried *(Yan Zhi)*

Names: *Yan Zhi Bu Gu Zhi, Yan Bu Gu Zhi, Yan Po Gu Zhi, Bu Gu Zhi*

Flavors & nature: Bitter, acrid and slightly salty; warm

Functions: Supplements the kidneys, strengthens yang, promotes the absorption of qi

Indications:

1. Asthma, cough due to the kidneys not absorbing

the qi with dyspnea on exertion, shortness of breath, fatigue, low back weakness...

2. Impotence, premature ejaculation due to kidney yang vacuity

3. Low back pain due to kidney yang vacuity

4. Enuresis, spermatorrhea due to kidney yang vacuity

5. Daybreak diarrhea due to spleen/kidney yang vacuity

Fructus Psoraleae Corylifoliae continued . . .

Typical combinations:

1. With Cortex Cinnamomi (*Rou Gui*), Lignum Aquilariae Agallochae (*Chen Xiang*), and dip calcined Magnetitum (*Cui Ci Shi*)

2. With wine[-processed] Rhizoma Curculiginis Orchioidis (*Jiu Xian Mao*) and processed Herba Epimedii (*Zhi Yin Yang Huo*)

3. With salt[-processed] Cortex Eucommiae Ulmoidis (*Yan Du Zhong*), salt[-processed] Radix Achyranthis Bidentatae (*Yan Huai Niu Xi*), and

salt[-processed] Radix Dipsaci (*Yan Xu Duan*)

4. With salt[-processed] Fructus Alpiniae Oxyphyllae (*Yan Yi Zhi Ren*), salt[-processed] Ootheca Mantidis (*Yan Sang Piao Xiao*), Fructus Rubi (*Fu Pen Zi*), and uncooked Endothelium Corneum Gigeriae Galli (*Sheng Ji Nei Jin*)

5. With roasted Fructus Myristicae Fragrantis (*Wei Rou Dou Kou*) and wine-steamed Fructus Schizandrae Chinensis (*Jiu Zheng Wu Wei Zi*) as in *Si Shen Wan* (Four Spirits Pills [313])

Dosage: 5-10g and up to 30g in severe cases

Cortex Eucommiae Ulmoidis *(Du Zhong)*

Uncooked *(Sheng)*

Name: *Sheng Du Zhong*

Flavors & nature: Sweet and slightly acrid; warm

Functions: Nourishes the liver, relaxes the sinews

Indications:

1. Vertigo, dizziness due to liver/kidney vacuity

2. Rheumatic complaints due to wind cold dampness and kidney vacuity

3. Sinew contracture due to internal wind caused by liver blood vacuity with tendonomuscular spasms...

Typical combinations:

1. With stir-fried Rhizoma Gastrodiae Elatae (*Chao Tian Ma*), uncooked Radix Achyranthis

Bidentatae (*Sheng Huai Niu Xi*), and Ramulus Uncariae Cum Uncis (*Gou Teng*) as in *Tian Ma Gou Teng Yin* (Gastrodia & Uncaria Drink [323])

2. With uncooked Radix Achyranthis Bidentatae (*Sheng Huai Niu Xi*), wine[-processed] Ramus Loranthi Seu Visci (*Jiu Sang Ji Sheng*), and Radix Angelicae Pubescentis (*Du Huo*) as in *Du Huo Ji Sheng Tang* (*Du Huo* & Loranthus Decoction [88])

3. With wine[-processed] Rhizoma Ligustici Wallichii (*Jiu Chuan Xiong*), Lumbricus (*Di Long*), prepared Radix Rehmanniae (*Shu Di Huang*), processed Radix Polygoni Multiflori (*Zhi He Shou Wu*), and wine[-processed] Radix Albus Paeoniae Lactiflorae (*Jiu Bai Shao Yao*)

Dosage: 10-15g and up to 30g in severe cases

Cortex Eucommiae Ulmoidis continued . . .

_____Salt Mix-fried **(Yan Zhi)**_____

Names: *Yan Zhi Du Zhong, Yan Du Zhong, Du Zhong*

Flavors & nature: Sweet and slightly salty; warm

Functions: Supplements the kidneys, strengthens the low back, quiets the fetus

Indications:

1. Low back pain due to A) kidney vacuity; B) traumatic injury (blood stasis); C) cold damp- ness; or D) wind dampness

2. Threatened spontaneous abortion, metrorrhagia during pregnancy due to either A) qi vacuity or B) kidney vacuity

3. Impotence, premature ejaculation, spermator- rhea due to kidney yang vacuity

Typical combinations:

1. A) With salt[-processed] Radix Dipsaci (*Yan*

Xu Duan) and wine[-processed] Cortex Radicis Acanthopanacis (*Jiu Wu Jia Pi*)
B) With wine[-processed] Radix Cyathulae (*Jiu Chuan Niu Xi*), stir-fried Resina Olibani (*Chao Ru Xiang*), and stir-fried Resina Myrrhae (*Chao Mo Yao*)
C) With wine[-processed] Radix Clematidis Chinensis (*Jiu Wei Ling Xian*) and wine[-pro- cessed] Radix Gentianae Macrophyllae (*Jiu Qin Jiao*)

2. A) With bran stir-fried Rhizoma Atractylodis Macrocephalae (*Fu Chao Bai Zhu*) and stir-fried Radix Astragali Membranacei (*Chao Huang Qi*)
B) With salt[-processed] Radix Dipsaci (*Yan Xu Duan*) and wine[-processed] Ramus Loranthi Seu Visci (*Jiu Sang Ji Sheng*)

3. With salt[-processed] Radix Morindae Off- icinalis (*Yan Ba Ji Tian*) and processed Herba Epimedii (*Zhi Yin Yang Huo*)

Dosage: 10-15g and up to 30g in severe cases

Rhizoma Cibotii Barometz *(Gou Ji)*

_____Uncooked **(Sheng)**_____

Names: *Sheng Gou Ji, Sheng Fu Jin*

Flavors & nature: Sweet and bitter; warm

Functions: Dispels wind dampness, disinhibits the joints

Indications: Rheumatic complaints due to either 1) wind cold dampness penetrating the network vessels and joints with joint pain, loss of mobility or 2) wind cold dampness and blood vacuity

Typical combinations:

1. With wine[-processed] Radix Clematidis Chinensis (*Jiu Wei Ling Xian*), Radix Angelicae Pubescentis (*Du Huo*), and Radix Et Rhizoma Notopterygii (*Qiang Huo*)

2. With wine[-processed] Radix Gentianae Macro- phyllae (*Jiu Qin Jiao*), steamed Fructus Chae- nomelis Lagenariae (*Zheng Mu Gua*), wine[-pro- cessed] Radix Angelicae Sinensis (*Jiu Dang Gui*), and prepared Radix Rehmanniae (*Shu Di Huang*) as in *Gou Ji Yin* (Cibotium Drink [115])

Dosage: 5-15g and up to 30g in severe cases

Rhizoma Cibotii Barometz continued . . .

_____**Sand Stir-fried (Sha Chao)**_____

Names: *Sha Chao Gou Ji, Chao Gou Ji*

Flavors & nature: Sweet and bitter; warm

Functions: Supplements the liver, strengthens the sinews and bones, restrains that which is escaping

Indications:

1. Low back pain due to liver/kidney vacuity with weak knees...

2. Enuresis, urinary incontinence, frequent urination due to kidney qi vacuity

3. Abnormal vaginal discharge due to kidney qi and *dai mai* vacuity with whitish, watery, abundant discharge...

Typical combinations:

1. With salt[-processed] Cortex Eucommiae Ulmoidis (*Yan Du Zhong*), salt[-processed] Radix Dipsaci (*Yan Xu Duan*), and salt[-processed] Radix Achyranthis Bidentatae (*Yan Huai Niu Xi*)

2. With salt[-processed] Fructus Alpiniae Oxyphyllae (*Yan Yi Zhi Ren*), salt[-processed] Radix Linderae Strychnifoliae (*Yan Wu Yao*), and steamed Fructus Corni Officinalis (*Zheng Shan Zhu Yu*)

3. With uncooked Semen Euryalis Ferocis (*Sheng Qian Shi*), Stamen Nelumbinis Nuciferae (*Lian Xu*), stir-fried Semen Gingkonis Bilobae (*Chao Bai Guo*), and Fructus Rubi (*Fu Pen Zi*)

Dosage: 5-15g and up to 30g in severe cases

Rhizoma Drynariae (*Gu Sui Bu*)

_____**Uncooked (Sheng)**_____

Names: *Sheng Gu Sui Bu, Sheng Bu Sui Gu*

Flavors & nature: Bitter; warm

Functions: Harmonizes the blood, treats alopecia

Indications: Alopecia due to wind dryness or qi stagnation and blood stasis

Typical combinations: Allow 25g of crushed Drynaria to soak in 100ml of 70% alcohol for 7 days. Apply locally 2-3 times per day.

Dosage: Applied locally, whatever amount necessary

_____**Sand Stir-fried (Sha Chao)**_____

Names: *Sha Chao Gu Sui Bu, Sha Chao Bu Sui Gu, Chao Gu Sui Bu, Chao Bu Sui Gu*

Flavors & nature: Bitter; warm

Functions: Supplements the kidneys, quickens the blood, stops bleeding, knits the sinews and bones

Indications:

1. Low back pain due to kidney qi vacuity

2. Tinnitus, deafness due to kidney qi vacuity

3. Traumatic injury, bone fracture, torn ligaments

Rhizoma Drynariae continued . . .

Typical combinations:

1. With salt[-processed] Cortex Eucommiae Ulmoidis (*Yan Du Zhong*), salt[-processed] Fructus Psoraleae Corylifoliae (*Yan Bu Gu Zhi*), and salt[-processed] Radix Dipsaci (*Yan Xu Duan*)

2. With dip calcined Magnetitum (*Cui Ci Shi*), Rhizoma Acori Graminei (*Shi Chang Pu*), stir-fried Radix Bupleuri (*Chao Chai Hu*), and pre-

pared Radix Rehmanniae (*Shu Di Huang*)

3. With wine[-processed] Radix Dipsaci (*Jiu Xu Duan*), vinegar dip calcined Pyritum (*Cu Cui Zi Ran Tong*), wine[-processed] Cortex Radicis Acanthopanacis (*Jiu Wu Jia Pi*), dip calcined Plastrum Testudinis (*Cui Gui Ban*), and stone-baked Eupolyphaga Seu Opisthoplatia (*Bei Zhe Chong*)

Dosage: 10-20g

Semen Trigonellae Foeni-graecae *(Hu Lu Ba)*

Uncooked *(Sheng)*

Names: *Hu Lu Ba, Sheng Hu Lu Ba, Sheng Hu Ba*

Flavors & nature: Sweet; warm

Functions: Scatters cold, eliminates dampness

Indications:

1. Abdominal and lateral costal distention due to vacuity cold of the kidneys with internal accumulation of cold dampness

2. Foot qi due to cold dampness with knee and leg pain...

Typical combinations:

1. With processed Radix Lateralis Praeparatus Aconiti Carmichaeli (*Zhi Fu Zi*) and processed Sulfur (*Zhi Liu Huang*) as in *Hu Lu Ba Wan* (Fenugreek Pills [I; 142])

2. With processed Fructus Evodiae Rutecarpae (*Zhi Wu Zhu Yu*), steamed Fructus Chaenomelis Lagenariae (*Zheng Mu Gua*), and uncooked Radix Cyathulae (*Sheng Chuan Niu Xi*)

Dosage: 5-10g

Salt Mix-fried *(Yan Zhi)*

Names: *Yan Zhi Hu Lu Ba, Yan Hu Lu Ba, Yan Hu Ba*

Flavors & nature: Bitter and slightly salty; warm

Functions: Warms the kidneys, strengthens yang

Indications:

1. Impotence, premature ejaculation, spermatorrhea due to kidney yang vacuity

2. Inguinal hernia, maladies of the scrotum or testicles due to kidney yang vacuity and accumu-

lation of internal cold with severe pain...

3. Dysmenorrhea due to kidney yang vacuity and vacuity cold of the *chong* and *ren*

4. Headache at the vertex due to kidney vacuity with head distention...

Typical combinations:

1. With salt[-processed] Radix Morindae Officinalis (*Yan Ba Ji Tian*), salt[-processed] Fructus Psoraleae Corylifoliae (*Yan Bu Gu Zhi*), and

Semen Trigonellae Foeni-graecae continued . . .

wine[-processed] Rhizoma Curculiginis Orchioidis (*Jiu Xian Mao*)

2. With salt[-processed] Fructus Foeniculi Vulgaris (*Yan Xiao Hui Xiang*) and stir-fried Fructus Meliae Toosendan (*Chao Chuan Lian Zi*) as in *Hu Lu Ba Wan* (Fenugreek Pills [II; 143])

3. With vinegar[-processed] Folium Artemisiae Argyii (*Cu Ai Ye*), processed Fructus Evodiae Rutecarpae (*Zhi Wu Zhu Yu*), and wine[-processed] Radix Angelicae Sinensis (*Jiu Dang Gui*)

4. With vinegar[-processed] Rhizoma Sparganii (*Cu San Leng*) and dry Rhizoma Zingiberis (*Gan Jiang*) as in *Hu Lu Ba San* (Fenugreek Powder [141])

Dosage: 5-10g

Cornu Cervi *(Lu Jiao)*

Uncooked *(Sheng)*[1]

Names: *Lu Jiao Pian, Lu Jiao Fen, Lu Jiao*

Flavors & nature: Salty; warm

Functions: Quickens the blood, disperses swelling, warms the kidneys, nourishes the essence

Indications:

1. Skin inflammation of the yin type which does not heal, tends to sink, and suppurates chronically...

2. Mastitis with either A) swelling and fixed, localized nodulations (in the inflammatory stage) or B) chronic suppuration, sores which do not heal

3. Low back pain due to kidney essence insufficiency with mental and physical apathy, darkness around the eyes...

4. Impotence, premature ejaculation due to kidney yang vacuity

Typical combinations:

1. With Cortex Cinnamomi (*Rou Gui*) and Fructus Gleditschiae Chinensis (*Zao Jiao*)

2. A) Herba Cum Radice Taraxaci Mongolici (*Pu Gong Ying*), uncooked Flos Lonicerae Japonicae (*Sheng Jin Yin Hua*), uncooked Fructus Forsythiae Suspensae (*Sheng Lian Qiao*), and Radix Trichosanthis Kirlowii (*Tian Hua Fen*)
B) With Flos Chrysanthemi Indici (*Ye Ju Hua*), Spina Gleditschiae Chinensis (*Zao Jiao Ci*), and Cortex Cinnamomi (*Rou Gui*)

3. With salt[-processed] Radix Achyranthis Bidentatae (*Yan Huai Niu Xi*) as in *Lu Jiao Wan* (Deer Antler Pills [211])

4. With salt[-processed] Semen Cuscutae (*Yan Tu Si Zi*) and steamed Fructus Corni Officinalis (*Zheng Shan Zhu Yu*)

Dosage: 5-10g in decoction and up to 30g in decoction in severe cases[2]; 1-3g in powder

Notes: 1. This refers to the slices (*Lu Jiao Pian*) or the powder (*Lu Jiao Fen*) of adult deer antler. 2. One should pay particular attention when using high doses of Deer Antler since there is possible risk of falling hair, vertigo, epistaxis, and bleeding gums. It is counseled to progressively raise the dose in decoction and not to go beyond 3g in pill or powder. This drawback is less severe than for Cornu Parvum Cervi (*Lu Rong*).

Cornu Cervi continued . . .

Gelatinum (Jiao)[1]

Names: *Lu Jiao Jiao, Bai Jiao*

Flavors & nature: Sweet and salty; warm

Functions: Supplements the kidneys, strengthens yang, nourishes the essence and blood, stops bleeding

Indications:

1. Impotence, premature ejaculation due to kidney yang vacuity

2. Spermatorrhea due to kidney yang and essence vacuity

3. Hemoptysis due to yin and yang vacuity

4. Hematuria, metrorrhagia due to kidney yang and essence vacuity

5. *Yong*, phlegmon or spreading, diffuse, deeply subcutaneous lesions causing multiple small pockets of pus, osteomylitis of the yin type which is sunken and with sterile suppuration...

Typical combinations:

1. With wine[-processed] Rhizoma Curculiginis

Orchioidis (*Jiu Xian Mao*) and processed Herba Epimedii (*Zhi Yin Yang Huo*)

2. With Fructus Rubi (*Fu Pen Zi*) and salt[-processed] Semen Plantaginis (*Yan Che Qian Zi*) as in *Lu Jiao Jiao San* (Deer Antler Glue Powder [209])

3. With uncooked, processed Radix Rehmanniae (*Zhi Sheng Di Huang*) as in *Lu Jiao Jiao Fang* (Deer Antler Glue Formula [208])

4. With prepared Radix Rehmanniae (*Shu Di Huang*) and Crinis Carbonisatus (*Xue Yu Tan*) as in *Lu Jiao Jiao Wan* (Deer Antler Glue Pills [210])

5. With Cortex Cinnamomi (*Rou Gui*) and stir-fried Semen Sinapis Albae (*Chao Bai Jie Zi*) as in *Yang He Tang* (Harmonize Yang Decoction [395])

Dosage: 5-10g and up to 15g in severe cases

Note: 1. Gelatinum Cornu Cervi (*Lu Jiao Jiao*) is a gelatin obtained by decocting Deer Antler (*Lu Jiao*) for a prolonged period of time.

Defatted (Shuang)[1]

Name: *Lu Jiao Shuang*

Flavors & nature: Salty; warm

Functions: Supplements the kidneys, strengthens yang, stops outflow (blood, stools, liquids, sperm...)

Indications:

1. Spermatorrhea due to kidney qi not securing

2. Abnormal vaginal discharge due to kidney yang vacuity with whitish, fluid, abundant discharge...

3. Diarrhea due to spleen/kidney vacuity with loose stools containing undigested food

4. Metrorrhagia due to *chong* and *ren* not securing

5. Strangury with chyluria due to kidney vacuity and accumulation of dampness

Typical combinations:

1. With calcined Concha Ostreae (*Duan Mu Li*) and calcined Os Draconis (*Duan Long Gu*)

Cornu Cervi continued . . .

2. With Semen Nelumbinis Nuciferae (*Lian Zi*), uncooked Semen Euryalis Ferocis (*Sheng Qian Shi*), and stir-fried Semen Ginkgonis Bilobae (*Chao Bai Guo*)

3. With salt[-processed] Fructus Psoraleae Corylifoliae (*Yan Bu Gu Zhi*), roasted Semen Myristicae Fragrantis (*Wei Rou Dou Kou*), and earth stir-fried Rhizoma Atractylodis Macrocephalae (*Tu Chao Bai Zhu*)

4. With stir-fried Os Sepiae Seu Sepiellae (*Chao Hai Piao Xiao*), carbonized Folium Et Petiolus Trachycarpi (*Zong Lu Tan*), and carbonized Radix Angelicae Sinensis (*Dang Gui Tan*)

5. With Rhizoma Acori Graminei (*Shi Chang Pu*), salt[-processed] Rhizoma Dioscoreae Hypoglaucae (*Yan Bei Xie*), uncooked Sclerotium Poriae Cocos (*Sheng Fu Ling*), and salt[-processed] Radix Morindae Officinalis (*Yan Ba Ji Tian*)

Dosage: 5-10g and up to 15g in severe cases

Note: 1. This refers to the powdered residue obtained after preparing Deer Antler Glue (*Lu Jiao Jiao*).

Herba Cistanchis (*Rou Cong Rong*)

Uncooked (*Sheng*)

Names: *Rou Cong Rong, Cong Rong, Dan Cong Rong, Xian Cong Rong, Da Yun*

Flavors & nature: Sweet, sour, and salty; warm

Functions: Supplements the kidneys, stops turbidity, moistens the intestines, frees the stools

Indications:

1. Urinary strangury with dribbling and dripping due to kidney vacuity

2. Constipation due to either A) blood vacuity with dry stools or B) yang vacuity with low back pain, aversion to cold...

Typical combinations:

1. With bran stir-fried Radix Dioscoreae Oppositae (*Fu Chao Shan Yao*), uncooked Sclerotium Poriae Cocos (*Sheng Fu Ling*), stir-fried Semen Cuscutae (*Chao Tu Si Zi*), Cornu Parvum Cervi (*Lu Rong*), and salt[-processed] Radix Morindae Officinalis (*Yan Ba Ji Tian*)

2. A) With uncooked Radix Angelicae Sinensis (*Sheng Dang Gui*), stir-fried Semen Cannabis Sativae (*Chao Huo Ma Ren*), and uncooked Radix Rehmanniae (*Sheng Di Huang*) as in *Cong Rong Run Chang Tang* (Cistanches Moisten the Intestines Decoction [58])

B) With salt[-processed] Radix Achyranthis Bidentatae (*Yan Huai Niu Xi*) and uncooked Radix Angelicae Sinensis (*Sheng Dang Gui*) as in *Ji Chuan Jian* (Benefit the River [Flow] Decoction [165])

Dosage: 10-20g and up to 30g in severe cases

Wine Mix-fried (*Jiu Zhi*)

Names: *Jiu Zhi Cong Rong, Jiu Rou Cong Rong*

Flavors & nature: Sweet, sour, salty and slightly acrid; warm

Functions: Supplements the kidneys, strengthens yang, strengthens the low back, nourishes the essence

Herba Cistanchis continued ...

Indications:

1. Impotence, premature ejaculation, spermatorrhea due to kidney yang vacuity

2. Low back pain due to yang and/or kidney essence vacuity

3. Infertility due to kidney yang and essence vacuity or cold in the uterus

Typical combinations:

1. Processed Herba Epimedii (*Zhi Yin Yang Huo*), salt[-processed] Radix Morindae Officinalis (*Yan* Ba Ji Tian), and Cortex Cinnamomi (*Rou Gui*)

2. With salt[-processed] Radix Dipsaci (*Yan Xu Duan*) and salt[-processed] Cortex Eucommiae Ulmoidis (*Yan Du Zhong*) as in *Rou Cong Rong Wan* (Cistanches Pills [266])

3. With processed Radix Lateralis Praeparatus Aconiti Carmichaeli (*Zhi Fu Zi*), processed Fructus Evodiae Rutecarpae (*Zhi Wu Zhu Yu*), wine[-processed] Radix Angelicae Sinensis (*Jiu Dang Gui*), and wine[-processed] Radix Albus Paeoniae Lactiflorae (*Jiu Bai Shao Yao*)

Dosage: 10-20g and up to 30g in severe cases

Semen Astragali *(Sha Yuan Zi)*

_____ Uncooked *(Sheng)*_____

Names: *Sheng Sha Yuan Zi, Sha Yuan Zi, Sha Yuan Ji Li, Tong Ji Li*

Flavors & nature: Sweet; warm

Functions: Nourishes the liver, brightens the eyes

Indications: Diminished visual acuity, blurred vision due to either 1) liver vacuity with vertigo, dizziness, headache or 2) liver/kidney blood and essence vacuity with weak low back and knees...

Typical combinations:

1. With Feces Vespertilionis Murini (*Ye Ming Sha*), uncooked Flos Chrysanthemi Morifolii (*Sheng Ju Hua*), and stir-fried Semen Cassiae Torae (*Chao Jue Ming Zi*)

2. With uncooked Fructus Ligustri Lucidi (*Sheng Nu Zhen Zi*), Fructus Lycii Chinensis (*Gou Qi Zi*), uncooked Semen Cuscutae (*Sheng Tu Si Zi*), prepared Radix Rehmanniae (*Shu Di Huang*), and processed Radix Polygoni Multiflori (*Zhi He Shou Wu*)

Dosage: 10-20g

_____ Salt Mix-fried *(Yan Zhi)*_____

Names: *Yan Zhi Sha Yuan Zi, Yan Sha Yuan Zi*

Flavors & nature: Sweet and slightly salty; warm

Functions: Supplements the kidneys, secures the essence, controls urination

Indications:

1. Low back pain due to A) kidney qi vacuity,; B) kidney yang vacuity; or C) kidney essence insufficiency

2. Spermatorrhea due to kidney qi not securing

3. Enuresis, urinary incontinence, nocturia due to A) kidney qi vacuity, kidney yang vacuity, or B) spleen qi vacuity

Semen Astragali continued . . .

Typical combinations:

1. A) With salt[-processed] Cortex Eucommiae Ulmoidis (*Yan Du Zhong*) and salt[-processed] Radix Dipsaci (*Yan Xu Duan*)
B) With processed Radix Lateralis Praeparatus Aconiti Carmichaeli (*Zhi Fu Zi*) and salt[-processed] Fructus Psoraleae Corylifoliae (*Yan Bu Gu Zhi*)
C) With Gelatinum Cornu Cervi (*Lu Jiao Jiao*) and salt[-processed] Semen Cuscutae (*Yan Tu Si Zi*)

2. With uncooked Semen Euryalis Ferocis (*Sheng Qian Shi*) and calcined Os Draconis (*Duan Long Gu*) as in *Jin Suo Gu Jing Wan* (Golden Lock Secure the Essence Pills [182])

3. A) With salt[-processed] Semen Cuscutae (*Yan Tu Si Zi*), salt[-processed] Fructus Alpiniae Oxyphyllae (*Yan Yi Zhi Ren*), and uncooked Endothelium Corneum Gigeriae Galli (*Sheng Ji Nei Jin*)
B) With Cortex Cinnamomi (*Rou Gui*) and processed Radix Lateralis Praeparatus Aconiti Carmichaeli (*Zhi Fu Zi*)
C) With stir-fried Radix Astragali Membranacei (*Chao Huang Qi*), honey mix-fried Radix Codonopsis Pilosulae (*Mi Zhi Dang Shen*), and honey mix-fried Rhizoma Cimicifugae (*Mi Zhi Sheng Ma*)

Dosage: 10-20g

Semen Cuscutae *(Tu Si Zi)*

—————————— Uncooked *(Sheng)*——————————

Names: *Tu Si Zi, Sheng Tu Si Zi*

Flavors & nature: Acrid and sweet; neutral

Functions: Nourishes the liver, brightens the eyes

Indications: Diminished visual acuity, blurred vision due to either 1) liver vacuity or 2) liver/-kidney essence insufficiency

Typical combinations:

1. With Feces Vespertilionis Murini (*Ye Ming Sha*), Flos Buddleiae Officinalis (*Mi Meng Hua*), uncooked Fructus Ligustri Lucidi (*Sheng Nu Zhen Zi*), and uncooked Flos Chrysanthemi Morifolii (*Sheng Ju Hua*)

2. With prepared Radix Rehmanniae (*Shi Di Huang*), Fructus Lycii Chinensis (*Gou Qi Zi*), and uncooked Semen Astragali (*Sheng Sha Yuan Zi*)

Dosage: 10-15g and up to 30g in severe cases

—————————— Mix-fried *(Zhi)*[1] ——————————

Names: *Zhi Tu Si Zi, Yan Tu Si Zi, Jiu Tu Si Zi, Tu Si Zi Bing*

Flavors & nature: Sweet, acrid, and slightly salty[1]; warm[1]

Functions: Supplements the kidneys, secures the essence, stops diarrhea, quiets the fetus, controls urination

Indications:

1. Impotence, premature ejaculation due to kidney yang and essence vacuity

2. Diarrhea due to spleen/kidney vacuity

3. Enuresis, urinary incontinence due to either A) heart and kidneys not communicating or

Semen Cuscutae continued . . .

B) kidney yang vacuity

4. Abnormal vaginal discharge due to spleen/-kidney vacuity

5. Low back pain due to either A) kidney qi vacuity or B) kidney yang vacuity

6. Threatened spontaneous abortion, metrorrhagia during pregnancy, *i.e.*, A) restless fetus due to kidney vacuity or B) restless fetus due to kidney vacuity with metrorrhagia during pregnancy

Typical combinations:

1. With wine[-processed] Herba Cistanchis (*Jiu Rou Cong Rong*), Cornu Cervi (*Lu Jiao*), and Placenta Hominis (*Zi He Che*)

2. With salt[-processed] Fructus Psoraleae Corylifoliae (*Yan Bu Gu Zhi*) and earth stir-fried Rhizoma Atractylodis Macrocephalae (*Tu Chao Bai Zhu*)

3. A) With Sclerotium Pararadicis Poriae Cocos (*Fu Shen*), processed Radix Polygalae Tenuifoliae (*Zhi Yuan Zhi*), Rhizoma Acori Graminei (*Shi Chang Pu*), and Semen Nelumbinis Nuciferae (*Lian Zi*)
B) With processed Radix Lateralis Praeparatus Aconiti Carmichaeli (*Zhi Fu Zi*), salt[-processed] Fructus Alpiniae Oxyphyllae (*Yan Yi Zhi Ren*), and salt[-processed] Ootheca Mantidis (*Yan Sang Piao Xiao*)

4. With Stamen Nelumbinis Nuciferae (*Lian Xu*), uncooked Semen Euryalis Ferocis (*Sheng Qian Shi*), and stir-fried Semen Ginkgonis Bilobae (*Chao Bai Guo*)

5. A) With salt[-processed] Radix Dipsaci (*Yan Xu Duan*) and salt[-processed] Cortex Eucommiae Ulmoidis (*Yan Du Zhong*)
B) With Cornu Parvum Cervi (*Lu Rong*), Cortex Cinnamomi (*Rou Gui*), and processed Radix Lateralis Praeparatus Aconiti Carmichaeli (*Zhi Fu Zi*)

6. A) With Ramus Loranthis Seu Visci (*Sang Ji Sheng*), salt[-processed] Radix Dipsaci (*Yan Xu Duan*), and salt[-processed] Cortex Eucommiae Ulmoidis (*Yan Du Zhong*)
B) With the same as above plus Pollen Typhae stir-fried Gelatinum Corii Asini (*Pu Huang Chao E Jiao*) and Herba Ecliptae Prostratae (*Han Lian Cao*)

Dosage: 10-15g and up to 30g in severe cases

Note: 1. If one wishes to supplement the kidneys harmoniously (*i.e.*, both yin and yang), salt mix-fried Cuscuta (*Yan Zhi Tu Si Zi*) is prescribed. If one wishes to supplement the kidneys and strengthen yang, wine[-processed] Cuscuta pancakes (*Jiu Tu Si Zi Bing*) are prescribed. Wine[-processed] Cuscuta pancake is obtained by first cooking the grains of Cuscuta. These are then crushed and mixed with rice wine and wheat bran which are then made into medicinal pancakes or *bing*.

Rhizoma Curculiginis Orchioidis *(Xian Mao)*

Uncooked *(Sheng)*

Names: *Xian Mao, Sheng Xian Mao*

Flavors & nature: Acrid and slightly sweet; warm; toxic

Functions: Scatters cold, eliminates dampness

Indications:

1. Rheumatic complaints due to cold dampness with cold, painful low back and knees, weak legs, sinews, and bones...

Rhizoma Curculiginis Orchioidis cont. . . .

2. *Yong* due to heat toxins, enduring *yong*, swelling without a head and dark in color...

Typical combinations:

1. With processed Radix Lateralis Praeparatus coniti Carmichaeli (*Zhi Fu Zi*), uncooked Rhizoma Cibotii Barometz (*Sheng Gou Ji*), and uncooked Cortex Eucommiae Ulmoidis (*Sheng Du Zhong*)

2. Apply locally either a powder or decoction of uncooked Curculigo

Dosage: 3-10g

Wine mix-fried (Jiu Zhi)

Names: *Jiu Zhi Xian Mao, Jiu Xian Mao*

Flavors & nature: Acrid and slightly sweet; warm; slightly toxic

Functions: Supplements the kidneys, strengthens yang

Indications:

1. Impotence, premature ejaculation, spermatorrhea due to kidney yang vacuity

2. Dizziness, vertigo due to liver/kidney vacuity

3. Urinary incontinence, nocturia, abundant urination due to kidney yang vacuity

4. Asthma, cough due to kidneys not absorbing qi

Typical combinations:

1. With processed Herba Epimedii (*Zhi Yin Yang Huo*), salt[-processed] Radix Morindae Officinalis (*Yan Ba Ji Tian*), and Herba Cynomorii Songarici (*Suo Yang*)

2. With Fructus Lycii Chinensis (*Gou Qi Zi*) and prepared Radix Rehmanniae (*Shu Di Huang*) as in *Xian Mao Wan* (Curculigo Pills [366])

3. With salt[-processed] Fructus Alpiniae Oxyphyllae (*Yan Yi Zhi Ren*), salt[-processed] Semen Cuscutae (*Yan Tu Si Zi*), and salt[-processed] Ootheca Mantidis (*Yan Sang Piao Xiao*)

4. With Lignum Aquilariae Agallochae (*Chen Xiang*), dip calcined Magnetitum (*Cui Ci Shi*), salt[-processed] Fructus Psoraleae Corylifoliae (*Yan Bu Gu Zhi*), Gecko (*Ge Jie*), and Radix Panacis Ginseng (*Ren Shen*)

Dosage: 3-10g

Radix Dipsaci (*Xu Duan*)

Uncooked (Sheng)

Names: *Sheng Xu Duan, Xu Duan, Chuan Duan*

Flavors & nature: Bitter and acrid; slightly warm

Functions: Dispels wind dampness, quickens the blood, disperses swelling

Indications:

1. Rheumatic complaints due to wind cold dampness and liver/kidney vacuity with weak low back, knees, and legs, joint and sinew pain...

2. Mastitis (inflammatory stage)

Radix Dipsaci continued . . .

Typical combinations:

1. With uncooked Radix Ledebouriellae Sesloidis (*Sheng Fang Feng*), uncooked Radix Achyranthis Bidentatae (*Sheng Huai Niu Xi*), and processed Radix Aconiti Carmichaeli (*Zhi Chuan Wu Tou*) as in *Xu Duan Wan* (Dipsacus Pills [386])

2. With Herba Cum Radice Taraxaci Mongolici (*Pu Gong Ying*) and Flos Chrysanthemi Indici (*Ye Ju Hua*)

Dosage: 10-15g

Wine Mix-fried (*Jiu Zhi*)

Names: *Jiu Zhi Xu Duan, Jiu Xu Duan*

Flavors & nature: Bitter and acrid; warm

Functions: Moves the blood, dispels blood stasis, knits the sinews and bones

Indications:

1. Agalactia due to qi stagnation, blood stasis, and blood vacuity

2. Postpartum vertigo due to blood stasis with severe abdominal pain, a sensation of cold and heat in the lower abdomen...

3. Bone fracture, torn ligaments, luxation with swelling, pain, hematoma...

Typical combinations:

1. With wine[-processed] Radix Angelicae Sinen-sis (*Jiu Dang Gui*), wine[-processed] Radix Ligustici Wallichii (*Jiu Chuan Xiong*), and dip calcined Squama Manitis Pentadactylis (*Cui Chuan Shan Jia*) as in *Ru Zhi Xia Xing Fang* (Breast Milk Descend & Move Formula [268])

2. With wine[-processed] Radix Angelicae Sinensis (*Jiu Dang Gui*), stir-fried Rhizoma Gastrodiae Elatae (*Chao Tian Ma*), and wine[-processed] Rhizoma Ligustici Wallichii (*Jiu Chuan Xiong*)

3. With stir-fried Rhizoma Drynariae (*Chao Gu Sui Bu*), calcined Pyritum (*Duan Zi Ran Tong*), stir-fried Resina Olibani (*Chao Ru Xiang*), and Sanguis Draconis (*Xue Jie*) as in *Jie Gu San* (Knit Bones Powder [177])

Dosage: 10-15g and 15-30g for broken bones and torn ligaments

Salt Mix-fried (*Yan Zhi*)

Names: *Yan Zhi Xu Duan, Yan Xu Duan*

Flavors & nature: Bitter, slightly acrid, and slightly salty; slightly warm

Functions: Supplements the kidneys, strengthens the sinews and bones, quiets the fetus, stops metrorrhagia

Indications:

1. Low back pain due to either A) kidney qi vacuity or B) kidney essence insufficiency

2. Atony of the lower limbs due to kidney vacuity

3. Metrorrhagia due to *chong* and *ren* not securing

4. Threatened spontaneous abortion due to kidney vacuity

Typical combinations:

1. A) With salt[-processed] Cortex Eucommiae Ulmoidis (*Yan Du Zhong*), wine[-processed] Ramus Loranthi Seu Visci (*Jiu Sang Ji Sheng*), and salt[-processed] Fructus Psoraleae Corylifoliae (*Yan Bu Gu Zhi*)

Radix Dipsaci continued . . .

B) With Gelatinum Cornu Cervi (*Lu Jiao Jiao*) and salt[-processed] Semen Cuscutae (*Yan Tu Si Zi*)

2. With salt[-processed] Cortex Eucommiae Ulmoidis (*Yan Du Zhong*), salt[-processed] Radix Achyranthis Bidentatae (*Yan Huai Niu Xi*), wine[-processed] Cortex Radicis Acanthopanacis (*Jiu Wu Jia Pi*), and wine[-processed] Ramus Loranthi Seu Visci (*Jiu Sang Ji Sheng*)

3. With Gelatinum Cornu Cervi (*Lu Jiao Jiao*), Pollen Typhae stir-fried Gelatinum Corii Asini (*Pu Huang Chao E Jiao*), Herba Ecliptae Prostratae (*Han Lian Cao*), and carbonized Folium Et Petiolus Trachycarpi (*Zong Lu Tan*)

4. With salt[-processed] Cortex Eucommiae Ulmoidis (*Yan Du Zhong*), Ramus Loranthi Seu Visci (*Sang Ji Sheng*), and salt[-processed] Semen Cuscutae (*Yan Tu Si Zi*)

Dosage: 10-15g

Fructus Alpiniae Oxyphyllae *(Yi Zhi Ren)*

Stir-fried [till] Scorched *(Chao Jiao)*

Names: *Yi Zhi Ren, Yi Zhi Zi, Chao Yi Zhi Ren*

Flavors & nature: Acrid; warm

Functions: Warms the spleen, stops diarrhea, restrains saliva

Indications:

1. Diarrhea, vomiting due to cold dampness in the spleen and stomach with epigastric and abdominal distention, cold extremities...

2. Hypersalivation due to spleen yang vacuity

Typical combinations:

1. With dry Rhizoma Zingiberis (*Gan Jiang*) and processed Radix Lateralis Praeparatus Aconiti Carmichaeli (*Zhi Fu Zi*)

2. With honey mix-fried Radix Codonopsis Pilosulae (*Mi Zhi Dang Shen*), dry Rhizoma Zingiberis (*Gan Jiang*), uncooked Sclerotium Poriae Cocos (*Sheng Fu Ling*), and bran stir-fried Rhizoma Atractylodis Macrocephalae (*Fu Chao Bai Zhu*)

Dosage: 5-10g and up to 15g in severe cases

Salt Mix-fried *(Yan Zhi)*

Names: *Yan Zhi Yi Zhi Ren, Yan Yi Zhi Ren*

Flavors & nature: Acrid and slightly salty; warm

Functions: Supplements the kidneys, strengthens yang, secures the essence, controls urination

Indications:

1. Enuresis, urinary incontinence, nocturia due to kidney yang vacuity

2. Spermatorrhea, premature ejaculation due to kidney qi not securing

3. Urinary strangury with dribbling and dripping due to kidney qi vacuity

4. Metrorrhagia due to kidney qi vacuity

5. Inguinal hernia, maladies of the scrotum or testicles due to kidney vacuity and accumulation of cold

Fructus Alpiniae Oxyphyllae continued . . .

Typical combinations:

1. With salt[-processed] Radix Linderae Strychnifoliae (*Yan Wu Yao*) and stir-fried Radix Dioscoreae Oppositae (*Chao Shan Yao*) as in *Suo Quan Wan* (Shut the Spring Pills [319])

2. With salt[-processed] Semen Cuscutae (*Yan Tu Si Zi*), Stamen Nelumbinis Nuciferae (*Lian Xu*), and salt[-processed] Fructus Psoraleae Corylifoliae (*Yan Bu Gu Zhi*)

3. With salt[-processed] Rhizoma Dioscoreae Hypoglaucae (*Yan Bei Xie*), uncooked Sclerotium Poriae Cocos (*Sheng Fu Ling*), and Rhizoma Acori Graminei (*Shi Chang Pu*)

4. With carbonized Radix Angelicae Sinensis (*Dang Gui Tan*), carbonized Folium Et Petiolus Trachycarpi (*Zong Lu Tan*), and stir-fried Os Sepiae Seu Sepiellae (*Chao Hai Piao Xiao*)

5. With salt[-processed] Fructus Foeniculi Vulgaris (*Yan Xiao Hui Xiang*) and vinegar[-processed] Pericarpium Viridis Citri Reticulatae (*Cu Qing Pi*) as in *Yi Zhi Ren Tang* (Alpinia Oxyphylla Decoction [407])

Dosage: 5-10g and up to 15g in severe cases

Herba Epimedii *(Yin Yang Huo)*

Uncooked (Sheng)

Names: *Sheng Yin Yang Huo, Sheng Xian Ling Pi, Yin Yang Huo, Xian Ling Pi*

Flavors & nature: Sweet and acrid; warm

Functions: Dispels wind, eliminates dampness

Indications: Rheumatic complaints due to cold dampness and kidney yang vacuity

Typical combinations: With uncooked Fructus Xanthii (*Sheng Cang Er Zi*), wine[-processed] Radix Clematidis Chinensis (*Jiu Wei Ling Xian*), and wine[-processed] Rhizoma Ligustici Wallichii (*Jiu Chuan Xiong*) as in *Xian Ling Pi San* (Epimedium Powder [365])

Dosage: 10-15g and up to 30g in severe cases

Mix-fried (Zhi)[¹]

Names: *Zhi Yin Yang Huo, Zhi Xian Ling Pi*

Flavors & nature: Sweet and slightly acrid; warm

Functions: Warms the kidneys, strengthens yang

Indications:

1. Impotence, premature ejaculation due to either A) kidney yin and yang vacuity with spermatorrhea or B) severe kidney yang vacuity

2. Infertility due to kidney yang vacuity and cold in the uterus

3. Low back pain due to kidney yang vacuity

4. Menopausal syndrome due to kidney yin and yang vacuity with arterial hypertension, hot flashes, irritability...

Typical combinations:

1. A) With Fructus Lycii Chinensis (*Gou Qi Zi*) and salt[-processed] Semen Astragali (*Yan Sha Yuan Zi*) as in *Yang Huo San Zi Tang* (Epimedium Three Seeds Decoction [396])

Herba Epimedii continued . . .

B) With Cornu Parvum Cervi (*Lu Rong*), processed Radix Lateralis Praeparatus Aconiti Carmichaeli (*Zhi Fu Zi*), and salt[-processed] Fructus Psoraleae Corylifoliae (*Yan Bu Gu Zhi*)

2. With Cortex Cinnamomi (*Rou Gui*), processed Radix Lateralis Praeparatus Aconiti Carmichaeli (*Zhi Fu Zi*), and processed Fructus Evodiae Rutecarpae (*Zhi Wu Zhu Yu*)

3. With salt[-processed] Cortex Eucommiae Ulmoidis (*Yan Du Zhong*), salt[-processed] Radix Dipsaci (*Yan Xu Duan*), and salt[-processed] Semen Cuscutae (*Yan Tu Si Zi*)

4. With wine[-processed] Rhizoma Curculiginis Orchioidis (*Jiu Xian Mao*), salt[-processed] Cortex Phellodendri (*Yan Huang Bai*), and salt[-processed] Rhizoma Anemarrhenae (*Yan Zhi Mu*) as in *Er Xian Tang* (Two Immortals Decoction [100])

Dosage: 10-15g and up to 30g in severe cases

Note: 1. To obtain processed Epimedium, one fries *Yin Yang Huo* with mutton fat.

19
Blood-supplementing Medicinals

Radix Albus Paeoniae Lactiflorae *(Bai Shao Yao)*

Uncooked *(Sheng)*

Names: *Sheng Bai Shao Yao, Sheng Bai Shao*

Flavors & nature: Bitter and sour; slightly cold

Functions: Settles the liver, downbears yang, nourishes the liver, restrains yin

Indications:

1. Vertigo due to liver blood vacuity in combination with liver yang rising with dizziness, hot flashes, tinnitus...

2. Clonic convulsions due to liver blood or yin vacuity in combination with internal wind

3. Night sweats, spontaneous perspiration due to A) disharmony between the constructive and defensive, B) yang vacuity, or C) yin vacuity

Typical combinations:

1. With uncooked Haematitum (*Sheng Dai Zhe Shi*) and uncooked Radix Achyranthis Bidentatae (*Sheng Huai Niu Xi*) as in *Zhen Gan Xi Feng*

Tang (Settle the Liver & Extinguish Wind Decoction [428])

2. With uncooked Plastrum Testudinis (*Sheng Gui Ban*), uncooked Radix Rehmanniae (*Sheng Di Huang*), and uncooked Gelatinum Corii Asini (*Sheng E Jiao*) as in *Da Ding Feng Zhu* (Great Stabilize Wind Pearls [62a])

3. A) With calcined Concha Ostreae (*Duan Mu Li*), calcined Os Draconis (*Duan Long Gu*), and stir-fried Ramulus Cinnamomi (*Chao Gui Zhi*) as in *Gui Zhi Jia Long Gu Mu Li Tang* (Cinnamon Twig Plus Dragon Bone & Oyster Shell Decoction [127])
B) With uncooked Radix Astragali Membranacei (*Sheng Huang Qi*), bran stir-fried Rhizoma Atractylodis Macrocephalae (*Fu Chao Bai Zhu*), and processed Radix Lateralis Praeparatus Aconiti Carmichaeli (*Zhi Fu Zi*)
C) With defatted Semen Biotae Orientalis (*Bai Zi Ren Shuang*), dip calcined Plastrum Testudinis (*Cui Gui Ban*), and uncooked Semen Zizyphi Spinosae (*Sheng Suan Zao Ren*)

Dosage: 10-15g and up to 30-60g in severe cases

Wine Mix-fried *(Jiu Zhi)*

Names: *Jiu Zhi Bai Shao, Jiu Bai Shao Yao, Bai Shao, Bai Shao Yao*

Flavors & nature: Bitter, sour, and slightly acrid; neutral

Functions: Nourishes liver blood, relaxes tension, stops pain

Indications:

1. Menstrual irregularity due to blood vacuity with

Radix Albus Paeoniae Lactiflorae continued . . .

scanty menstruation, shortened cycles, possible metrorrhagia...

2. Dysmenorrhea due to blood vacuity and blood stasis of the liver with pain in the lower abdomen...

3. Epigastric and abdominal pain due to vacuity cold in the middle burner with pain ameliorated by heat and pressure...

4. Chest and lateral costal pain due to liver blood vacuity and liver qi stagnation

5. Pain in the extremities due to liver blood vacuity

Typical combinations:

1. With prepared Radix Rehmanniae (*Shu Di Huang*) as in *Si Wu Tang* (Four Materials Decoction [315])

2. With wine[-processed] Radix Ligustici Wallichii (*Jiu Chuan Xiong*), wine[-processed] Radix Angelicae Sinensis (*Jiu Dang Gui*), and wine[-processed] Caulis Millettiae Seu Spatholobi (*Jiu Ji Xue Teng*)

3. With stir-fried Ramulus Cinnamomi (*Chao Gui Zhi*) and mix-fried Radix Glycyrrhizae (*Zhi Gan Cao*) as in *Xiao Jian Zhong Tang* (Minor Fortify the Middle Decoction [376])

4. With wine[-processed] Radix Angelicae Sinensis (*Jiu Dang Gui*) and vinegar[-processed] Radix Bupleuri (*Cu Chai Hu*) as in *Xiao Yao San* (Rambling Powder [380])

5. With mix-fried Radix Glycyrrhizae (*Zhi Gan Cao*) as in *Shao Yao Gan Cao Tang* (Peony & Licorice Decoction [284])

Dosage: 5-15g and up to 15-30g in severe cases

_____**Stir-fried [till] Yellow (Chao Huang)**_____

Names: *Chao Bai Shao Yao, Chao Bai Shao*

Flavors & nature: Bitter, sour, and astringent; neutral

Functions: Soothes the liver, harmonizes the spleen, stops diarrhea

Indications:

1. Alternating diarrhea and constipation due to liver/spleen disharmony with irritability, a tendency to depression, lateral costal pain, loss of appetite, abdominal pain, fatigue...

2. Painful diarrhea due to liver/spleen disharmony with abdominal pain which persists after defecation...

3. Dysentery due to either A) spleen qi vacuity[1] or B) damp heat in the large intestine

Typical combinations:

1. With stir-fried Radix Bupleuri (*Chao Chai Hu*) and bran stir-fried Rhizoma Atractylodis Macrocephalae (*Fu Chao Bai Zhu*) as in *Xiao Yao San* (Rambling Powder [380])

2. With earth stir-fried Rhizoma Atractylodis Macrocephalae (*Tu Chao Bai Zhu*) and carbonized Radix Ledebouriellae Sesloidis (*Fang Feng Tan*) as in *Tong Xie Yao Fang* (Painful Diarrhea Essential Formula [333])

3. A) With roasted Semen Myristicae Fragrantis (*Wei Rou Dou Kou*), roasted Fructus Terminaliae Chebulae (*Wei He Zi*), and roasted Radix Saussureae Seu Vladimiriae (*Wei Mu Xiang*)
B) With uncooked Rhizoma Coptidis Chinensis (*Sheng Huang Lian*) and stir-fried Semen Arecae

**Radix Albus Paeoniae Lactiflorae
continued . . .**

Catechu (*Chao Bing Lang*) as in *Shao Yao Tang*
(Peony Decoction [285])

Dosage: 5-15g and up to 15-30g in severe cases

Note: 1. For this indication, carbonized Peony (*Bai Shao Yao Tan*) is prescribed.

Radix Angelicae Sinensis *(Dang Gui)*

Uncooked *(Sheng)*

Names: *Dang Gui, Sheng Dang Gui*

Flavors & nature: Sweet and acrid; warm

Functions: Nourishes the blood, moistens the
intestines, downbears counterflow lung qi

Indications:

1. Blood vacuity[1] due to A) spleen qi vacuity;
B) cold in the blood; or C) heat in the blood

2. Diminished visual acuity, vertigo due to liver
blood vacuity

3. Constipation due to blood vacuity or fluid vacuity of the large intestine

4. Cough due to counterflow lung qi

Typical combinations:

1. A) with stir-fried Radix Astragali Membranacei
(*Chao Huang Qi*) as in *Dang Gui Bu Xue Tang*
(*Dang Gui* Supplement the Blood Decoction [73])

B) With stir-fried Ramulus Cinnamomi (*Chao Gui
Zhi*) as in *Dang Gui Si Ni Tang* (*Dang Gui* Four
Counterflows Decoction [79])
C) With uncooked Radix Rehmanniae (*Sheng Di
Huang*) as in *Qin Lian Si Wu Tang* (Scutellaria &
Coptis Four Materials Decoction [249])

2. With wine[-processed] Radix Albus Paeoniae
Lactiflorae (*Jiu Bai Shao Yao*) as in *Gui Shao Di
Huang Wan* (*Dang Gui*, Peony & Rehmannia Pills
[122])

3. With stir-fried Semen Cannabis Sativae (*Chao
Huo Ma Ren*) as in *Run Chang Wan*
(Moisten the Intestines Pills [269])

4. With uncooked Fructus Perillae Frutescentis
(*Sheng Zi Su Zi*) as in *Su Zi Jiang Qi Tang* (Perilla
Seed Downbear the Qi Decoction [316])

Dosage: 5-15g and up to 30g in severe cases

Note: 1. For this indication, wine mix-fried Radix
Angelicae Sinensis (*Jiu Zhi Dang Gui*) can be prescribed if one wishes to also quicken and/or warm the
blood.

Earth Stir-fried *(Tu Chao)*

Names: *Tu Chao Dang Gui, Chao Dang Gui*

Flavors & nature: Sweet and slightly acrid; warm

Functions: Nourishes the blood, quickens the
blood, but does not promote defecation or slow
the digestion

Indications:

1. Blood vacuity accompanied by loose stools or
diarrhea due to spleen vacuity or disharmony of
the middle burner accompanied by blood vacuity

2. Blood stasis and/or blood vacuity at the same
time as vacuity cold of the middle burner with
abdominal pain, loose stools...

Radix Angelicae Sinensis continued . . .

Typical combinations:

1. With stir-fried Ramulus Cinnamomi (*Chao Gui Zhi*), uncooked Rhizoma Zingiberis (*Sheng Jiang*), and stir-fried Radix Albus Paeoniae Lactiflorae (*Chao Bai Shao Yao*) as in *Dang Gui Jian Zhong Tang* (*Dang Gui* Fortify the Center Decoction [74])

2. With uncooked Rhizoma Zingiberis (*Sheng Jiang*) and Mutton (*Yang Rou*) as in *Dang Gui Sheng Jiang Yang Rou Tang* (*Dang Gui*, Fresh Ginger & Mutton Decoction [78])

Dosage: 5-15g

_____Wine Mix-fried (*Jiu Zhi*)_____

Names: *Jiu Zhi Dang Gui, Jiu Dang Gui*

Flavors & nature: Sweet and acrid; warm

Functions: Nourishes the blood, quickens the blood, dispels blood stasis

Indications:

1. Menstrual irregularity due to blood vacuity

2. Dysmenorrhea due to blood vacuity and blood stasis

3. Amenorrhea due to either A) qi and blood vacuity or B) qi stagnation and blood stasis

4. Postpartum abdominal pain due to cold in the uterus and blood stasis

5. Traumatic injury with pain, hematoma, swelling...

6. Rheumatic complaints due to wind cold dampness blocking the circulation of qi and blood in the network vessels with joint pain, loss of mobility, numbness of the extremities...

Typical combinations:

1. With prepared Radix Rehmanniae (*Shu Di Huang*) as in *Si Wu Tang* (Four Materials Decoction [315])

2. With uncooked Semen Pruni Persicae (*Sheng Tao Ren*) and Flos Carthami Tinctorii (*Hong Hua*) as in *Tao Hong Si Wu Tang* (Persica & Carthamus Four Materials Decoction [321])

3. A) With uncooked Radix Codonopsis Pilosulae (*Sheng Dang Shen*) and prepared Radix Rehmanniae (*Shu Di Huang*) as in *Ba Zhen Tang* (Eight Pearls Decoction [4])
B) With wine[-processed] Radix Cyathulae (*Jiu Chuan Niu Xi*) and uncooked Fructus Citri Seu Ponciri (*Sheng Zhi Ke*) as in *Xue Fu Zhu Yu Tang* (Blood Mansion Dispel Stasis Decoction [393])

4. With blast-fried Rhizoma Zingiberis (*Pao Jiang*) and Flos Carthami Tinctorii (*Hong Hua*) as in *Sheng Hua Tang* (Engendering & Transforming Decoction [294])

5. With vinegar[-processed] Squama Manitis Pentadactylis (*Cu Chuan Shan Jia*) and wine[-processed] Radix Et Rhizoma Rhei (*Jiu Da Huang*) as in *Fu Yuan Huo Xue Tang* (Restore the Source & Quicken the Blood Decoction [106])

6. With Radix Et Rhizoma Notopterygii (*Qiang Huo*) and Radix Angelicae Pubescentis (*Du Huo*) as in *Juan Bi Tang* (Alleviate *Bi* Decoction [192])

Dosage: 5-15g and up to 30g in severe cases

Radix Angelicae Sinensis continued . . .

_____Stir-fried [till] Carbonized *(Chao Tan)*_____

Name: *Dang Gui Tan*

Flavors & nature: Sweet, acrid, and slightly astringent; warm

Functions: Harmonizes the blood, stops bleeding

Indications: Metrorrhagia, menorrhagia due to

chong and *ren* not securing

Typical combinations: With carbonized Folium Et Petiolus Trachycarpi (*Zong Lu Tan*) and calcined Os Draconis (*Duan Long Gu*) as in *Dang Gui San* (*Dang Gui* Powder [II; 77])

Dosage: 5-15g

_____*Dang Gui* Roots are Composed of Four Distinct Parts_____

1. *Dang Gui Tou*

Th head of *Dang Gui* means the uppermost extremity of the root. It quickens the blood and stops bleeding. This part is often prepared by stir-frying [till] carbonized (*Chao Tan*) in order to reinforce its hemostatic action.

2. *Dang Gui Shen*

The body of *Dang Gui* means the main part of the root. It nourishes the blood.

3. *Dang Gui Wei*

The tails of *Dang Gui* mean the secondary roots of the lower extremity of the [main] root. They

quicken the blood and break blood stasis. This part is often prepared by wine mix-frying (*Jiu Zhi*) in order to reinforce its blood-quickening action.

4. *Dang Gui Xu*

The beard of *Dang Gui* means the rootlets of the root. They quicken the blood and free the network vessels. This part is often prepared by wine mix-frying in order to reinforce its blood-quickening and network vessel freeing actions.

Quan Dang Gui or whole *Dang Gui* corresponds to all the above four parts together. It both quickens the blood and nourishes the blood thus harmonizing the blood.

Gelatinum Corii Asini *(E Jiao)*

_____Uncooked *(Sheng)*_____

Names: *E Jiao, Yuan E Jiao, Chen E Jiao, Lu E Jiao*

Flavors & nature: Sweet; neutral

Functions: Nourishes the blood, enriches yin, moistens dryness

Indications:

1. Blood vacuity with anemia, heart palpitations, vertigo, a pale complexion...

2. Insomnia, vexation due to blood vacuity accompanied by vacuity heat

3. Spasms, trembling in the extremities due to liver blood or yin vacuity generating liver wind

4. Constipation due to blood vacuity or large intestine dryness

Gelatinum Corii Asini continued . . .

Typical combinations:

1. With prepared Radix Rehmanniae (*Shu Di Huang*), wine[-processed] Radix Angelicae Sinensis (*Jiu Dang Gui*), wine[-processed] Radix Albus Paeoniae Lactiflorae (*Jiu Bai Shao Yao*), stir-fried Radix Astragali Membranacei (*Chao Huang Qi*), and uncooked Radix Codonopsis Pilosulae (*Sheng Dang Shen*)

2 With uncooked Rhizoma Coptidis Chinensis (*Sheng Huang Lian*) as in *Huang Lian E Jiao Tang* (Coptis & Donkey Skin Glue Decoction [151])

3. With uncooked Radix Albus Paeoniae Lactiflorae (*Sheng Bai Shao Yao*) and Ramulus Uncariae Cum Uncis (*Gou Teng*) as in *E Jiao Ji Zi Huang Tang* (Donkey Skin Glue & Chicken Egg Yolk Decoction [90])

4. With uncooked Fructus Citri Seu Ponciri (*Sheng Zhi Ke*)

Dosage: 5-10g and up to 30g in severe cases

_____Powdered Concha Cyclinae Stir-fried (*Ge Fen Chao*)¹ _____

Name: *Ge Fen Chao E Jiao*

Flavors & nature: Sweet and slightly salty; neutral

Functions: Nourishes the lungs, moistens dryness

Indications: Dry cough due to either 1) lung yin vacuity with scanty, difficult to expectorate phlegm possibly streaked with blood, a dry, sore throat or 2) damage by external warmth and dryness (*wen zao*) with dry throat and nose, little mucus, thirst, fever, chills...

Typical combinations:

1. With honey mix-fried Fructus Aristolochiae (*Mi Zhi Ma Dou Ling*), Semen Pruni Armeniacae (*Xing Ren*), and mix-fried Radix Glycyrrhizae (*Zhi Gan Cao*) as in *Bu Fei E Jiao Tang* (Supplement the Lungs Donkey Skin Glue Decoction [32])

2. With uncooked Folium Mori Albi (*Sheng Sang Ye*) and uncooked Semen Pruni Armeniacae (*Sheng Xing Ren*) as in *Qing Zao Jiu Fei Tang* (Clear Dryness & Rescue the Lungs Decoction [260])

Dosage: 5-10g and up to 30g in severe cases

Note: 1. *E Jiao* is fried on a bed of powdered Concha Cyclinae (*Hai Ge Ke*). This reinforces its expectorant effect for treating phlegm dryness.

_____Pollen Typhae Stir-fried (*Pu Huang Chao*)¹ _____

Name: *Pu Huang Chao E Jiao*

Flavors & nature: Sweet and neutral

Functions: Nourishes the blood, stops bleeding, harmonizes the network vessels

Indications:

1. Hemoptysis due to heat damaging the lung network vessels

2. Epistaxis due to liver/lung heat

3. Hematemesis due to heat damaging the stomach network vessels

4. Bloody stools due to damp heat or heat in the large intestine

5. Hematuria, stranguria with hematuria due to damp heat in the bladder

Gelatinum Corii Asini continued . . .

6. Metrorrhagia during pregnancy, metrorrhagia due to blood vacuity

Typical combinations:

1. With uncooked Cacumen Biotae Orientalis (*Sheng Ce Bai Ye*) and uncooked Rhizoma Imperatae Cylindricae (*Sheng Bai Mao Gen*)

2. With carbonized Radix Rubiae Cordifoliae (*Qian Cao Gen Tan*) and Herba Ecliptae Prostratae (*Han Lian Cao*)

3. With Rhizoma Bletillae Striatae (*Bai Ji*) and Radix Pseudoginseng (*San Qi*)

4. With carbonized Flos Immaturus Sophorae Japonicae (*Huai Hua Tan*) and uncooked Radix Sanguisorbae (*Sheng Di Yu*)

5. With carbonized Nodus Nelumbinis Nuciferae (*Ou Jie Tan*), Herba carbonized Cephalanoploris Segeti (*Xiao Ji Tan*), and Folium Pyrossiae (*Shi Wei*)

6. With carbonized Folium Artemisiae Argyii (*Ai Ye Tan*) and carbonized Radix Angelicae Sinensis (*Dang Gui Tan*) as in *Jiao Ai Tang* (Donkey Skin Glue & Artemisia Argyium Decoction [173])

Dosage: 5-10g and up to 30g in severe cases

Note: 1. *E Jiao* is fried with Pollen Typhae (*Pu Huang*). This reinforces its hemostatic action.

Radix Polygoni Multiflori *(He Shou Wu)*

_____ Uncooked *(Sheng)* _____

Names: *Sheng He Shou Wu, Sheng Shou Wu*

Flavors & nature: Bitter, sweet, and astringent; neutral

Functions: Moistens the intestines, frees the stool, resolves toxins, softens nodulations

Indications:

1. Constipation due to blood vacuity and large intestine dryness

2. Skin inflammation due to damp heat and wind toxins with pain, pruritus...

3. Subcutaneous nodules, scrofula due to accumulation of phlegm heat in the neck or due to liver fire which congeals fluids and engenders phlegm, which then stagnates in the neck

Typical combinations:

1. With stir-fried Semen Cannabis Sativae (*Chao Huo Ma Ren*), roasted Semen Myristicae Fragrantis (*Wei Rou Dou Kou*), and Semen Sesami Indici (*Hei Zhi Ma*)

2. With Cortex Radicis Dictamni (*Bai Xian Pi*), Radix Sophorae Flavescentis (*Ku Shen*), uncooked Herba Schizonepetae Tenuifoliae (*Sheng Jing Jie*), and uncooked Flos Lonicerae Japonicae (*Sheng Jin Yin Hua*) as in *He Shou Wu Tang* (Polygonum Multiflorum Decoction [133])

3. With Spica Prunellae Vulgaris (*Xiao Ku Cao*), Bulbus Fritillariae Thunbergii (*Zhe Bei Mu*), Fructus Gleditschiae Chinensis (*Zao Jiao*), and Thallus Algae (*Kun Bu*)

Dosage: 10-15g

Radix Polygoni Multiflori continued . . .

_____**Processed** _(Zhi)_[1]_____

Names: _Zhi He Shou Wu, He Shou Wu, Shou Wu_

Flavors & nature: Sweet, bitter, and astringent; warm

Functions: Supplements the liver and kidneys, nourishes the blood and essence

Indications:

1. Premature greying of the hair due to liver/-kidney essence insufficiency

2. Vertigo, tinnitus, deafness due to liver/kidney vacuity

3. Diminished visual acuity, blurred vision due to liver blood vacuity

4. Low back pain, weak lower limbs due to kidney essence insufficiency

Typical combinations:

1. With Fructus Lycii Chinensis (_Gou Qi Zi_), salt[-processed] Semen Cuscutae (_Yan Tu Si Zi_), and salt[-processed] Fructus Psoraleae Cory-lifoliae (_Yan Bu Gu Zhi_) as in _Qi Bao Mei Ran Dan_ (Seven Treasures Beautiful Beard Elixir [235])

2. With wine-steamed Fructus Ligustri Lucidi (_Jiu Zheng Nu Zhen Zi_), prepared Radix Rehmanniae (_Shu Di Huang_), Fructus Lycii Chinensis (_Gou Qi Zi_), and Herba Ecliptae Prostratae (_Han Lian Cao_)

3. With uncooked Semen Cuscutae (_Sheng Tu Si Zi_), Fructus Lycii Chinensis (_Gou Qi Zi_), uncooked Fructus Ligustri Lucidi (_Sheng Nu Zhen Zi_), and uncooked Semen Astragali (_Sheng Sha Yuan Zi_)

4. With salt[-processed] Cortex Eucommiae Ulmoidis (_Yan Du Zhong_), prepared Radix Rehmanniae (_Shu Di Huang_), salt[-processed] Radix Achyranthis Bidentatae (_Yan Huai Niu Xi_), and wine[-processed] Cortex Radicis Acanthopanacis (_Jiu Wu Jia Pi_)

Dosage: 10-15g and up to 30g in severe cases

Note: 1. _He Shou Wu_ is cooked in the steam of black soybean juice (_Hei Dou_) and yellow rice wine.

20
Yin-supplementing Medicinals

Bulbus Lilii (Bai He)

Uncooked (Sheng)

Names: *Bai He, Sheng Bai He*

Flavors & nature: Sweet and slightly bitter; slightly cold

Functions: Clears the heart, quiets the spirit

Indications:

1. Vexation due to a warm disease damaging heart yin with palpitations, agitation, insomnia...

2. Insomnia due to heart and kidneys not communicating with abundant dreams

Typical combinations:

1. With uncooked Rhizoma Anemarrhenae (*Sheng Zhi Mu*) as in *Bai He Zhi Mu Tang* (Lily & Anemarrhena Decoction [13]) or uncooked Radix Rehmanniae (*Sheng Di Huang*) as in *Bai He Di Huang Tang* (Lily & Rehmannia Decoction [11])

2. With uncooked Semen Zizyphi Spinosae (*Sheng Suan Zao Ren*), processed Radix Polygalae Tenuifoliae (*Zhi Yuan Zhi*), and Cinnabar[-processed] Sclerotium Pararadicis Poriae Cocos (*Zhu Sha Ban Fu Shen*)

Dosage: 10-30g

Honey Mix-fried (Mi Zhi)

Names: *Mi Zhi Bai He, Zhi Bai He, Mi Bai He*

Flavors & nature: Sweet and slightly bitter; neutral

Functions: Moistens the lungs, stops cough

Indications:

1. Cough due to heat damaging lung fluids with phlegm streaked with blood...

2. Hemoptysis due to lung/kidney yin vacuity with dry cough, evening fever, night sweats, a dry, sore throat...

Typical combinations:

1. With uncooked Flos Tussilaginis Farfarae (*Sheng Kuan Dong Hua*) as in *Bai Hua Gao* (White Flower Paste [16])

2. With prepared Radix Rehmanniae (*Shu Di Huang*), Radix Scrophulariae Ningpoensis (*Xuan Shen*), uncooked Tuber Ophiopogonis Japonicae (*Sheng Mai Men Dong*), and honey mix-fried Radix Platycodi Grandiflori (*Mi Zhi Jie Geng*) as in *Bai He Gu Jin Tang* (Lily Secure Metal Decoction [12])

Dosage: 15-30g

Carapax Amydae Sinensis (Bie Jia)

Name: *Sheng Bie Jia*

Flavors & nature: Salty; slightly cold

Functions: Enriches yin, clears heat, settles the liver, downbears yang

Indications:

1. Evening fever either A) due to vacuity heat caused by liver/kidney yin vacuity with night sweats, a dry throat and mouth, thirst, steaming bone fever, insomnia or B) following a warm disease which has damaged the fluids and humors with thirst, emaciation, a red tongue with scanty coating, a rapid (*shu*) pulse...

2. Spasms of the hands and feet, involuntary trembling of the hands and feet after a warm disease which has damaged liver yin and engendered internal wind...

Typical combinations:

1. A) With salt[-processed] Rhizoma Anemarrhenae (*Yan Zhi Mu*) and Cortex Radicis Lycii (*Di Gu Pi*) as in *Qing Gu San* (Clear the Bones Powder [251])
B) With Amyda tortoise blood [processed] Herba Artemisiae Apiaceae (*Bei Xue Ban Qing Hao*) and uncooked Cortex Radicis Moutan (*Sheng Mu Dan Pi*) as in *Qing Hao Bei Jia Tang* (Artemisia Apiacea & Carapax Amydae Decoction [252])

2. With uncooked Radix Albus Paeoniae Lactiflorae (*Sheng Bai Shao Yao*), uncooked Concha Ostreae (*Sheng Mu Li*), and uncooked Radix Rehmanniae (*Sheng Di Huang*) as in *Er Jia Fu Mai Tang* (Two Carapaces Restore the Pulse Decoction [97])

Dosage: 15-30g

Names: *Bie Jia, Zhi Bie Jia, Cu Bie Jia*

Flavors & nature: Salty and slightly sour; neutral

Functions: Softens the hard, scatters nodulations, eliminates masses

Indications:

1. Abdominal masses due to either A) stagnation of phlegm, qi, and blood or B) malaria with lateral costal masses...

2. Amenorrhea due to blood stasis with lower abdominal pain...

Typical combinations:

1. A) With vinegar[-processed] Rhizoma Sparganii (*Cu San Leng*), vinegar[-processed] Rhizoma Curcumae Zedoariae (*Cu E Zhu*), vinegar[-processed] Pericarpium Viridis Citri Reticulatae (*Cu Qing Pi*), and clear Rhizoma Pinelliae Ternatae (*Qing Ban Xia*)
B) With uncooked Radix Bupleuri (*Sheng Chai Hu*), stir-fried Fructus Amomi Tsao-ko (*Chao Cao Guo*), uncooked Radix Scutellariae Baicalensis (*Sheng Huang Qin*), wine[-processed] Radix Albus Paeoniae Lactiflorae (*Jiu Bai Shao Yao*), uncooked Semen Pruni Persicae (*Sheng Tao Ren*), stone-baked Eupolyphaga Seu Opisthoplatia (*Bei Zhe Chong*), and uncooked Pericarpium Viridis Citri Reticulatae (*Sheng Qing Pi*)

2. With wine[-processed] Radix Angelicae Sinensis (*Jiu Dang Gui*), Flos Carthami Tinctorii (*Hong Hua*), vinegar[-processed] Rhizoma Sparganii (*Cu San Leng*), and vinegar[-processed] Rhizoma Cyperi Rotundi (*Cu Xiang Fu*)

Dosage: 15-30g

Carapax Amydae Sinensis continued . . .

Gelatin (Jiao)[1]

Name: *Bie Jia Jiao*

Flavors & nature: Salty; neutral

Functions: Enriches yin, clears vacuity heat, supplements the blood, stops bleeding

Indications:

1. Hemoptysis due to vacuity heat caused by lung/kidney yin vacuity with cough, red cheeks, night sweats...

2. Metrorrhagia due to blood vacuity and vacuity heat disturbing the *chong* and *ren*

Typical combinations:

1. With uncooked Radix Rehmanniae (*Sheng Di Huang*), uncooked Tuber Ophiopogonis Japonicae (*Sheng Mai Men Dong*), honey mix-fried Radix Adenophorae Strictae (*Mi Zhi Nan Sha Shen*), Cortex Radicis Lycii (*Di Gu Pi*), and salt[-processed] Rhizoma Anemarrhenae (*Yan Zhi Mu*)

2. With carbonized Radix Angelicae Sinensis (*Dang Gui Tan*), uncooked Radix Albus Paeoniae Lactiflorae (*Sheng Bai Shao Yao*), uncooked Radix Rehmanniae (*Sheng Di Huang*), and carbonized Radix Rubiae Cordifoliae (*Qian Cao Gen Tan*)

Dosage: 5-10g and up to 30g in severe cases

Note: 1. This refers to the gelatin obtained by prolonged boiling of Carapax Amydae Sinensis using certain other ingredients, such as Alumen (*Bai Fan*), rice wine, and sugar.

Radix Rehmanniae (Di Huang)

Fresh (Xian)[1]

Names: *Xian Di Huang, Xian Sheng Di*

Flavors & nature: Sweet and bitter; cold

Functions: Clears heat, cools the blood, engenders fluids, stops thirst

Indications:

1. Fever[2] due to either A) replete heat in the qi and blood levels with high fever, thirst, agitation, epistaxis or B) replete heat in the blood level with high fever aggravated at night, hemorrhages...

2. Thirst due to a warm disease or internal heat damaging the fluids and humors

3. Rheumatic complaints due to heat (*re bi*) with red, very painful, swollen, hot joints...

Typical combinations:

1. A) With uncooked Gypsum Fibrosum (*Sheng Shi Gao*), uncooked Rhizoma Anemarrhenae (*Sheng Zhi Mu*), and Radix Scrophulariae Ningpoensis (*Xuan Shen*)
B) With Cornu Rhinocerotis (*Xi Jiao*) [substitute Cornu Bubali, *Shui Niu Jiao*], uncooked Cortex Radicis Moutan (*Sheng Mu Dan Pi*), and uncooked Radix Rubrus Paeoniae Lactiflorae (*Sheng Chi Shao Yao*) as in *Xi Jiao Di Huang Tang* (Rhinoceros Horn & Rehmannia Decoction [362])

2. With Radix Trichosanthis Kirlowii (*Tian Hua Fen*), stir-fried Rhizoma Anemarrhenae (*Chao Zhi Mu*), Radix Scrophulariae Ningpoensis (*Xuan Shen*), and uncooked Rhizoma Polygonati Odorati (*Sheng Yu Zhu*)

Radix Rehmanniae continued . . .

3. With uncooked Ramulus Mori Albi (*Sheng Sang Zhi*), Caulis Lonicerae Japonicae (*Ren Dong Teng*), Lumbricus (*Di Long*), and Caulis Sargentodoxae (*Hong Teng*)

Dosage: 15-30g

Notes: 1. This refers to the fresh, uncooked root. 2. For this indication, uncooked Radix Rehmanniae (*Sheng Di Huang*) can be used. However, it is less powerful and, in case of excessive heat, a large dose must be prescribed, such as 20-30g.

Fresh Juice (*Xian Zhi*)

Names: *Di Huang Zhi, Xian Di Huang Zhi*

Flavors & nature: Sweet and slightly bitter; cold

Functions: Clears heat, stops bleeding

Indications:

1. Hemoptysis due to either A) replete head agitating the blood or B) heat in the blood level

2. Postpartum metrorrhagia due to heat in the blood and blood stasis with incessant metrorrhagia, vexation...

Typical combinations:

1. A) With wine[-processed] Radix Et Rhizoma Rhei (*Jiu Da Huang*)
B) With Gelatinum Cornu Cervi (*Lu Jiao Jiao*) and Infant's Urine (*Tong Bian*) as in *Di Huang Yin* (Rehmannia Drink [84])

2. With Succus Herba Leonuri Heterophylli (*Yi Mu Cao Zhi*) and Rice Wine (*Huang Jiu*) as in *Di Huang Jiu* (Rehmannia Wine [83])

Dosage: 15-30g and up to 60g in severe cases

Dry Uncooked (*Gan Sheng*)[1]

Names: *Sheng Di Huang, Gan Di Huang, Sheng Di, Di Huang*

Flavors & nature: Sweet and slightly bitter; cool

Functions: Enriches yin, clears heat

Indications:

1. Fever[2] due to yin vacuity with dry mouth and throat, a red tongue with scant coating, a fine (*xi*), rapid (*shu*) pulse...

2. Hemorrhage[2] due to vacuity heat in the blood with dry mouth and throat, a red tongue, a rapid (*shu*) pulse...

3. Constipation due to yin vacuity

Typical combinations:

1. With Radix Scrophulariae Ningpoensis (*Xuan Shen*), uncooked Tuber Ophiopogonis Japonicae (*Sheng Mai Men Dong*), and Cortex Radicis Lycii (*Di Gu Pi*)

2. With uncooked Rhizoma Imperatae Cylindricae (*Sheng Bai Mao Gen*), uncooked Folium Nelumbinis Nuciferae (*Sheng He Ye*), and uncooked Folium Artemisiae Argyii (*Sheng Ai Ye*) as in *Si Sheng Wan* (Four Uncooked [Ingredients] Pills [314])

3. With Radix Scrophulariae Ningpoensis (*Xuan Shen*) and uncooked Tuber Ophiopogonis Japonicae (*Sheng Mai Men Dong*) as in *Zeng Ye Tang* (Increase Humors Decoction [427])

Dosage: 10-20g and up to 30g in severe cases

Notes: 1. This refers to the crude, dried root. 2. For fevers or hemorrhages due to heat in the blood level, fresh Rehmannia (*Xian Di Huang*) is more powerful than uncooked Rehmannia (*Sheng Di Huang*). In any case, the latter can also be prescribed but at a dosage of between 20-30g.

Radix Rehmanniae continued . . .

_____Dry Stir-fried [till] Scorched *(Gan Chao Jiao)*[1]_____

Names: *Chao Sheng Di Huang, Chao Sheng Di, Chao Di Huang*

Flavors & nature: Sweet and slightly bitter; cool tending to neutral

Functions: Enriches yin, nourishes the blood

Indications:

1. Fever due to blood vacuity with pale complexion, pale nails...

2. Threatened spontaneous abortion due to qi and blood vacuity with abdominal pain, metrorrhagia...

3. Blood vacuity with pale complexion, nails, and tongue, insomnia, abundant dreams, poor memory...

Typical combinations:

1. With uncooked Radix Angelicae Sinensis (*Sheng Dang Gui*), honey mix-fried Radix Cynanchi Atrati (*Mi Zhi Bai Wei*), and stir-fried Radix Astragali Membranacei (*Chao Huang Qi*)

2. With prepared Radix Rehmanniae (*Shu Di Huang*), stir-fried Radix Albus Paeoniae Lactiflorae (*Chao Bai Shao Yao*), bran stir-fried Rhizoma Atractylodis Macrocephalae (*Fu Chao Bai Zhu*), and Fructus Amomi (*Sha Ren*)

3. With prepared Radix Rehmanniae (*Shu Di Huang*) as in *Er Huang Wan* (Two Yellows Pills [96])

Dosage: 10-20g

Note: 1. This refers to the crude, dried root which has been stir-fried till brown. This method of preparation reinforces its blood-supplementing action. In addition, the plant is less heavy to digest. This then permits better assimilation of its active principles.

Addendum: If blood vacuity is associated with spleen qi vacuity with lack of appetite, slow digestion, distention, loose stools, etc., one should prescribe either wine[-processed] uncooked Rehmannia (*Jiu Sheng Di Huang*) fried with rice wine or ginger[-processed] uncooked Rehmannia (*Jiang Sheng Di Huang*) fried with ginger juice.

_____Dry Stir-fried [till] Carbonized *(Gan Chao Tan)*[1]_____

Names: *Sheng Di Huang Tan, Sheng Di Tan, Di Huang Tan*

Flavors & nature: Sweet, bitter, and slightly astringent; cool tending to neutral

Functions: Enriches yin, stops bleeding

Indications:

1. Hemoptysis, epistaxis, pyorrhea[2] due to vacuity heat damaging the network vessels

2. Bloody stools[2] due to evil heat damaging the network vessels of the intestines with stools

streaked with blood or hemorrhaging of fresh, red blood...

3. Hematuria[2] due to damp heat damaging the network vessels of the bladder

4. Metrorrhagia, metrorrhagia during pregnancy[2] due to heat in the uterus disturbing the *chong* and *ren*

Typical combinations:

1. With uncooked Cacumen Biotae Orientalis (*Sheng Ce Bai Ye*), Herba Ecliptae Prostratae (*Han Lian Cao*), carbonized Folium Et Petiolus

Radix Rehmanniae continued . . .

Trachycarpi (*Zong Lu Tan*), and carbonized Radix Rubiae Cordifoliae (*Qian Cao Gen Tan*)

2. With carbonized Flos Immaturus Sophorae Japonicae (*Huai Hua Tan*), uncooked Radix Sanguisorbae (*Sheng Di Yu*), uncooked Cacumen Biotae Orientalis (*Sheng Ce Bai Ye*), and uncooked Rhizoma Coptidis Chinensis (*Sheng Huang Lian*)

3. With uncooked Rhizoma Imperatae Cylindricae (*Sheng Bai Mao Gen*), carbonized Herba Cephalanoploris Segeti (*Xiao Ji Tan*), carbonized Radix Rubiae Cordifoliae (*Qian Cao Gen Tan*), and salt[-processed] Semen Plantaginis (*Yan Che Qian Zi*)

4. With Pollen Typhae stir-fried Gelatinum Corii Asini (*Pu Huang Chao E Jiao*), Herba Ecliptae Prostratae (*Han Lian Cao*), uncooked Radix Albus Paeoniae Lactiflorae (*Sheng Bai Shao Yao*), and stir-fried Cortex Ailanthi Altissimi (*Chao Chun Gen Pi*)

Dosage: 10-20g and up to 30g in severe cases

Notes: 1. This refers to the crude, dried root which is stir-fried till black. 2. When bleeding is due to heat in the blood level, it is necessary to prescribe uncooked Radix Rehmanniae (*Sheng Di Huang*) or, even better, fresh Radix Rehmanniae (*Xian Di Huang*).

_____Prepared *(Shu)*[1]_____

Names: *Shu Di Huang, Da Shu Di, Shu Di*

Flavors & nature: Sweet; slightly warm

Functions: Supplements yin, supplements the blood, supplements the essence, supplements the kidneys

Indications: Yin vacuity[2] 1) of the liver and kidneys; 2) with low back pain and weak knees; 3) with spermatorrhea and premature ejaculation; 4) with tinnitus and deafness; 5) with vertigo and dizziness; 6) with night sweats, evening fever, heat in the five hearts; and 7) with toothache

Typical combinations:

1. With steamed Fructus Corni Officinalis (*Zheng Shan Zhu Yu*) as in *Liu Wei Di Huang Wan* (Six Flavors Rehmannia Pills [204])

2. With salt[-processed] Radix Achyranthis Bidentatae (*Yan Huai Niu Xi*) and dip calcined Plastrum Testudinis (*Cui Gui Ban*) as in *Hu Qian Wan* (Hidden Tiger Pills [144])

3. With salt[-processed] Rhizoma Anemarrhenae (*Yan Zhi Mu*) and salt[-processed] Cortex Phello-

dendri (*Yan Huang Bai*) as in *Zhi Bai Di Huang Wan* (Anemarrhena & Phellodendron Rehmannia Pills [431])

4. With stir-fried Radix Bupleuri (*Chao Chai Hu*) and dip calcined Magnetitum (*Cui Ci Shi*) as in *Er Long Zuo Ci Wan* (Deafness Left [Kidney] Good Pills [98])

5. With salt[-processed] Radix Achyranthis Bidentatae (*Yan Huai Niu Xi*) and Gelatinum Plastri Testudinis (*Gui Ban Jiao*) as in *Zuo Gui Wan* (Restorethe Left [Kidney] Pills [451])

6. With uncooked Radix Rehmanniae (*Sheng Di Huang*) and salt[-processed] Cortex Phellodendri (*Yan Huang Bai*) as in *Dang Gui Liu Huang Tang* (*Dang Gui* Six Yellows Decoction [75])

7. With uncooked Gypsum Fibrosum (*Sheng Shi Gao*) and uncooked Radix Achyranthis Bidentatae (*Sheng Huai Niu Xi*) as in *Yu Nu Jian* (Jade Maiden Decoction [416])

Dosage: 10-30g and up to 30-60g in severe cases

Radix Rehmanniae continued . . .

Notes: 1. This refers to the crude, dried root which is cooked in rice wine steam. 2. If yin vacuity is associated with phlegm dampness, the preparation ginger mix-fried prepared Radix Rehmanniae (*Jiang Zhi Shu Di Huang*) can be prescribed. If yin vacuity is associated with spleen vacuity and qi stagnation, prepared Rehmannia is often prescribed with Fructus Amomi (*Sha Ren*) or Pericarpium Citri Reticulatae (*Chen Pi*).

_____Prepared Stir-fried [till] Scorched (Shu Chao Jiao)[1] _____

Names: *Chao Shu Di Huang, Chao Shu Di*

Flavors & nature: Sweet; warm

Functions: Nourishes the blood, nourishes the constructive qi, enriches yin

Indications: Blood vacuity with 1) anemia, a pale complexion, pale nails, pale lips, 2) headache, vertigo, 3) palpitations, insomnia, 4) diminished visual acuity, blurred vision, or 5) menstrual irregularity...

Typical combinations:

1. With wine[-processed] Radix Angelicae Sinensis (*Jiu Dang Gui*) and stir-fried Radix Astragali Membranacei (*Chao Huang Qi*)

2. With uncooked Radix Albus Paeoniae Lactiflorae (*Sheng Bai Shao Yao*) and Radix Panacis Ginseng (*Ren Shen*) as in *Ba Zhen Tang* (Eight Pearls Decoction [4])

3. With Arillus Euphoriae Longanae (*Long Yan Rou*) and uncooked Semen Zizyphi Spinosae (*Sheng Suan Zao Ren*) as in *Gui Pi Tang* (Return the Spleen Decoction [121])

4. With uncooked Radix Albus Paeoniae Lactiflorae (*Sheng Bai Shao Yao*) and salt[-processed] Semen Plantaginis (*Yan Che Qian Zi*) as in *Yang Gan Wan* (Nourish the Liver Pills [394])

5. With wine[-processed] Radix Angelicae Sinensis (*Jiu Dang Gui*) and wine[-processed] Radix Albus Paeoniae Lactiflorae (*Jiu Bai Shao Yao*) as in *Si Wu Tang* (Four Materials Decoction [315])

Dosage: 10-30g and up to 60g in severe cases

Note: 1. This method of preparing *Shu Di Huang* makes it more easily digestible and, therefore, more easily assimilated. It is also a more specific supplement for the blood. In addition, stir-fried prepared Rehmannia being warmer, this preparation is prescribed in formulas which supplement yin and yang, such as *Shen Qi Wan* (Kidney Qi Pills [291]), *You Gui Wan* (Return the Right [Kidney] Pills), *You Gui Yin* (Return the Right [Kidney] Drink), etc.

_____Prepared Stir-fried [till] Carbonized (Shu Chao Tan)[1] _____

Names: *Shu Di Huang Tan, Shu Di Tan*

Flavors & nature: Sweet and slightly astringent; warm

Functions: Supplements the blood, stops bleeding

Indications: Metrorrhagia due to either 1) *chong* and *ren* insufficiency or 2) qi and blood vacuity

Typical combinations:

1. With carbonized Folium Artemisiae Argyii (*Ai Ye Tan*), blast-fried Rhizoma Zingiberis (*Pao Jiang*), uncooked Cacumen Biotae Orientalis (*Sheng Ce Bai Ye*), and carbonized Folium Et Petiolus Trachycarpi (*Zong Lu Tan*)

2. With stir-fried Radix Astragali Membranacei (*Chao Huang Qi*), honey mix-fried Radix Codonopsis Pilosulae (*Mi Zhi Dang Shen*), carbonized Folium Et Petiolus Trachycarpi (*Zong Lu Tan*), and Crinis Carbonisatus (*Xue Yu Tan*)

Dosage: 10-20g and up to 30g in severe cases

Note: 1. This refers to prepared Rehmannia stir-fried till black.

Plastrum Testudinis (Gui Ban)

Uncooked (Sheng)

Names: *Sheng Gui Ban, Sheng Kan Ban*

Flavors & nature: Sweet and salty; cold

Functions: Enriches yin, downbears yang

Indications:

1. Vertigo due to liver/kidney yin vacuity which generates liver yang rising with headache, tinnitus, deafness...

2. Clonic convulsions due to a warm disease which has damaged yin and hence engendered internal wind

Typical combinations:

1. With uncooked Radix Achyranthis Bidentatae (*Sheng Huai Niu Xi*), uncooked Haematitum (*Sheng Dai Zhe Shi*), and uncooked Concha Ostreae (*Sheng Mu Li*) as in *Zhen Gan Xi Feng Tang* (Settle the Liver & Extinguish Wind Decoction [428])

2. With uncooked Radix Albus Paeoniae Lactiflorae (*Sheng Bai Shao Yao*), uncooked Tuber Ophiopogonis Japonicae (*Sheng Mai Men Dong*), uncooked Carapax Amydae Sinensis (*Sheng Bie Jia*), and uncooked Concha Ostreae (*Sheng Mu Li*) as in *Da Ding Feng Zhu* (Great Stabilize Wind Pearls [62a])

Dosage: 15-30g

Vinegar Dip Calcined (Cu Cui)[1]

Names: *Gui Ban, Xuan Wu Ban, Zhi Gui Ban, Cu Cui Ban*

Flavors & nature: Sweet, salty, and slightly sour; cold tending to neutral

Functions: Supplements yin, the kidneys, and the heart, strengthens the sinews and bones, clears vacuity heat

Indications:

1. Night sweats, bone-steaming fever due to
A) vacuity heat caused by yin vacuity or B) vacuity heat caused by yin and qi vacuity

2. Atony, weak legs, knees, and lower back due to liver/kidney vacuity

3. Heart palpitations, insomnia, poor memory due to heart yin vacuity

Typical combinations:

1. A) With salt[-processed] Rhizoma Anemarrhenae (*Yan Zhi Mu*), salt[-processed] Cortex Phellodendri (*Yan Huang Bai*), and prepared Radix Rehmanniae (*Shu Di Huang*) as in *Da Bu Yin Wan* (Great Supplement Yin Pills [59])
B) With Radix Panacis Ginseng (*Ren Shen*), salt[-processed] Cortex Phellodendri (*Yan Huang Bai*), and uncooked Tuber Asparagi Cochinensis (*Sheng Tian Men Dong*) as in *Da Zao Wan* (Great Creation Pills [70])

2. With sand stir-fried Os Tigridis (*Sha Chao Hu Gu*)[2], salt[-processed] Radix Achyranthis Bidentatae (*Yan Huai Niu Xi*), and prepared Radix Rehmanniae (*Shu Di Huang*) as in *Hu Qian Wan* (Hidden Tiger Pills [144])

3. With uncooked Os Draconis (*Sheng Long Gu*) and processed Radix Polygalae Tenuifoliae (*Zhi Yuan Zhi*) as in *Zhen Zhong Dan* (Pillow Elixir [430])

Dosage: 15-30g

Notes: 1. Vinegar dip calcined Plastrum Testudinis is obtained by heating the *Gui Ban* till red hot and then

Plastrum Testudinis continued . . .

plunging it while still hot into a vinegar solution. This operation is repeated several times. 2. It is Blue Poppy

Press' opinion that medicinals obtained from endangered species, such as tigers, should not be used. Pig bone can be used as effectively in this formula.

_____ Gelatin *(Jiao)*[1] _____

Name: *Gui Ban Jiao*

Flavors & nature: Sweet and salty; neutral

Functions: Enriches yin, supplements the essence, nourishes the blood, stops bleeding

Indications:

1. Impotence, spermatorrhea due to kidney essence, yin, and yang vacuity with weak low back, tinnitus, diminished visual acuity...

2. Low back pain due to kidney yin and essence vacuity

3. Metrorrhagia due to *chong* and *ren* insufficiency or kidney essence insufficiency

Typical combinations:

1. With Gelatinum Cornu Cervi (*Lu Jiao Jiao*), Fructus Lycii Chinensis (*Gou Qi Zi*), and Radix Panacis Ginseng (*Ren Shen*)

2. With salt[-processed] Radix Achyranthis Bidentatae (*Yan Huai Niu Xi*), salt[-processed] Cortex Eucommiae Ulmoidis (*Yan Du Zhong*), and salt[-processed] Radix Dipsaci (*Yan Xu Duan*)

3. With prepared Radix Rehmanniae (*Shu Di Huang*), carbonized Radix Angelicae Sinensis (*Dang Gui Tan*), calcined Os Draconis (*Duan Long Gu*), and carbonized Radix Rubiae Cordifoliae (*Qian Cao Gen Tan*)

Dosage: 5-15g and up to 30g in severe cases

Note: 1. This refers to a gelatin obtained by prolonged cooking of *Gui Ban*.

Tuber Ophiopogonis Japonicae *(Mai Men Dong)*

_____ Uncooked *(Sheng)* _____

Names: *Mai Men Dong, Mai Dong, Cun Mai Dong, Sheng Mai Dong*

Flavors & nature: Sweet and slightly bitter; slightly cold

Functions: Enriches yin, moistens the lungs, nourishes the stomach, moistens the intestines

Indications:

1. Cough due to A) external dryness damaging the lungs or B) lung yin vacuity

2. Pulmonary tuberculosis due to lung yin vacuity

3. Sore throat due to vacuity heat

4. Thirst due to a warm disease damaging stomach fluids with dry mouth and throat, a red tongue with no coating...

5. Constipation due to large intestine dryness caused by yin vacuity...

Typical combinations:

1. A) With uncooked Gypsum Fibrosum (*Sheng Shi Gao*) and Concha Cyclinae stir-fried Gelatinum Corii Asini (*Ge Fen Chao E Jiao*) as in *Qing Zao Jiu Fei Tang* (Clear Dryness & Rescue

Tuber Ophiopogonis Japonicae continued . . .

the Lungs Decoction [260])
B) With honey mix-fried Bulbus Lilii (*Mi Zhi Bai He*) and prepared Radix Rehmanniae (*Shu Di Huang*) as in *Bai He Gu Jin Tang* (Lily Secure Metal Decoction [12]_

2. With honey mix-fried Radix Platycodi Grandiflori (*Mi Zhi Jie Geng*) and Herba Artemisiae Apiaceae (*Qing Hao*) as in *Mai Men Dong Tang* (Ophiopogon Decoction [219])

3. With Radix Scrophulariae Ningpoensis (*Xuan Shen*) and Radix Platycodi Grandiflori (*Jie Geng*) as in *Xuan Mai Gan Jie Tang* (Scrophularia, Ophiopogon, Licorice & Platycodon Decoction [391])

4. With Radix Glehniae Littoralis (*Bei Sha Shen*) and uncooked Rhizoma Polygonati Odorati (*Sheng Yu Zhu*) as in *Yi Wei Tang* (Boost the Stomach Decoction [404])

5. With Radix Scrophulariae Ningpoensis (*Xuan Shen*) as in *Zeng Ye Tang* (Increase Humors Decoction [427])

Dosage: 5-15g and up to 30g in severe cases

Cinnabar (*Zhu Sha*)

Names: *Zhu Sha Ban Mai Dong, Zhu Mai Dong*

Flavors & nature: Sweet and slightly bitter; cold

Functions: Clears the heart, resolves vexation

Indications:

1. Vexation due to evil heat penetrating the constructive level (*ying fen*) with fever, thirst...

2. Insomnia due to a warm disease which has damaged heart yin with vexation...

3. Heart palpitations due to heat qi and yin vacuity with a bound (*jie*) or regularly interrupted (*dai*) pulse...

Typical combinations:

1. With uncooked Rhizoma Coptidis Chinensis (*Sheng Huang Lian*), Radix Scrophulariae Ningpoensis (*Xuan Shen*), and uncooked Radix Rehmanniae (*Sheng Di Huang*) as in *Qing Ying Tang* (Clear the Constructive Decoction [259])

2. With uncooked Bulbus Lilii (*Sheng Bai He*), pig blood [processed] Radix Salviae Miltiorrhizae (*Zhu Xue Ban Dan Shen*), and uncooked Semen Zizyphi Spinosae (*Sheng Suan Zao Ren*)

3. With uncooked Radix Rehmanniae (*Sheng Di Huang*), mix-fried Radix Glycyrrhizae (*Zhi Gan Cao*), and Radix Panacis Ginseng (*Ren Shen*) as in *Zhi Gan Cao Tang* (Mix-fried Licorice Decoction [432])

Dosage: 5-15g

Fructus Ligustri Lucidi *(Nu Zhen Zi)*

Uncooked *(Sheng)*

Names: *Sheng Nu Zhen Zi, Sheng Nu Zhen*

Flavors & nature: Bitter and slightly sweet; slightly cold

Functions: Clears the liver, moistens dryness, brightens the eyes

Indications:

1. Photophobia due to heat penetrating the liver channel with red, painful eyes...

2. Constipation due to either A) large intestine dryness or blood vacuity or B) heat in the stomach and large intestine

Typical combinations:

1. With uncooked Semen Cassiae Torae (*Sheng Jue Ming Zi*), Flos Buddleiae Officinalis (*Mi Meng Hua*), and uncooked Flos Chrysanthemi Morifolii (*Sheng Ju Hua*)

2. A) With uncooked Radix Polygoni Multiflori (*Sheng He Shou Wu*) and stir-fried Semen Cannabis Sativae (*Chao Huo Ma Ren*)
B) With uncooked Radix Et Rhizoma Rhei (*Sheng Da Huang*) and Mirabilitum (*Mang Xiao*)

Dosage: 10-15g and up to 30g in severe cases

Wine-steamed *(Jiu Zheng)*

Names: *Nu Zhen Zi, Nu Zhen Shi, Jiu Nu Zhen, Zhi Nu Zhen*

Flavors & nature: Sweet and slightly bitter; neutral

Functions: Enriches yin, supplements the liver and kidneys

Indications:

1. Premature greying of the hair due to kidney essence insufficiency

2. Diminished visual acuity due to liver/kidney yin vacuity with photophobia, blurred vision...

3. Vertigo, tinnitus, deafness due to liver/kidney yin vacuity

4. Low back and knee weakness due to liver/-kidney yin vacuity

Typical combinations:

1. With processed Radix Polygoni Multiflori (*Zhi He Shou Wu*), prepared Radix Rehmanniae (*Shu Di Huang*), and Placenta Hominis (*Zi He Che*)

2. With Fructus Lycii Chinensis (*Gou Qi Zi*), uncooked Semen Cuscutae (*Sheng Tu Si Zi*), and uncooked Semen Astragali (*Sheng Sha Yuan Zi*)

3. With Herba Ecliptae Prostratae (*Han Lian Cao*) as in *Er Zhi Wan* (Two Ultimates Pills [101])

4. With salt[-processed] Cortex Eucommiae Ulmoidis (*Yan Du Zhong*), salt[-processed] Radix Achyranthis Bidentatae (*Yan Huai Niu Xi*), salt[-processed] Radix Dipsaci (*Yan Xu Duan*), and prepared Radix Rehmanniae (*Shu Di Huang*)

Dosage: 10-15g and up to 30g in severe cases

Rhizoma Polygonati Odorati *(Yu Zhu)*

Uncooked *(Sheng)*

Names: *Yu Zhu, Sheng Yu Zhu, Fei Yu Zhu, Wei Rui, Lou Rui*

Functions: Engenders fluids, stops thirst

Indications:

1. Common cold, flu accompanied by chronic yin vacuity preceding the external affection

2. Thirst due to affection of the fluids and humors by external dryness with a dry mouth and tongue or due to replete stomach heat

Typical combinations:

1. With Herba Menthae Haplocalycis (*Bo He*), uncooked Radix Platycodi Grandiflori (*Sheng Jie Geng*), and Semen Praeparatum Sojae (*Dan Dou Chi*) as in *Jia Jian Lou Rui Tang* (Additions & Subtractions Polygonatum Decoction [169])

2. With Radix Glehniae Littoralis (*Bei Sha Shen*) and uncooked Tuber Ophiopogonis Japonicae (*Sheng Mai Men Dong*) as in *Yu Zhu Mai Men Dong Tang* (Solomon Seal & Ophiopogon Decoction [421])

Dosage: 10-15g and up to 60g in severe cases

Steamed *(Zheng)*

Names: *Zheng Yu Zhu, Zheng Lou Rui, Zhi Yu Zhu, Zhi Wei Rui*

Flavors & nature: Sweet; neutral

Functions: Enriches yin, supplements the qi

Indications:

1. Warm disease which has damaged yin, *i.e.*, the consequences of a warm disease which has dried fluids and humors with dry mouth and throat, a red tongue with no coating...

2. Dry cough due to external dryness attacking the lungs with dry throat, sticky, difficult to expectorate phlegm, fever...

3. Chronic fever due to qi and yin vacuity with emaciation, spontaneous perspiration and/or night sweats, fatigue, low but constant fever...

Typical combinations:

1. With uncooked Radix Rehmanniae (*Sheng Di Huang*) and Radix Glehniae Littoralis (*Bei Sha Shen*) as in *Yi Wei Tang* (Boost the Stomach Decoction [404])

2. With uncooked Gypsum Fibrosum (*Sheng Shi Gao*), uncooked Semen Pruni Armeniacae (*Sheng Xing Ren*), and honey mix-fried Herba Ephedrae (*Mi Zhi Ma Huang*) as in *Wei Rui Tang* (Solomon Seal Decoction [339])

3. With stir-fried Radix Astragali Membranacei (*Chao Huang Qi*), uncooked Radix Angelicae Sinensis (*Sheng Dang Gui*), and Cortex Radicis Lycii (*Di Gu Pi*)

Dosage: 10-15g and up to 60g in severe cases

21
Astringent Medicinals

Hallyositum Rubrum *(Chi Shi Zhi)*

_____**Uncooked** *(Sheng)*_____

Names: *Chi Shi Zhi, Sheng Chi Shi Zhi*

Flavors & nature: Sweet, sour, and astringent; warm

Functions: Absorbs dampness, engenders new tissue, stops bleeding

Indications:

1. Sores which will not heal over, with sterile suppuration...

2. Bleeding due to traumatic injury

Typical combinations:

1. With dip calcined Smithsonitum (*Cui Lu Gan Shi*) and uncooked Os Sepiae Seu Sepiellae (*Sheng Hai Piao Xiao*). Reduce these three substances to powder and apply locally.

2. With Galla Rhi Chinensis (*Wu Bei Zi*) and Colophonia (*Song Xiang*). Reduce these three substances to powder and apply locally with a tight bandage.

Dosage: Use externally whatever amount is needed.

_____**Calcined** *(Duan)*_____

Name: *Duan Chi Shi Zhi*

Flavors & nature: Sweet and astringent; warm

Functions: Restrains that which is escaping, stops bleeding, stops diarrhea

Indications:

1. Melena due to damage of the large intestine network vessels with dark, purple blood in the stools...

2. Metrorrhagia, menorrhagia due to *chong* and *ren* not securing

3. Persistent dysentery due to attack by cold in the *shao yin* with bloody, purulent stools...

4. Chronic diarrhea due to spleen and stomach yang vacuity with fatigue, cold limbs...

5. Spermatorrhea due to kidneys not securing

6. Abnormal vaginal discharge due to accumulation internally of cold dampness with clear, fluid, and abundant vaginal discharge...

Typical combinations:

1. With Terra Flava Usta (*Fu Long Gan*), carbonized Nodus Nelumbinis Nuciferae (*Ou Jie Tan*), and carbonized Folium Et Petiolus Trachycarpi (*Zong Lu Tan*)

2. With uncooked Cacumen Biotae Orientalis (*Sheng Ce Bai Ye*) and stir-fried Os Sepiae Seu Sepiellae (*Chao Hai Piao Xiao*) as in *Chi Shi Zhi San* (Hallyositum Rubrum Powder [48])

Hallyositum Rubrum continued . . .

3. With dry Rhizoma Zingiberis (*Gan Jiang*) as in *Tao Hua Tang* (Hallyositum Decoction [322]. *Tao Hua* is another name for Hallyositum.)

4. With processed Radix Lateralis Praeparatus Aconiti Carmichaeli (*Zhi Fu Zi*) and earth stir-fried Rhizoma Atractylodis Macrocephalae (*Tu Chao Bai Zhu*) as in *Da Tao Hua Tang* (Major Hallyositum Decoction [67])

5. With uncooked Semen Euryalis Ferocis (*Sheng Qian Shi*) and Fructus Rosae Laevigatae (*Jin Ying Zi*)

6. With stir-fried Rhizoma Atractylodis (*Chao Cang Zhu*) and stir-fried Semen Ginkgonis Bilobae (*Chao Bai Guo*)

Dosage: 10-20g

Cortex Ailanthi Altissimi *(Chun Gen Pi)*

Uncooked *(Sheng)*

Names: *Chun Gen Pi, Chun Bai Pi, Chu Gen Pi, Sheng Chun Gen*

Flavors & nature: Bitter and astringent; cold

Functions: Clears heat, dries dampness, stops abnormal vaginal discharge

Indications:

1. Abnormal vaginal discharge due to damp heat in the lower burner with yellowish, sticky vaginal discharge...

2. Urinary stangury with dribbling and dripping due to damp heat

3. Mycoses due to damp heat

Typical combinations:

1. With uncooked Cortex Phellodendri (*Sheng Huang Bai*), stir-fried Radix Angelicae Dahuricae (*Chao Bai Zhi*), and Rhizoma Smilacis Glabrae (*Tu Fu Ling*)

2. With salt[-processed] Rhizoma Dioscoreae Hypoglaucae (*Yan Bei Xie*) and uncooked Sclerotium Poriae Cocos (*Sheng Fu Ling*)

3. Make a decoction of Ailanthus and apply the cooled liquid locally.

Dosage: 5-12g

Stir-fried [till] Yellow *(Chao Huang)*

Names: *Chao Chun Gen Pi, Chao Chu Gen Pi, Chao Chun Bai Pi*

Flavors & nature: Bitter and astringent; cold tending to neutral

Functions: Secures the intestines, stops diarrhea, secures the menstruation, stops bleeding

Indications:

1. Chronic diarrhea due to either A) spleen and

stomach vacuity or B) damp heat in the large intestine

2. Persistent dysentery due to large intestine damp heat

3. Metrorrhagia due to either A) liver fire disturbing the *chong* and *ren* with vexation[1] or B) *chong* and *ren* not securing

Cortex Ailanthi Altissimi continued . . .

Typical combinations:

1. A) With earth stir-fried Rhizoma Atractylodis Macrocephalae (*Tu Chao Bai Zhu*) and earth stir-fried Radix Dioscoreae Oppositae (*Tu Chao Shan Yao*)
B) With uncooked Rhizoma Coptidis Chinensis (*Sheng Huang Lian*) and stir-fried Semen Plantaginis (*Chao Che Qian Zi*)

2. With Radix Pulsatillae Chinensis (*Bai Tou Weng*) and Herba Portulacae Oleraceae (*Ma Chi Xian*)

3. A) With uncooked Radix Scutellariae Baicalensis (*Sheng Huang Qin*) and uncooked Radix Albus Paeoniae Lactiflorae (*Sheng Bai Shao Yao*) as in *Gu Jing Wan* (Secure the Menses Pills [118])
B) With carbonized Radix Rubiae Cordifoliae (*Qian Cao Gen Tan*), carbonized Folium Et Petiolus Trachycarpi (*Zong Lu Tan*), and stir-fried Os Sepiae Seu Sepiellae (*Chao Hai Piao Xiao*)

Dosage: 5-12g

Note: 1. In this case, one can prescribe uncooked Ailanthus (*Sheng Chun Gen Pi*).

Os Sepiae Seu Sepiellae *(Hai Piao Xiao)*

Uncooked *(Sheng)*

Names: *Hai Piao Xiao, Wu Zei Gu, Sheng Hai Piao Xiao*

Flavors & nature: Salty; slightly warm

Functions: Stops stomach hyperacidity, stops pain, eliminates dampness, promotes the healing of sores

Indications:

1. Stomach acidity and pain due to disharmony of the stomach with vomiting or acid regurgitation...

2. Sores which do not heal over, purulent sores, bleeding sores

3. Pruritus due to damp heat

Typical combinations:

1. With Bulbus Fritillariae Thunbergii (*Zhe Bei Mu*) and uncooked Radix Glycyrrhizae (*Sheng Gan Cao*) as in *Wu Bei San* (Sepia & Fritillaria Powder [337])

2. With dip calcined Smithsonitum (*Cui Lu Gan Shi*). Reduce to a powder these two substances and apply locally.

3. With uncooked Rhizoma Coptidis Chinensis (*Sheng Huang Lian*), uncooked Cortex Phellodendri (*Sheng Huang Bai*), and Pulvis Indigonis (*Qing Dai*). Reduce to a powder these four substances and apply locally.

Dosage: 6-15g and up to 30g for severe stomach acidity and pain

_____Bran Stir-fried *(Fu Chao)*_____

Names: *Chao Hai Piao Xiao, Chao Wu Zei Gu*

Flavors & nature: Salty and slightly astringent; slightly warm

Functions: Secures the essence, stops abnormal vaginal discharge, stops bleeding

Indications:

1. Metrorrhagia due to the *chong* and *ren* not securing

2. Abnormal vaginal discharge due to accumulation of dampness in the lower burner with reddish discharge...

3. Spermatorrhea due to the kidneys not securing

Typical combinations:

1. With carbonized Radix Rubiae Cordifoliae (*Qian Cao Gen Tan*) and carbonized Folium Et Petiolus Trachycarpi (*Zong Lu Tan*) as in *Gu Chong Tang* (Secure the *Chong* Decoction [117])

2. With stir-fried Radix Angelicae Dahuricae (*Chao Bai Zhi*) and Crinis Carbonisatus (*Xue Yu Tan*) as in *Bai Zhi San* (Angelica Powder [21])

3. With uncooked Semen Euryalis Ferocis (*Sheng Qian Shi*), salt[-processed] Semen Cuscutae (*Yan Tu Si Zi*), and Fructus Rosae Laevigatae (*Jin Ying Zi*)

Dosage: 6-15g and up to 30g in severe cases

Fructus Terminaliae Chebulae *(He Zi)*

_____Uncooked *(Sheng)*_____

Names: *Sheng He Zi, Sheng He Zi Rou, Sheng He Li Le*

Flavors & nature: Bitter, sour, and astringent; slightly warm

Functions: Secures the lungs, soothes the throat

Indications:

1. Chronic cough due to lung qi and/or yin vacuity with asthmatic breathing, shortness of breath...

2. Aphonia, hoarse voice due to lung yin vacuity with a dry, possibly painful throat, possible cough...

Typical combinations:

1. With uncooked Semen Pruni Armeniacae (*Sheng Xing Ren*) and stir-fried Semen Trichosanthis Kirlowii (*Chao Gua Lou Ren*) as in *He Li Le Wan* (Terminalia Pills [132])

2. With honey mix-fried Radix Platycodi Grandiflori (*Mi Zhi Jie Geng*) and uncooked Radix Glycyrrhizae (*Sheng Gan Cao*) as in *He Zi Qing Yin Tang* (Terminalia Clear the Voice Decoction [135])

Dosage: 5-10g and up to 15g in severe cases

Fructus Terminaliae Chebulae continued . . .

_____**Bran Stir-fried** *(Fu Chao)*[1] _____

Names: *He Zi, He Zi Rou, He Li Le, Chao He Zi, Wei He Zi*

Flavors & nature: Bitter, sour, and astringent; warm

Functions: Secures the intestines, stops diarrhea

Indications:

1. Chronic diarrhea due to middle burner yang vacuity

2. Persistent dysentery due to damage of the stomach and intestines with slightly bloody dysentery, abdominal pain...

3. Rectal prolapse due to middle burner qi fall with chronic diarrhea...

Typical combinations:

1. With dry Rhizoma Zingiberis (*Gan Jiang*) and

uncooked Pericarpium Papaveris Somniferi (*Sheng Ying Su Ke*) as in *He Zi Pi San* (Terminalia Powder [134])

2. With uncooked Rhizoma Coptidis Chinensis (*Sheng Huang Lian*) and roasted Radix Saussureae Seu Vladimiriae (*Wei Mu Xiang*) as in *He Zi San* (Terminalia Powder [136])

3. With stir-fried Radix Astragali Membranacei (*Chao Huang Qi*), earth stir-fried Rhizoma Atractylodis Macrocephalae (*Tu Chao Bai Zhu*), honey mix-fried Rhizoma Cimicifugae (*Mi Zhi Sheng Ma*), roasted Radix Puerariae (*Wei Ge Gen*), and stir-fried Radix Bupleuri (*Chao Chai Hu*)

Dosage: 5-10g and up to 15g in severe cases

Note: 1. One can also use roasted Terminalia (*Wei He Zi*).

Addendum: The astringent action of Terminalia is also used in case of abnormal vaginal discharge, spermatorrhea, urinary incontinence, and metrorrhagia.

Semen Euryalis Ferocis *(Qian Shi)*

_____**Uncooked** *(Sheng)* _____

Names: *Qian Shi, Nan Qian Shi, Bei Qian Shi, Sheng Qian Shi*

Flavors & nature: Sweet and astringent; neutral

Functions: Secures the kidneys, secures the essence

Indications:

1. Spermatorrhea due to kidneys not securing with weak low back...

2. Enuresis, urinary incontinence due to kidney qi vacuity with abundant, frequent urination, nocturia...

3. Urinary strangury with dribbling and dripping due to spleen/kidney vacuity

4. Abnormal vaginal discharge due to either A) spleen/kidney vacuity or B) damp heat

Typical combinations:

1. With Fructus Rosae Laevigatae (*Jin Ying Zi*) as in *Shui Tu Er Xian Dan* (Water & Earth Two Immortals Elixir [308])

2. With salt[-processed] Ootheca Mantidis (*Yan Sang Piao Xiao*) and salt[-processed] Fructus Alpiniae Oxyphyllae (*Yan Yi Zhi Ren*)

Semen Euryalis Ferocis continued . . .

3. With uncooked Sclerotium Poriae Cocos (*Sheng Fu Ling*) as in *Fen Qing Wan* (Separate the Clear Pills [105])

4. A) With bran stir-fried Radix Dioscoreae Oppositae (*Fu Chao Shan Yao*), bran stir-fried Rhizoma Atractylodis Macrocephalae (*Fu Chao Bai Zhu*), and Semen Ginkgonis Bilobae (*Bai Guo*)

B) With uncooked Cortex Phellodendri (*Sheng Huang Bai*) and stir-fried Semen Plantaginis (*Chao Che Qian Zi*) as in *Yi Huang San* (Treat Yellow Powder [400])

Dosage: 10-15g and up to 30g in severe cases

_____**Bran Stir-fried** *(Fu Chao)*[1]_____

Names: *Chao Qian Shi, Fu Chao Qian Shi*

Flavors & nature: Sweet and astringent; slightly warm

Functions: Supplements the spleen, stops diarrhea

Indications:

1. Diarrhea due to spleen and stomach vacuity with lack of appetite, fatigue...

2. Infantile malnutrition syndrome (*gan ji*) due to spleen and stomach vacuity with emaciation, abdominal distention and bloating...

Typical combinations:

1. With earth stir-fried Rhizoma Atractylodis Macrocephalae (*Tu Chao Bai Zhu*), earth stir-fried Radix Dioscoreae Oppositae (*Tu Chao Shan Yao*), earth stir-fried Semen Dolichoris Lablab (*Tu Chao Bai Bian Dou*), and rice stir-fried Radix Codonopsis Pilosulae (*Mi Chao Dang Shen*)

2. With bran stir-fried Rhizoma Atractylodis Macrocephalae (*Fu Chao Bai Zhu*) and stir-fried Fructus Quisqualis Indicae (*Chao Shi Jun Zi*)

Dosage: 10-15g and up to 30g in severe cases

Note: 1. One can also use stir-fried [till] yellow Euryales (*Chao Huang Qian Shi*).

Ootheca Mantidis *(Sang Piao Xiao)*

_____**Bran Stir-fried** *(Fu Chao)*_____

Names: *Sang Piao Xiao, Tang Lang Zi, Chao Sang Piao Xiao*

Flavors & nature: Sweet and slightly salty; neutral

Functions: Restrains that which is escaping, stops abnormal vaginal discharge

Indications:

1. Abnormal vaginal discharge due to spleen/kidney vacuity with whitish, fluid, abundant vaginal discharge...

2. Urinary strangury with dribbling and dripping due to spleen/kidney vacuity

Typical combinations:

1. With uncooked Semen Euryalis Ferocis (*Sheng Qian Shi*), stir-fried Radix Dioscoreae Oppositae (*Chao Shan Yao*), and stir-fried Semen Ginkgonis Bilobae (*Chao Bai Guo*)

2. With uncooked Sclerotium Poriae Cocos (*Sheng Fu Ling*) and salt[-processed] Rhizoma Dioscoreae Hypoglaucae (*Yan Bei Xie*)

Dosage: 5-10g and up to 30g in severe cases

Ootheca Mantidis continued . . .

Names: *Yan Zhi Sang Piao Xiao, Yan Sang Piao Xiao, Yan Sang Xiao*

Flavors & nature: Sweet and salty; neutral

Functions: Supplements the kidneys, secures the essence, controls urination

Indications:

1. Spermatorrhea due to either A) heart and kidneys not communicating or B) kidneys not securing

2. Impotence due to kidney yang vacuity

3. Enuresis, urinary incontinence due to either A) kidney qi vacuity or B) heart and kidneys not communicating

Typical combinations:

1. A) With calcined Os Draconis (*Duan Long Gu*) and processed Radix Polygalae Tenuifoliae (*Zhi Yuan Zhi*) as in *Sang Piao Xiao San* (Mantis Egg Case Powder [278])

B) With steamed Fructus Corni Officinalis (*Zheng Shan Zhu Yu*), uncooked Semen Euryalis Ferocis (*Sheng Qian Shi*), and Fructus Rosae Laevigatae (*Jin Ying Zi*)

2. With wine[-processed] Herba Cistanchis (*Jiu Rou Cong Rong*), processed Herba Epimedii (*Zhi Yin Yang Huo*), and wine[-processed] Rhizoma Curculiginis Orchioidis (*Jiu Xian Mao*)

3. A) With salt[-processed] Fructus Alpiniae Oxyphyllae (*Yan Yi Zhi Ren*) and salt[-processed] Fructus Psoraleae Corylifoliae (*Yan Bu Gu Zhi*)
B) With calcined Os Draconis (*Duan Long Gu*) and Sclerotium Pararadicis Poriae Cocos (*Fu Shen*) as in *Sang Piao Xiao San* (Mantis Egg Case Powder [278])

Dosage: 5-10g and up to 30g in severe cases

Fructus Corni Officinalis *(Shan Zhu Yu)*

Names: *Sheng Zhu Yu, Sheng Shan Zhu Yu, Sheng Yu Rou*

Flavors & nature: Sour and astringent; neutral

Functions: Restrains yin, stops perspiration

Indications:

1. Spontaneous perspiration due to either A) qi vacuity with fatigue, shortness of breath, sweating on slight exertion or B) yang desertion with cold sweat, cold limbs, a faint (*wei*) pulse...

2. Night sweats due to vacuity heat caused by yin vacuity with evening fever, heat in the five hearts...

Typical combinations:

1. A) With uncooked Radix Astragali Membranacei (*Sheng Huang Qi*), uncooked Rhizoma Atractylodis Macrocephalae (*Sheng Bai Zhu*), honey mix-fried Radix Codonopsis Pilosulae (*Mi Zhi Dang Shen*), and Radix Ephedrae (*Ma Huang Gen*)

Fructus Corni Officinalis continued . . .

B) With processed Radix Lateralis Praeparatus Aconiti Carmichaeli (*Zhi Fu Zi*), Radix Panacis Ginseng (*Ren Shen*), uncooked Radix Astragali Membranacei (*Sheng Huang Qi*), and uncooked Fructus Schizandrae Chinensis (*Sheng Wu Wei Zi*)

2. With uncooked Radix Albus Paeoniae Lactiflorae (*Sheng Bai Shao Yao*), uncooked Fructus Schizandrae Chinensis (*Sheng Wu Wei Zi*), dip calcined Plastrum Testudinis (*Cui Gui Ban*), and uncooked Semen Zizyphi Spinosae (*Sheng Suan Zao Ren*)

Dosage: 6-12g and up to 30g in severe cases

_____ Steamed *(Zheng)*_____

Names: *Shan Zhu Yu, Shan Yu Rou, Zheng Yu Rou, Yu Rou*

Flavors & nature: Sour and astringent; slightly warm

Functions: Supplements the kidneys, secures the essence, secures menstruation, controls urination

Indications:

1. Impotence due to kidney yin and yang or essence vacuity with weak lower back, mental apathy...

2. Spermatorrhea due to kidney qi not securing

3. Enuresis, urinary incontinence due to kidney qi vacuity

4. Menorrhagia due to kidney qi vacuity and deficiency of the *chong* and *ren*

Typical combinations:

1. With salt[-processed] Radix Morindae Officinalis (*Yan Ba Ji Tian*), processed Herba Epimedii (*Zhi Yin Yang Huo*), and Cornu Parvum Cervi (*Lu Rong*)

2. With uncooked Semen Euryalis Ferocis (*Sheng Qian Shi*), Fructus Rosae Laevigatae (*Jin Ying Zi*), and stir-fried Semen Cuscutae (*Chao Tu Si Zi*)

3. With salt[-processed] Fructus Alpiniae Oxyphyllae (*Yan Yi Zhi Ren*) and salt[-processed] Ootheca Mantidis (*Yan Sang Piao Xiao*)

4. With carbonized Folium Et Petiolus Trachycarpi (*Zong Lu Tan*) and carbonized Radix Rubiae Cordifoliae (*Qian Cao Gen Tan*) as in *Gu Chong Tang* (Secure the *Chong* Decoction [117])

Dosage: 6-12g and up to 30g in severe cases

_____ Wine-steamed *(Jiu Zheng)*[1] _____

Names: *Jiu Yu Rou, Jiu Shan Zhu Yu*

Flavors & nature: Sour, astringent, and slightly acrid; warm

Functions: Supplements the liver and kidneys, warms the kidneys, opens the network vessels

Indications:

1. Low back pain due to liver/kidney vacuity with weak knees, mental apathy...

2. Lateral costal pain due to liver yin vacuity

3. Vertigo, tinnitus due to liver/kidney yin vacuity resulting in liver yang rising

Typical combinations:

1. With salt[-processed] Cortex Eucommiae Ulmoidis (*Yan Du Zhong*), salt[-processed] Radix Dipsaci (*Yan Xu Duan*), and Caulis Millettiae Seu Spatholobi (*Ji Xue Teng*)

Fructus Corni Officinalis continued . . .

2. With wine[-processed] Radix Albus Paeoniae Lactiflorae (*Jiu Bai Shao Yao*) and stir-fried Fructus Meliae Toosendan (*Chao Chuan Lian Zi*)

3. With Fructus Lycii Chinensis (*Gou Qi Zi*), wine-steamed Fructus Ligustri Lucidi (*Jiu Zheng Nu Zhen Zi*), stir-fried Flos Chrysanthemi Morifolii (*Chao Ju Hua*), and Fructus Tribuli Terrestris (*Bai Ji Li*)

Dosage: 6-12g and up to 30g in severe cases

Note: 1. This refers to Cornus cooked in rice wine steam.

Concha Arcae *(Wa Leng Zi)*

_____Uncooked *(Sheng)*_____

Names: *Wa Leng Zi, Wa Long Zi, Sheng Wa Leng Zi, Sheng Wa Leng*

Flavors & nature: Salty; neutral

Functions: Dispels blood stasis, dissipates phlegm, softens the hard, scatters nodulations

Indications:

1. Abdominal masses due to blood stasis with palpable, fixed, possibly painful mass...

2. Subcutaneous nodules, scrofula due to accumulation of phlegm in the channels or neck

Typical combinations:

1. With vinegar[-processed] Rhizoma Sparganii (*Cu San Leng*), vinegar[-processed] Rhizoma Curcumae Zedoariae (*Cu E Zhu*), uncooked Semen Pruni Persicae (*Sheng Tao Ren*), and vinegar[-processed] Carapax Amydae Sinensis (*Cu Bie Jia*)

2. With Bulbus Fritillariae Thunbergii (*Zhe Bei Mu*), Herba Sargassii (*Hai Zao*), and Thallus Algae (*Kun Bu*)

Dosage: 10-15g

_____Calcined *(Duan)*_____

Names: *Duan Wa Leng Zi, Duan Wa Long Zi, Duan Wa Leng*

Flavors & nature: Salty and slightly astringent; neutral

Functions: Harmonizes the stomach, stops pain, stops stomach hyperacidity

Indications:

1. Stomach acidity and pain due to liver/stomach disharmony with vomiting or acid regurgitation...

2. Clamoring stomach, *i.e.*, *cao za*, due to stomach heat with a sensation of emptiness, hunger,

burning, and discomfort in the epigastrium, acid regurgitation...

Typical combinations:

1. With uncooked Os Sepiae Seu Sepiellae (*Sheng Hai Piao Xiao*), wine[-processed] Rhizoma Corydalis Yanhusuo (*Jiu Yan Hu Suo*), and uncooked Radix Glycyrrhizae (*Sheng Gan Cao*)

2. With stir-fried Fructus Gardeniae Jasminoidis (*Chao Zhi Zi*) and ginger[-processed] Caulis In Taeniis Bambusae (*Jiang Zhu Ru*)

Dosage: 10-15g and up to 20g in severe cases

Fructus Pruni Mume (*Wu Mei*)

Uncooked (*Sheng*)

Names: *Wu Mei, Da Wu Mei, Sheng Wu Mei*

Flavors & nature: Sour; slightly warm

Functions: Engenders fluids and humors, stops thirst, secures the lungs, stops cough, calms ascarids

Indications:

1. Thirst due to yin vacuity

2. Chronic cough due to lung qi and/or yin vacuity with permanent cough which will not heal...

3. Ascariasis[1] with abdominal pain

Typical combinations:

1. With uncooked Tuber Ophiopogonis Japonicae (*Sheng Mai Men Dong*), Radix Trichosanthis Kirlowii (*Tian Hua Fen*), and uncooked Radix Puerariae (*Sheng Ge Gen*) as in *Yu Quan Wan* (Jade Spring Pills [418])

2. With uncooked Semen Pruni Armeniacae (*Sheng Xing Ren*), uncooked Gelatinum Corii Asini (*Sheng E Jiao*), and honey mix-fried Pericarpium Papaveris Somniferi (*Mi Zhi Ying Su Ke*) as in *Yi Fu San* (One Administration Powder [398])

3. With stir-fried Pericarpium Zanthoxyli Bungeani (*Chao Hua Jiao*) add in *Wu Mei Wan* (Mume Pills [350])

Dosage: 6-12g and up to 30-60g in severe cases, notably for painful ascariasis

Note: 1. Mume does not eliminate parasites but anesthetizes them, thus calming abdominal pain due to ascariasis. This is the reason why, for this indication, this ingredient should always be combined with those which eliminate ascarids.

Stir-fried [till] Carbonized (*Chao Tan*)

Name: *Wu Mei Tan*

Flavors & nature: Sour and astringent; warm

Functions: Secures the intestines, stops diarrhea, stops bleeding

Indications:

1. Chronic diarrhea due to spleen vacuity

2. Persistent dysentery due to disharmony of the intestines with abdominal pain, slightly bloody stools, loss of appetite...

3. Bloody stools due to either A) large intestine heat or B) large intestine cold

4. Metrorrhagia due to *chong* and *ren* not securing

Typical combinations:

1. With stir-fried Fructus Terminaliae Chebulae (*Chao He Zi*), earth stir-fried Rhizoma Atractylodis Macrocephalae (*Tu Chao Bai Zhu*), and earth stir-fried Radix Dioscoreae Oppositae (*Tu Chao Shan Yao*)

2. With roasted Semen Myristicae Fragrantis (*Wei Rou Dou Kou*), uncooked Rhizoma Coptidis Chinensis (*Sheng Huang Lian*), and roasted Radix Saussureae Seu Vladimiriae (*Wei Mu Xiang*)

3. A) With uncooked Cacumen Biotae Orientalis (*Sheng Ce Bai Ye*), carbonized Folium Et Petiolus Trachycarpi (*Zong Lu Tan*), and uncooked Radix

Fructus Pruni Mume continued . . .

Rehmanniae (*Sheng Di Huang*)
B) With uncooked Cacumen Biotae Orientalis (*Sheng Ce Bai Ye*), carbonized Folium Et Petiolus Trachycarpi (*Zong Lu Tan*), and blast-fried Rhizoma Zingiberis (*Pao Jiang*)

4. With stir-fried Os Sepiae Seu Sepiellae (*Chao Hai Piao Xiao*), carbonized Radix Rubiae Cordifoliae (*Qian Cao Gen Tan*), and carbonized Radix Angelicae Sinensis (*Dang Gui Tan*)

Dosage: 6-12g and up to 30g in severe cases

Fructus Schizandrae Chinensis *(Wu Wei Zi)*

Uncooked *(Sheng)*

Names: *Wu Wei Zi, Sheng Wu Wei Zi, Bei Wu Wei*

Flavors & nature: Sour; warm

Functions: Supplements the qi, secures the lungs, stops cough, stops perspiration, engenders fluids and humors, stops thirst

Indications:

1. Perspiration due to defensive qi vacuity

2. Thirst due to a warm disease (with abundant perspiration) having damaged the qi and yin with a dry mouth, palpitations, insomnia, shortness of breath, fatigue...

3. Chronic cough due to lung qi vacuity with shortness of breath, weak cough, weak voice, sweating on slight exertion...

4. Heart palpitations, insomnia, poor memory due to heart qi and yin vacuity with night sweats...

Typical combinations:

1. With Radix Panacis Ginseng (*Ren Shen*), bran stir-fried Rhizoma Atractylodis Macrocephalae (*Fu Chao Bai Zhu*), and defatted Semen Biotae Orientalis (*Bai Zi Ren Shuang*) as in *Bai Zi Ren Wan* (Biota Seed Pills [24])

2. With Radix Panacis Ginseng (*Ren Shen*) and uncooked Tuber Ophiopogonis Japonicae (*Sheng Mai Men Dong*) as in *Sheng Mai San* (Engender the Pulse Powder [298])

3. With honey mix-fried Radix Astragali Membranacei (*Mi Zhi Huang Qi*), bran stir-fried Rhizoma Atractylodis Macrocephalae (*Fu Chao Bai Zhu*), Radix Panacis Ginseng (*Ren Shen*), and uncooked Fructus Terminaliae Chebulae (*Sheng He Zi*)

4. With defatted Semen Biotae Orientalis (*Bai Zi Ren Shuang*), uncooked Semen Zizyphi Spinosae (*Sheng Suan Zao Ren*), and Radix Panacis Ginseng (*Ren Shen*) as in *Tian Wang Bu Xin Dan* (Heavenly Emperor Supplement the Heart Elixir [326])

Dosage: 3-10g and up to 15g in severe cases

Fructus Schizandrae Chinensis continued . . .

Wine-steamed (Jiu Zheng)[1]

Names: *Jiu Zheng Wu Wei, Jiu Wu Wei Zi*

Flavors & nature: Sour and slightly acrid; warm

Functions: Supplements the kidneys, secures the essence, warms the lungs and kidneys, stops cough

Indications:

1. Spermatorrhea due to qi vacuity of the kidneys which are not securing or kidney yang vacuity

2. Cough due to lung yang vacuity with shortness of breath, aversion to cold, whitish, fluid phlegm...

Typical combinations:

1. With steamed Fructus Corni Officinalis (*Zheng Shan Zhu Yu*), Fructus Rosae Laevigatae (*Jin Ying Zi*), and uncooked Semen Euryalis Ferocis (*Sheng Qian Shi*)

2. With honey mix-fried Herba Cum Radice Asari (*Mi Zhi Xi Xin*), dry Rhizoma Zingiberis (*Gan Jiang*), and uncooked Sclerotium Poriae Cocos (*Sheng Fu Ling*) as in *Wu Wei Xi Xin Tang* (Schizandra & Asarum Decoction [357])

Dosage: 3-10g and up to 15g in severe cases

Note: 1. This refers to cooking in rice wine steam.

Vinegar-steamed (Cu Zheng)[1]

Names: *Cu Zheng Wu Wei, Cu Wu Wei Zi*

Flavors & nature: Sour; warm

Functions: Secures the lungs, stops diarrhea, has a strong astringing action

Indications:

1. Cockcrow diarrhea due to spleen/kidney yang vacuity with lack of appetite, loose stools with undigested food in them, fatigue, aversion to cold...

2. Cough[2] due to either A) lung qi and yin vacuity with weak, dry, chronic cough, asthmatic breathing, spontaneous perspiration or B) lung/kidney yin vacuity with chronic cough, asthmatic breathing, night sweats, spermatorrhea...

Typical combinations:

1. With roasted Semen Myristicae Fragrantis (*Wei Rou Dou Kou*) and salt[-processed] Fructus Psoraleae Corylifoliae (*Yan Bu Gu Zhi*) as in *Si Shen Wan* (Four Spirits Pills [313])

2. A) With uncooked Fructus Pruni Mume (*Sheng Wu Mei*), honey mix-fried Pericarpium Papaveris Somniferi (*Mi Zhi Ying Su Ke*), uncooked Gelatinum Corii Asini (*Sheng E Jiao*), Radix Panacis Ginseng (*Ren Shen*), and honey mix-fried Flos Tussilaginis Farfarae (*Mi Zhi Kuan Dong Hua*) as in *Jiu Xian San* (Nine Immortals Powder [186]) B) With steamed Fructus Corni Officinalis (*Zheng Shan Zhu Yu*) and prepared Radix Rehmanniae (*Shu Di Huang*) as in *Du Qi Wan* (Capital Qi Pill [89])

Dosage: 3-10g and up to 15g in severe cases

Notes: 1. This refers to cooking in vinegar steam. 2. If this is a dry cough due to severe lung yin vacuity, then honey mix-fried Schizandra (*Mi Zhi Wu Wei Zi*) is prescribed.

Addendum: There are two types of Schizandra. Northern Schizandra (*Bei Wu Wei Zi*), Schizandra Chinensis Baill., corresponds to the Schizandra commonly used in clinic and studied in detail above. Southern Schizandra (*Nan Wu Wei Zi*), Schizandra Sphenanthera Rehd. et Wils., rectifies the qi, eliminates dampness, and transforms phlegm. It is used, for example, in *Xiao Qing Long Tang* (Minor Blue Dragon Decoction [377]).

Pericarpium Papaveris Somniferi (Ying Su Ke)

Uncooked (Sheng)

Names: *Ying Su Ke, Yu Mi Ke, Sheng Ying Su Ke*

Flavors & nature: Sour and astringent; neutral

Functions: Secures the intestines, stops diarrhea, stops pain

Indications:

1. Chronic diarrhea due to spleen and stomach vacuity

2. Incessant dysentery due to disharmony of the intestines with abdominal pain, loss of appetite...

3. Epigastric pain due to spleen and stomach vacuity

4. Pain of the sinews and bones due to blood vacuity and wind dampness

Typical combinations:

1. With stir-fried Fructus Terminaliae Chebulae (*Chao He Zi*), earth stir-fried Rhizoma Atractylodis Macrocephalae (*Tu Chao Bai Zhu*), and earth stir-fried Radix Dioscoreae Oppositae (*Tu Chao Shan Yao*)

2. With uncooked Rhizoma Coptidis Chinensis (*Sheng Huang Lian*) and roasted Radix Saussureae Seu Vladimiriae (*Wei Mu Xiang*) as in *Mu Xiang San* (Saussurea Powder [226])

3. With Fructus Amomi (*Sha Ren*) and mix-fried Radix Glycyrrhizae (*Zhi Gan Cao*)

4. With wine[-processed] Radix Angelicae Sinensis (*Jiu Dang Gui*), wine[-processed] Radix Albus Paeoniae Lactiflorae (*Jiu Bai Shao Yao*), and stir-fried Ramulus Cinnamomi (*Chao Gui Zhi*)

Dosage: 2-8g and up to 15g in severe cases

Honey Mix-fried (Mi Zhi)

Names: *Mi Zhi Ying Su Ke, Mi Ying Su Ke, Mi Zhi Yu Mi Ke*

Flavors & nature: Sour, astringent, and slightly sweet; neutral

Functions: Secures the lungs, stops cough

Indications: Cough due to 1) lung qi vacuity with weak cough, asthmatic breathing, spontaneous perspiration or 2) lung yin vacuity with dry mouth and throat, a red tongue with no coating, dry cough...

Typical combinations:

1. With honey mix-fried Radix Astragali Membranacei (*Mi Zhi Huang Qi*), Radix Panacis Ginseng (*Ren Shen*), uncooked Radix Dioscoreae Oppositae (*Sheng Shan Yao*), Gecko (*Ge Jie*), uncooked Fructus Schizandrae Chinensis (*Sheng Wu Wei Zi*), and uncooked Fructus Terminaliae Chebulae (*Sheng He Zi*)

2. With uncooked Tuber Ophiopogonis Japonicae (*Sheng Mai Men Dong*), honey mix-fried Bulbus Lilii (*Mi Zhi Bai He*), uncooked Gelatinum Corii Asini (*Sheng E Jiao*), and uncooked Fructus Terminaliae Chebulae (*Sheng He Zi*)

Dosage: 5-10g

Limonitum (Yu Yu Liang)

Uncooked (Sheng)

Names: *Yu Yu Liang, Yu Liang Shi, Sheng Yu Yu Liang*

Flavors & nature: Sweet and astringent; slightly cold

Functions: Secures the intestines, stops diarrhea, stops abnormal vaginal discharge

Indications:

1. Chronic diarrhea due to disharmony of the intestines

2. Incessant dysentery due to spleen and stomach yang vacuity

3. Abnormal vaginal discharge due to spleen/kidney vacuity with clear, fluid, abundant discharge

Typical combinations:

1. With calcined Hallyositum Rubrum (*Duan Chi Shi Zhi*) as in *Chi Shi Zhi Yu Yu Liang Tang* (Hallyositum & Limonitum Decoction [49])

2. With dry Rhizoma Zingiberis (*Gan Jiang*), earth stir-fried Rhizoma Atractylodis Macrocephalae (*Tu Chao Bai Zhu*), and roasted Radix Saussureae Seu Vladimiriae (*Wei Mu Xiang*)

3. With stir-fried Rhizoma Atractylodis (*Chao Cang Zhu*), stir-fried Radix Dioscoreae Oppositae (*Chao Shan Yao*), stir-fried Semen Ginkgonis Bilobae (*Chao Bai Guo*), and uncooked Semen Euryalis Ferocis (*Sheng Qian Shi*)

Dosage: 10-20g

Calcined (Duan)

Names: *Duan Yu Yu Liang, Duan Yu Liang Shi*

Flavors & nature: Sweet and astringent; neutral

Functions: Stops bleeding

Indications:

1. Melena due to spleen yang vacuity

2. Metrorrhagia, menorrhagia due to *chong* and *ren* not securing

Typical combinations:

1. With dry Rhizoma Zingiberis (*Gan Jiang*), stir-fried Os Sepiae Seu Sepiellae (*Chao Hai Piao Xiao*), and carbonized Folium Et Petiolus Trachycarpi (*Zong Lu Tan*)

2. With carbonized Radix Angelicae Sinensis (*Dang Gui Tan*), uncooked Cacumen Biotae Orientalis (*Sheng Ce Bai Ye*), and Terra Flava Usta (*Fu Long Gan*)

Dosage: 10-20g

22
Other Prepared Medicinal Substances

Medicinal Substances Either Systematically or Occasionally Prepared

Certain medicinal substances are systematically prepared with unique processes of transformation. Such unique preparation permits one to profit from the different functions and indications of such medicinals. These medicinals are (in principle) available on the market and are ready to use. Other medicinals are prepared only occasionally according to the habits of certain practitioners or according to the customs of certain areas of production. The following list gives some characteristic examples.

Fructus Tribuli Terrestris (Bai Ji Li)

Salt mix-fried Tribulus (*Yan Zhi Bai Ji Li*) allows for the better treatment of vertigo and eye diseases which are due to liver/kidney vacuity causing internal wind.

Radix Angelicae Dahuricae (Bai Zhi)

Stir-fried [till] yellow Angelica (*Chao Huang Bai Zhi*) allows one to lessen the function of dispelling external wind of uncooked Angelica (*Sheng Bai Zhi*). It also is better for drying dampness for treating abnormal vaginal discharge.

Rhizoma Dioscoreae Hypoglaucae (Bei Xie)

Bran stir-fried Dioscorea Hypoglauca (*Fu Chao Bei Xie*) permits better fortification of the spleen and stomach and transformation of dampness.

Wine mix-fried Dioscorea Hypoglauca (*Jiu Zhi Bei Xie*) permits better dispelling of wind damp-

ness, opening of the network vessels, and treatment of *bi* and low back pain.

Salt mix-fried Dioscorea Hypoglauca (*Yan Zhi Bei Xie*) allows one to guide its therapeutic action to the kidneys in order to treat strangury with chyluria or dribbling and dripping due to kidney vacuity.

Semen Alpiniae Katsumadai (Cao Dou Kou)

Ginger mix-fried Alpinia Katsumada (*Jiang Zhi Cao Dou Kou*) permits better warming of the middle burner and stopping of vomiting.

Roasted Alpinia Katsumada (*Wei Cao Dou Kou*) permits better warming of the middle burner for the treatment of diarrhea.

Rhizoma Alpiniae Officinari (Gao Liang Jiang)

Earth stir-fried Alpinia Officinarum (*Tu Chao Gao Liang Jiang*) permits better warming of the stomach and stopping of diarrhea due to middle burner vacuity cold.

Evodia stir-fried Alpinia Officinarum (*Wu Yu Chao Gao Liang Jiang*)[1] permits better warming of the stomach and stopping vomiting due to stomach cold.

---

[1] This refers to Alpinia Officinarum which is fried with a decoction of Fructus Evodiae Rutecarpae (*Wu Zhu Yu*).

Fructus Lycii Chinensis (Gou Qi Zi)

Stir-fried [till] yellow Lycium (*Chao Huang Gou Qi Zi*) allows one to lessen the moistening nature of uncooked Lycium (*Sheng Gou Qi Zi*) when one wishes to supplement yin in the presence of spleen/stomach vacuity with loose or liquid stools.

Salt mix-fried Lycium (*Yan Zhi Gou Qi Zi*) allows one to guide the therapeutic action of this medicinal to the kidneys in order to nourish kidney essence.

Tuber Curcumae (Guan Yu Jin)

Vinegar mix-fried Curcuma (*Cu Zhi Guan Yu Jin*) permits better quickening of the qi, resolution of liver depression (*gan yu*), and treatment of pain in the chest, lateral costal regions, and breasts...

Folium Nelumbinis Nuciferae (He Ye)

Carbonized Lotus Leaves (*He Ye Tan*) permit better stopping of bleeding, such as epistaxis, melena, metrorrhagia...

Talcum (Hua Shi)

Water-ground Talcum (*Shui Fei Hua Shi*) allows it to be pulverized. Crude Talcum is not used.

Semen Citri Reticulatae (Ju He)

Salt mix-fried Orange Seeds (*Yan Zhi Ju He*) permit better treatment of *shan*, i.e., inguinal hernia, severe periumbilical pain, maladies of the scrotum or testicles. Uncooked Orange Seeds (*Sheng Ju He*) are only seldom used for external application.

Radix Sophorae Flavescentis (Ku Shen)

Stir-fried [till] scorched Sophora (*Chao Jiao Ku Shen*) allows one to lessen the cold nature and bitter flavor of uncooked Sophora (*Sheng Ku Shen*) in order to protect the stomach and to guide

its therapeutic action to the level of the blood, there to better treat dysentery with bloody stools.

Semen Litchi Chinensis (Li Zhi He)

Salt mix-fried Litchi (*Yan Zhi Li Zhi He*) permits better treatment of *shan*, i.e., inguinal hernia, severe periumbilical pain, maladies of the scrotum or testicles. Uncooked Litchi (*Sheng Li Zhi He*) is seldom used.

Semen Nelumbinis Nuciferae (Lian Zi)

Stir-fried [till] yellow Lotus Seeds (*Chao Huang Lian Zi*) allows one to warm the nature of uncooked Lotus Seeds (*Sheng Lian Zi*) and to reinforce their astringent action in order to better treat diarrhea due to spleen vacuity. For this indication, uncooked Lotus Seeds (*Sheng Lian Zi*) are not used.

Radix Gentianae Scabrae (Long Dan Cao)

Stir-fried [till] yellow Gentiana Scabra (*Chao Huang Long Dan Cao*) allows one to lessen the cold nature and bitter taste of uncooked Gentiana Scabra (*Sheng Long Dan Cao*) so as to protect the stomach, yin, and blood.[2]

Wine mix-fried Gentiana Scabra (*Jiu Zhi Long Dan Cao*) permits one to guide the therapeutic action of this medicinal to the upper body in order to better treat eyes diseases, deafness, tinnitus, of a bitter taste in the mouth. In addition, this permits the quickening of the blood and qi when liver fire has its origin in liver qi stagnation.

Smithsonitum (Lu Gan Shi)

Dip calcined Smithsonitum (*Cui Lu Gan Shi*) facilitates its pulverization. Uncooked Smithsonitum (*Sheng Lu Gan Shi*) is not used.

---

[2] Traditionally, Radix Gentianae Scabrae, Caulis Akebiae Mutong, and Fructus Gardeniae Jasminoidis are considered the three bitterest plants in the Chinese materia medica.

Sulfur (Liu Huang)

Processed Sulfur (*Zhi Liu Huang*)[3] allows one to reduce the toxicity of uncooked Sulfur (*Sheng Liu Huang*) in order to use it orally to strengthen yang and augment the lifegate fire.

Radix Aristolochiae Fangchi (Mu Fang Ji)

Wine mix-fried Aristolochia Fangchi (*Jiu Zhi Mu Fang Ji*) permits better dispelling of wind dampness, opening of the network vessels, and treatment of *bi*.

Caulis Akebiae Mutong (Mu Tong)

Stir-fried [till] scorched Akebia (*Chao Jiao Mu Tong*) permits one to lessen the cold nature and bitter taste of uncooked Akebia (*Sheng Mu Tong*) in order to protect the stomach and disinhibit urination without weakening the *yuan qi*.[2]

Radix Adenophorae Strictae (Nan Sha Shen)

Honey mix-fried Adenophora (*Mi Zhi Nan Sha Shen*) permits better moistening and nourishing of lung yin.

Radix Gentianae Macrophyllae (Qin Jiao)

Wine mix-fried Gentiana Macrophylla (*Jiu Zhi Qin Jiao*) permits better dispelling of wind dampness, opening of the network vessels, and treatment of *bi*.

Cortex Fraxini (Qin Pi)

Carbonized Fraxinus (*Qin Pi Tan*) permits one to lessen the cold nature of uncooked Fraxinus (*Sheng Qin Pi*), to guide its therapeutic action to the level of the blood, and to reinforce its astringent property in order to

treat dysentery with bloody, purulent stools.

Herba Artemisiae Apiaceae (Qing Hao)

Amyda tortoise blood [processed] Artemisia Apiacea (*Bie Xue Ban Qing Hao*)[4] permits better clearing of vacuity heat or treatment of malaria.

Semen Myristicae Fragrantis (Rou Dou Kou)

Roasted Nutmeg (*Wei Rou Dou Kou*) allows one to eliminate the irritating character of uncooked Nutmeg (*Sheng Rou Dou Kou*) and to remove the oil from the seed in order to promote its anti-diarrhetic action.

Ramus Loranthi Seu Visci (Sang Ji Sheng)

Wine mix-fried Loranthus (*Jiu Zhi Sang Ji Sheng*) permits better dispelling of wind dampness, opening of the network vessels, and treatment of *bi*.

Fructus Amomi (Sha Ren)

Ginger mix-fried Amomum (*Jiang Zhi Sha Ren*) permits better warming of the middle burner and stopping of vomiting.

Rhizoma Belamcandae (She Gan)

Stir-fried [till] yellow Belamcanda (*Chao Huang She Gan*) allows one to lessen the cold nature and bitter flavor of uncooked Belamcanda (*Sheng She Gan*) in order to clear heat and resolve toxins in the presence of qi vacuity or spleen/stomach vacuity.

Herba Lycopodii (Shen Jin Cao)

Wine mix-fried Lycopodium (*Jiu Zhi Shen Jin Cao*) permits better dispelling of wind, cold,

---

[3] Sulfur is boiled with tofu (*Dou Fu*).

[4] This refers to Artemisia Apiacea which is prepared with the blood of the Amydae Sinensis tortoise.

dampness, opening of the network vessels, and treatment of *bi*.

Rhizoma Acori Graminei (Shi Chang Pu)

Ginger mix-fried Acorus (*Jiang Zhi Shi Chang Pu*) permits better elimination of phlegm and stimulates the appetite.

Fructus Quisqualis Indicae (Shi Jun Zi)

Stir-fried [till] yellow Quisqualis (*Chao Huang Shi Jun Zi*) allows one to lessen the toxicity of uncooked Quisqualis (*Sheng Shi Jun Zi*) and to better fortify the spleen in the treatment of intestinal parasites in infants and infantile malnutrition (*gan ji*).

Tuber Asparagi Cochinensis (Tian Men Dong)

Honey mix-fried Asparagus (*Mi Zhi Tian Men Dong*) permits better moistening and nourishing of lung yin.

Cinnabar[-processed] Asparagus (*Zhu Sha Ban Tian Men Dong*)[5] permits better treatment of insomnia and restless spirit due to kidney yin vacuity.

Realgar (Xiong Huang)

Water-ground Realgar (*Shui Fei Xiong Huang*) permits its pulverization. Crude Realgar is not used.

Radix Stellariae Dichotomae (Yin Chai Hu)

Stir-fried [till] scorched Stellaria (*Chao Jiao Yin Chai Hu*) allows for better stopping of bleeding due to vacuity heat.

Amyda tortoise blood [processed] Stellaria (*Bie Xue Yin Chai Hu*) allows for better clearing of vacuity heat and elimination of steaming-bones fever.

Margarita (Zhen Zhu)

Water-ground Pearl (*Shui Fei Zhen Zhu*) permits its pulverization. Crude Pearl is not used.

Cinnabar (Zhu Sha)

Water-ground Cinnabar (*Shui Fei Zhu Sha*) permits its pulverization. Crude Cinnabar is not used.

Pyritum (Zi Ran Tong)

Vinegar dip calcined Pyritum (*Cu Cui Zi Ran Tong*) allows for better dispelling of blood stasis, stopping pain, and facilitates its pulverization. Uncooked Pyritum (*Sheng Zi Ran Tong*) is not used.

Folium Et Petiolus Trachycarpi (Zong Lu Pi)

Carbonized Trachycarpus (*Zong Lu Tan*) reinforces this medicinal's astringent action and allows for better stopping of bleeding. Uncooked Trachycarpus (*Sheng Zong Lu Pi*) is never used.

---

[5] This refers to powdered Cinnabar, which is mixed with Asparagus Cochinensis.

Medicinal Substances Systematically Prepared Because of Their Side Effects

Numerous medicinal substances are transformed in order to reduce their toxicity, their side effects, or their drastic action, thus benefitting from their therapeutic actions at the same time as protecting the organism.

Semen Crotonis Tiglii *(Ba Dou)*

Defatted Croton (*Ba Dou Shuang*) allows one to eliminate the extremely toxic oil from the seed, thus moderating the drastic purgative action of uncooked Croton (*Sheng Ba Dou*).

Semen Ginkgonis Bilobae *(Bai Guo)*

Stir-fried [till] yellow Ginkgo (*Chao Huang Bai Guo*) allows one to lessen the toxicity of uncooked Ginkgo (*Sheng Bai Guo*).

Semen Sinapis Albae *(Bai Jie Zi)*

Stir-fried [till] yellow Mustard Seed (*Chao Huang Bai Jie Zi*) allows one to lessen the drying character and dispersing nature of uncooked Mustard Seed (*Sheng Bai Jie Zi*), therefore preserving yin.

Mylabris *(Ban Mao)*

Rice stir-frying Mylabris (*Mi Chao Ban Mao*) allows one to lessen the toxicity and disagreeable odor of uncooked Mylabris (*Sheng Ban Mao*).

Radix Dichroae Febrifugae *(Chang Shan)*

Bran stir-fried (*Fu Chao*), wine mix-fried (*Jiu Zhi*), or vinegar mix-fried Dichroa (*Cu Zhi Chang Shan*) allow one to avoid the vomiting and nausea caused by uncooked Dichroa (*Sheng Chang Shan*).

Corium Erinacei *(Ci Wei Pi)*

Sand stir-fried (*Sha Chao*) or Talcum Powder stir-fried Hedgehog Skin (*Hua Shi Fen Chao Ci Wei Pi*)[6] allows one to lessen the disagreeable odor of uncooked Hedgehog Skin (*Sheng Ci Wei Pi*) and renders this remedy appropriate for consumption.

Lacca Sinica Excciccata *(Gan Qi)*

Calcined Lacquer (*Duan Gan Qi*) allows one to lessen the toxicity of uncooked Lacquer (*Sheng Gan Qi*).

Pericarpium Zanthoxyli Bungeani *(Hua Jiao)*

Stir-fried [till] yellow Pericarpium Zanthoxyli (*Chao Huang Hua Jiao*) allows one to lessen the toxicity, acrid flavor, and very dispersing nature of uncooked Pericarpium Zanthoxyli (*Sheng Hua Jiao*).

Semen Cannabis Sativae *(Huo Ma Ren)*

Stir-fried [till] yellow Cannabis (*Chao Huang Huo Ma Ren*) allows one to lessen the toxicity of uncooked Cannabis (*Sheng Huo Ma Ren*).

Radix Euphorbiae Pekinensis *(Jing Da Ji)*

Vinegar mix-fried Euphorbia Pekinensis (*Cu Zhi Jing Da Ji*) allows one to lessen the toxicity and drastic action of uncooked Euphorbiae Pekinensis (*Sheng Jing Da Ji*).

---

[6] This refers to the frying of medicinal substances with powdered Talcum.

Semen Euphorbiae Lathyridis *(Qian Jin Zi)*

Defatted Euphorbiae Lathyris (*Qian Jin Zi Shuang*) allows one to eliminate the toxic oil from the seed and to moderate the drastic purgative action of uncooked Euphorbia Lathyris (*Sheng Qian Jin Zi*).

Radix Phytolaccae *(Shang Lu)*

Vinegar mix-fried Phytolacca (*Cu Zhi Shang Lu*) allows one to lessen the toxicity and drastic action of uncooked Phytolacca (*Sheng Shang Lu*).

Hirudo *(Shui Zhi)*

Talcum Powder stir-fried Hirudo (*Hua Shi Fen Chao Shui Zhi*)[6] allows one to lessen the toxicity and disagreeable odor of uncooked Hirudo (*Sheng Shui Zhi*).

Scolopendra Subspinipes *(Wu Gong)*

Stone-baked Centipede (*Bei Wu Gong*) allows one to lessen the toxicity and facilitate the pulverization and preservation of uncooked Centipede (*Sheng Wu Gong*).

Flos Daphnis Genkwae *(Yuan Hua)*

Vinegar mix-fried Daphnes Genkwa (*Cu Zhi Yuan Hua*) allows one to lessen the toxicity and drastic action of uncooked Daphnes Genkwa (*Sheng Yuan Hua*).

Semen Pruni *(Yu Li Ren)*

Stir-fried [till] yellow Prune Seed (*Chao Huang Yu Li Ren*) allows one to lessen the descending and purgative actions of uncooked Prune Seed (*Sheng Yu Li Ren*) in order to enable it to be used for constipation in the aged or postpartum.

Eupolyphaga Seu Opisthoplatia *(Zhe Chong)*

Stone-baked Eupolyphaga (*Bei Zhe Chong*) allows one to lessen the toxicity and facilitates the pulverization and preservation of uncooked Eupolyphaga (*Sheng Zhe Chong*).

23
Glossary of the Principal Methods of Processing

Each process of preparation has already been explained in the section on theory. For the details of these processes, see the chapter titled "Methods of Preparing the Chinese Materia Medica." [This glossary is based on Nigel Wiseman's *Glossary of Chinese Medical Terms and Acupuncture Points.*]

Bei: stone-baked
Chao Huang: stir-fried [till] yellow
Chao Jiao: stir-fried [till] scorched
Chao Tan: stir-fried [till] carbonized
Chao: stir-fried
Cu Cui: vinegar dip calcined
Cu Zheng: vinegar-steamed
Cu Zhi: vinegar mix-fried
Cui: dip calcined
Dan: scalded
Duan: calcined
Fu Chao: bran stir-fried
Gan Cao Zhi: Licorice mix-fried
Gan: dry
Ge Fen Chao: Concha Cyclinae powder stir-fried
Hong: baked
Hua Shi Fen Chao: Talcum Powder stir-fried
Jiang Zhi or ***Jiang Zhi Zhi***: Ginger mix-fried or ginger juice mix-fried
Jiao: gelatin / 焦 jiāo: burnt, scorched
Jiu Zheng: wine-steamed
Jiu Zhi: wine mix-fried
Mi Chao: rice stir-fried
Mi Zhi: honey mix-fried
Pao Zhi: drug processing
Pao: blast-fried
Pu Huang Fen Chao: Pollen Typhae powder stir-fried
Qing Dai or ***Qing Dai Ban***: Indigo[-processed]
Sha Chao: sand stir-fried
Sheng: uncooked

Shu: prepared
Shuang: defatted
Tu Chao: earth stir-fried
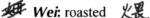 ***Wei***: roasted 火畏
Xian: fresh
Yan Zhi: salt mix-fried
You Zhi: oil mix-fried
Zheng: steamed
Zhi: processed
Zhi: juice
Zhu Sha or ***Zhu Sha Ban***: Cinnabar[-processed]
Zhu: boiled

24
Glossary of Traditional Formulas

1. *An Shen Ding Zhi Wan* (Quiet the Spirit & Stabilize the Will Pills): Sclerotium Poriae Cocos (*Fu Ling*), Sclerotium Pararadicis Poriae Cocos (*Fu Shen*), Radix Panacis Ginseng (*Ren Shen*), Radix Polygalae Tenuifoliae (*Yuan Zhi*), Dens Draconis (*Long Chi*), Rhizoma Acori Graminei (*Shi Chang Pu*)

2. *An Shen Wan* (Quiet the Spirit Pills): Rhizoma Coptidis Chinensis (*Huang Lian*), Cinnabar (*Zhu Sha*), uncooked Radix Rehmanniae (*Sheng Di Huang*), Radix Angelicae Sinensis (*Dang Gui*), Radix Glycyrrhizae (*Gan Cao*)

3. *Ba Ji Wan* (Morinda Pills): Radix Morindae Officinalis (*Ba Ji Tian*), Radix Achyranthis Bidentatae (*Huai Niu Xi*), Radix Et Rhizoma Notopterygii (*Qiang Huo*), Cortex Cinnamomi (*Rou Gui*), Cortex Radicis Acanthopanacis (*Wu Jia Pi*), Cortex Eucommiae Ulmoidis (*Du Zhong*), dry Rhizoma Zingiberis (*Gan Jiang*)

4. *Ba Zhen Tang* (Eight Pearls Decoction): Prepared Radix Rehmanniae (*Shu Di Huang*), Radix Albus Paeoniae Lactiflorae (*Bai Shao Yao*), Radix Angelicae Sinensis (*Dang Gui*), Radix Ligustici Wallichii (*Chuan Xiong*), Radix Codonopsis Pilosulae (*Dang Shen*), Rhizoma Atractylodis Macrocephalae (*Bai Zhu*), Sclerotium Poriae Cocos (*Fu Ling*), mix-fried Radix Glycyrrhizae (*Zhi Gan Cao*)

5. *Ba Zheng San* (Eight Righteous [Medicinals] Powder): Caulis Akebiae Mutong (*Mu Tong*), Herba Dianthi (*Qu Mai*), Radix Et Rhizoma Rhei (*Da Huang*), Semen Plantaginis (*Che Qian Zi*), Talcum (*Hua Shi*), Fructus Gardeniae Jasminoidis (*Shan Zhi Zi*), Herba Polygoni Avicularis (*Bian Xu*), Medulla Junci Effusi (*Deng Xin Cao*), Radix Glycyrrhizae (*Gan Cao*)

6. *Bai Bu Gao* (Stemona Paste): Radix Stemonae (*Bai Bu*), Cortex Radicis Dictamni (*Bai Xian Pi*), Cortex Phellodendri (*Huang Bai*), Realgar (*Xiong Huang*)

7. *Bai Bu Jian* (Stemona Decoction): Radix Stemonae (*Bai Bu*), Radix Asteris Tatarici (*Zi Wan*), Radix Cynanchi Stautonii (*Bai Qian*), Radix Adenophorae Strictae (*Nan Sha Shen*), Bulbus Fritillariae Cirrhosae (*Chuan Bei Mu*), Pericarpium Citri Reticulatae (*Chen Pi*), Radix Glycyrrhizae (*Gan Cao*)

8. *Bai Bu Tang* (Stemona Decoction): Radix Stemonae (*Bai Bu*), Tuber Ophiopogonis Japonicae (*Mai Men Dong*), Radix Adenophorae Strictae (*Nan Sha Shen*), Cortex Radicis Mori Albi (*Sang Bai Pi*), Bulbus Lilii (*Bai He*), Sclerotium Poriae Cocos (*Fu Ling*), Cortex Radicis Lycii (*Di Gu Pi*), Semen Coicis Lachryma-jobi (*Yi Yi Ren*), Radix Astragali Membranacei (*Huang Qi*)

9. *Bai Bu Wan* (Stemona Pills): Radix Stemonae (*Bai Bu*), Herba Ephedrae (*Ma Huang*), Semen Pruni Armeniacae (*Xing Ren*), Radix Glycyrrhizae (*Gan Cao*)

10. *Bai Fu Yin* (Typhonium Drink): Rhizoma Typhonii (*Bai Fu Zi*), Rhizoma Pinelliae Ternatae (*Ban Xia*), Rhizoma Gastrodiae Elatae (*Tian Ma*), Rhizoma Arisaematis (*Tian Nan Xing*), Radix Aconiti Carmichaeli (*Chuan Wu Tou*), Buthus Martensi (*Quan Xie*), Bombyx Batryticatus (*Jiang Can*), Pericarpium Citri Reticulatae (*Chen Pi*), Radix Saussureae Seu Vladimiriae (*Mu Xiang*)

11. *Bai He Di Huang Tang* (Lily & Rehmannia Decoction): Bulbus Lilii (*Bai He*), uncooked Radix Rehmanniae (*Sheng Di Huang*)

12. *Bai He Gu Jin Tang* (Lily Secure Metal Decoction): Bulbus Lilii (*Bai He*), uncooked Radix Rehmanniae (*Sheng Di Huang*), prepared Radix Rehmanniae (*Shu Di Huang*), Tuber Ophiopogonis Japonicae (*Mai Men Dong*), Rhizoma Anemarrhenae (*Zhi Mu*), Radix Scrophulariae Ningpoensis (*Xuan Shen*), Radix Platycodi Grandiflori (*Jie Geng*), Radix Angelicae Sinensis (*Dang Gui*), Radix Albus Paeoniae Lactiflorae (*Bai Shao Yao*), Radix Glycyrrhizae (*Gan Cao*)

13. *Bai He Zhi Mu Tang* (Lily & Anemarrhena Decoction): Bulbus Lilii (*Bai He*), Rhizoma Anemarrhenae (*Zhi Mu*)

14. *Bai Hu Jia Cang Zhu Tang* (White Tiger Plus Atractylodes Decoction): Gypsum Fibrosum (*Shi Gao*), Rhizoma Anemarrhenae (*Zhi Mu*), mix-fried Radix Glycyrrhizae (*Zhi Gan Cao*), Semen Oryzae Sativae (*Geng Mi*), Rhizoma Atractylodis (*Cang Zhu*)

15. *Bai Hu Tang* (White Tiger Decoction): Gypsum Fibrosum (*Shi Gao*), Rhizoma Anemarrhenae (*Zhi Mu*), mix-fried Radix Glycyrrhizae (*Zhi Gan Cao*), Semen Oryzae Sativae (*Geng Mi*)

16. *Bai Hua Gao* (White Flower Paste): Bulbus Lilii (*Bai He*), Flos Tussilaginis Farfarae (*Kuan Dong Hua*)

16a. *Bai Hua She Jiu* (Agkistrodon Wine): Agkistrodon Seu Bungarus (*Bai Hua She*), Buthus Martensi (*Quan Xie*), Radix Angelicae Sinensis (*Dang Gui*), Radix Ledebouriellae Sesloidis (*Fang Feng*), Radix Et Rhizoma Notopterygii (*Qiang Huo*), Radix Angelicae Pubescentis (*Du Huo*), Radix Angelicae Dahuricae (*Bai Zhi*), Rhizoma Gastrodiae Elatae (*Tian Ma*), Radix Rubrus Paeoniae Lactiflorae (*Chi Shao Yao*), Radix Glycyrrhizae (*Gan Cao*), Rhizoma Cimicifugae (*Sheng Ma*)

17. *Bai Jiang Can San* (White Silkworm Powder): Bombyx Batryticatus (*Jiang Can*), Folium Mori Albi (*Sang Ye*), Herba Schizonepetae Tenuifoliae (*Jing Jie*), Herba Equiseti Hiemalis (*Mu Zei*), Herba Cum Radice Asari (*Xi Xin*), Flos Inulae (*Xuan Fu Hua*), Radix Glycyrrhizae (*Gan Cao*)

18. *Bai Tou Weng Tang* (Pulsatilla Decoction): Radix Pulsatillae Chinensis (*Bai Tou Weng*), Cortex Phellodendri (*Huang Bai*), Rhizoma Coptidis Chinensis (*Huang Lian*), Cortex Fraxini (*Qin Pi*)

19. *Bai Wei Tang* (Cynanchus Atratus Decoction): Radix Cynanchi Atrati (*Bai Wei*), Radix Angelicae Sinensis (*Dang Gui*), Radix Panacis Ginseng (*Ren Shen*), mix-fried Radix Glycyrrhizae (*Zhi Gan Cao*)

20. *Bai Ye Tang* (Cacumen Biotae Decoction): Cacumen Biotae Orientalis (*Ce Bai Ye*), dry Rhizoma Zingiberis (*Gan Jiang*), Folium Artemisiae Argyii (*Ai Ye*), Feces Praeparatus Equus Caballi (*Ma Tong*)

21. *Bai Zhi San* (Angelica Powder): Radix Angelicae Dahuricae (*Bai Zhi*), Os Sepiae Seu Sepiellae (*Hai Piao Xiao*), Crinis Carbonisatus (*Xue Yu Tan*)

22. *Bai Zhu Fu Zi Tang* (Atractylodes & Aconite Decoction): Rhizoma Atractylodis Macrocephalae (*Bai Zhu*), Radix Lateralis Praeparatus Aconiti Carmichaeli (*Fu Zi*), Rhizoma Atractylodis (*Cang Zhu*), Pericarpium Citri Reticulatae (*Chen Pi*), Cortex Magnoliae Officinalis (*Hou Po*), Rhizoma Pinelliae Ternatae (*Ban Xia*), Sclerotium Poriae Cocos (*Fu Ling*), Rhizoma Alismatis (*Ze Xie*), Sclerotium Polypori Umbellati (*Zhu Ling*), Cortex Cinnamomi (*Rou Gui*), uncooked Rhizoma Zingiberis (*Sheng Jiang*)

23. *Bai Zhu San* (Atractylodes Powder): Rhizoma Atractylodis Macrocephalae (*Bai Zhu*), Pericarpium Arecae Catechu (*Da Fu Pi*), Cortex Sclerotii Poriae Cocos (*Fu Ling Pi*), uncooked Cortex Rhizomatis Zingiberis (*Sheng Jiang Pi*), Pericarpium Citri Reticulatae (*Chen Pi*)

24. *Bai Zi Ren Wan* (Biota Seed Pills): Semen

Biotae Orientalis (*Bai Zi Ren*), Concha Ostreae (*Mu Li*), Fructus Schizandrae Chinensis (*Wu Wei Zi*), Rhizoma Atractylodis Macrocephalae (*Bai Zhu*), Radix Panacis Ginseng (*Ren Shen*), Rhizoma Pinelliae Ternatae (*Ban Xia*), Radix Ephedrae (*Ma Huang Gen*)

25. *Bai Zi Yang Xin Wan* (Biota Seed Nourish the Heart Pills): Semen Biotae Orientalis (*Bai Zi Ren*), Fructus Lycii Chinensis (*Gou Qi Zi*), Tuber Ophiopogonis Japonicae (*Mai Men Dong*), Radix Angelicae Sinensis (*Dang Gui*), Rhizoma Acori Graminei (*Shi Chang Pu*), Sclerotium Pararadicis Poriae Cocos (*Fu Shen*), Radix Scrophulariae Ningpoensis (*Xuan Shen*), prepared Radix Rehmanniae (*Shu Di Huang*), mix-fried Radix Glycyrrhizae (*Zhi Gan Cao*)

26. *Ban Xia Bai Zhu Tian Ma Tang* (Pinellia, Atractylodes & Gastrodia Decoction): Rhizoma Pinelliae Ternatae (*Ban Xia*), Rhizoma Atractylodis Macrocephalae (*Bai Zhu*), Rhizoma Gastrodiae Elatae (*Tian Ma*), Sclerotium Poriae Cocos (*Fu Ling*), Pericarpium Citri Reticulatae (*Chen Pi*), mix-fried Radix Glycyrrhizae (*Zhi Gan Cao*)

27. *Ban Xia Hou Po Tang* (Pinellia & Magnolia Decoction): Rhizoma Pinelliae Ternatae (*Ban Xia*), Cortex Magnoliae Officinalis (*Hou Po*), Folium Perillae Frutescentis (*Zi Su Ye*), Sclerotium Poriae Cocos (*Fu Ling*), uncooked Rhizoma Zingiberis (*Sheng Jiang*)

27a. *Ban Xia Shu Mi Tang* (Pinellia & Millet Decoction): Rhizoma Pinelliae Ternatae (*Ban Xia*), Semen Panici Miliacei (*Shu Mi*)

28. *Ban Xia Xie Xin Tang* (Pinellia Drain the Heart Decoction): Rhizoma Pinelliae Ternatae (*Ban Xia*), Radix Scutellariae Baicalensis (*Huang Qin*), Rhizoma Coptidis Chinensis (*Huang Lian*), Radix Panacis Ginseng (*Ren Shen*), dry Rhizoma Zingiberis (*Gan Jiang*), Fructus Zizyphi Jujubae (*Da Zao*), mix-fried Radix Glycyrrhizae (*Zhi Gan Cao*)

29. *Bao He Wan* (Protect Harmony Pills): Semen Raphani Sativi (*Lai Fu Zi*), Massa Medica Fermentata (*Shen Qu*), Fructus Germinatus Hordei Vulgaris (*Mai Ya*), Rhizoma Pinelliae Ternatae (*Ban Xia*), Pericarpium Citri Reticulatae (*Chen Pi*), Fructus Crataegi (*Shan Zha*), Sclerotium Poriae Cocos (*Fu Ling*), Fructus Forsythiae Suspensae (*Lian Qiao*)

30. *Bi Xiao Wan* (Compelling Results Pills): Fructus Meliae Toosendan (*Chuan Lian Zi*), Radix Gentianae Scabrae (*Long Dan Cao*), Herba Artemisiae Capillaris (*Yin Chen Hao*), Fructus Gardeniae Jasminoidis (*Shan Zhi Zi*), Radix Scutellariae Baicalensis (*Huang Qin*)

31. *Bing Peng San* (Borneol & Borax Powder): Borneol (*Bing Pian*), Cinnabar (*Zhu Sha*), Mirabilitum (*Mang Xiao*), Borax (*Peng Sha*)

32. *Bu Fei E Jiao Tang* (Supplement the Lungs Donkey Skin Glue Decoction): Gelatinum Corii Asini (*E Jiao*), Fructus Arctii Lappae (*Niu Bang Zi*), Fructus Aristolochiae (*Ma Dou Ling*), Semen Pruni Armeniacae (*Xing Ren*), Semen Oryzae Sativae (*Geng Mi*), mix-fried Radix Glycyrrhizae (*Zhi Gan Cao*)

33. *Bu Fei Tang* (Supplement the Lungs Decoction): Radix Codonopsis Pilosulae (*Dang Shen*), Radix Astragali Membranacei (*Huang Qi*), Fructus Schizandrae Chinensis (*Wu Wei Zi*), Radix Asteris Tatarici (*Zi Wan*), Cortex Radicis Mori Albi (*Sang Bai Pi*), prepared Radix Rehmanniae (*Shu Di Huang*)

34. *Bu Gu Zhi Wan* (Psoralea Pills): Fructus Psoraleae Corylifoliae (*Bu Gu Zhi*), Semen Cuscutae (*Tu Si Zi*), Semen Juglandis Regiae (*Hu Tao Ren*), Lignum Aquilariae Agallochae (*Chen Xiang*)

35. *Bu Huan Jin Zheng Qi San* (More Valuable than Gold Righteous Qi Powder): Herba Agastachis Seu Pogostemi (*Huo Xiang*), Rhizoma Atractylodis (*Cang Zhu*), Cortex Magnoliae Officinalis (*Hou Po*), Pericarpium Citri Reticulatae

(*Chen Pi*), Rhizoma Pinelliae Ternatae (*Ban Xia*), uncooked Rhizoma Zingiberis (*Sheng Jiang*), Fructus Zizyphi Jujubae (*Da Zao*), mix-fried Radix Glycyrrhizae (*Zhi Gan Cao*)

36. *Bu Wang San* (No Forgetting Powder): Radix Panacis Ginseng (*Ren Shen*), Radix Polygalae Tenuifoliae (*Yuan Zhi*), Sclerotium Poriae Cocos (*Fu Ling*), Sclerotium Pararadicis Poriae Cocos (*Fu Shen*), Rhizoma Acori Graminei (*Shi Chang Pu*)

37. *Bu Yang Huan Wu Tang* (Supplement Yang & Slacken (*i.e.*, Relax) the Five [Viscera] Decoction): Radix Astragali Membranacei (*Huang Qi*), Lumbricus (*Di Long*), Radix Ligustici Wallichii (*Chuan Xiong*), Radix Angelicae Sinensis (*Dang Gui*), Flos Carthami Tinctorii (*Hong Hua*), Semen Pruni Persicae (*Tao Ren*), Radix Rubrus Paeoniae Lactiflorae (*Chi Shao Yao*)

38. *Bu Zhong Yi Qi Tang* (Supplement the Center & Boost the Qi Decoction): Radix Astragali Membranacei (*Huang Qi*), Rhizoma Atractylodis Macrocephalae (*Bai Zhu*), Radix Angelicae Sinensis (*Dang Gui*), Rhizoma Cimicifugae (*Sheng Ma*), Radix Panacis Ginseng (*Ren Shen*), Pericarpium Citri Reticulatae (*Chen Pi*), Radix Bupleuri (*Chai Hu*), mix-fried Radix Glycyrrhizae (*Zhi Gan Cao*)

39. *Cang Er San* (Xanthium Powder): Fructus Xanthii (*Cang Er Zi*), Flos Magnoliae Officinalis (*Xin Yi Hua*), Radix Angelicae Dahuricae (*Bai Zhi*), Herba Menthae Haplocalycis (*Bo He*)

40. *Cao Guo Yin* (Amomum Tsao-ko Drink): Fructus Amomi Tsao-ko (*Cao Guo*), Radix Dichroae Febrifugae (*Chang Shan*), Rhizoma Anemarrhenae (*Zhi Mu*), Fructus Pruni Mume (*Wu Mei*), Semen Arecae Catechu (*Bing Lang*), Squama Manitis Pentadactylis (*Chuan Shan Jia*), Radix Glycyrrhizae (*Gan Cao*)

41. *Ce Bai Chun Gen Wan* (Cacumen Biotae & Ailanthus Pills): Cacumen Biotae Orientalis (*Ce Bai Ye*), Cortex Ailanthi Altissimi (*Chun Gen Pi*), Rhizoma Atractylodis Macrocephalae (*Bai Zhu*), Radix Albus Paeoniae Lactiflorae (*Bai Shao Yao*), Radix Angelicae Dahuricae (*Bai Zhi*), Rhizoma Cyperi Rotundi (*Xiang Fu*), Rhizoma Coptidis Chinensis (*Huang Lian*), Cortex Phellodendri (*Huang Bai*)

42. *Ce Bai San* (Cacumen Biotae Powder): Cacumen Biotae Orientalis (*Ce Bai Ye*), Flos Immaturus Sophorae Japonicae (*Huai Hua*)

43. *Chai Ge Jie Ji Tang* (Bupleurum & Pueraria Resolve the Muscles Decoction): Radix Bupleuri (*Chai Hu*), Radix Puerariae (*Ge Gen*), Radix Et Rhizoma Notopterygii (*Qiang Huo*), Radix Angelicae Dahuricae (*Bai Zhi*), Radix Platycodi Grandiflori (*Jie Geng*), Gypsum Fibrosum (*Shi Gao*), Radix Albus Paeoniae Lactiflorae (*Bai Shao Yao*), Radix Scutellariae Baicalensis (*Huang Qin*), uncooked Rhizoma Zingiberis (*Sheng Jiang*), Fructus Zizyphi Jujubae (*Da Zao*), Radix Glycyrrhizae (*Gan Cao*)

44. *Chai Hu Shu Gan San* (Bupleurum Course the Liver Powder): Radix Bupleuri (*Chai Hu*), Rhizoma Cyperi Rotundi (*Xiang Fu*), Radix Albus Paeoniae Lactiflorae (*Bai Shao Yao*), Radix Ligustici Wallichii (*Chuan Xiong*), Pericarpium Citri Reticulatae (*Chen Pi*), Fructus Immaturus Citri Seu Ponciri (*Zhi Shi*), mix-fried Radix Glycyrrhizae (*Zhi Gan Cao*)

45. *Chan Hua San* (Cicada & Chrysanthemum Powder): Periostracum Cicadae (*Chan Tui*), Flos Chrysanthemi Morifolii (*Ju Hua*), Fructus Viticis (*Man Jing Zi*), Scapus Et Inflorescentia Eriocaulonis Buergeriani (*Gu Jing Cao*), Fructus Tribuli Terrestris (*Bai Ji Li*), Radix Ledebouriellae Sesloidis (*Fang Feng*), Semen Cassiae Torae (*Cao Jue Ming*), Flos Buddleiae Officinalis (*Mi Meng Hua*), Radix Et Rhizoma Notopterygii (*Qiang Huo*), Radix Scutellariae Baicalensis (*Huang Qin*), Fructus Gardeniae Jasminoidis (*Shan Zhi Zi*), Radix Glycyrrhizae (*Gan Cao*), Radix Ligustici Wallichii (*Chuan Xiong*), Herba Equiseti

Hiemalis (*Mu Zei*), Herba Schizonepetae Tenui-foliae (*Jing Jie*)

46. *Che Qian San* (Plantago Powder): Semen Plantaginis (*Che Qian Zi*), Flos Buddleiae Officinalis (*Mi Meng Hua*), Radix Et Rhizoma Notopterygii (*Qiang Huo*), Fructus Tribuli Terrestris (*Bai Ji Li*), Radix Scutellariae Baicalensis (*Huang Qin*), Flos Chrysanthemi Morifolii (*Ju Hua*), Radix Gentianae Scabrae (*Long Dan Cao*), Radix Glycyrrhizae (*Gan Cao*), Semen Cassiae Torae (*Jue Ming Zi*)

47. *Cheng Shi Juan Bi Tang* (Master Cheng's Alleviate *Bi* Decoction): Radix Et Rhizoma Notopterygii (*Qiang Huo*), Radix Angelicae Pubescentis (*Du Huo*), Cortex Cinnamomi (*Rou Gui*), Radix Gentianae Macrophyllae (*Qin Jiao*), Radix Angelicae Sinensis (*Dang Gui*), Radix Ligustici Wallichii (*Chuan Xiong*), Radix Glycyrrhizae (*Gan Cao*), Caulis Piperis (*Hai Feng Teng*), Ramulus Mori Albi (*Sang Zhi*), Resina Olibani (*Ru Xiang*), Radix Saussureae Seu Vladimiriae (*Mu Xiang*)

48. *Chi Shi Zhi San* (Hallyositum Rubrum Powder): Hallyositum Rubrum (*Chi Shi Zhi*), Cacumen Biotae Orientalis (*Ce Bai Ye*), Os Sepiae Seu Sepiellae (*Hai Piao Xiao*)

49. *Chi Shi Zhi Yu Yu Liang Tang* (Hallyositum & Limonitum Decoction): Hallyositum Rubrum (*Chi Shi Zhi*), Limonitum (*Yu Yu Liang*)

49a. *Chu Wen Hua Du Tang* (Eliminate Warm [Disease] & Transform Toxins Decoction): Folium Mori Albi (*Sang Ye*), Radix Puerariae (*Ge Gen*), Flos Lonicerae Japonicae (*Jin Yin Hua*), Bulbus Fritillariae Cirrhosae (*Chuan Bei Mu*), uncooked Radix Rehmanniae (*Sheng Di Huang*), Caulis Akebiae Mutong (*Mu Tong*), Herba Menthae Haplocalycis (*Bo He*), Radix Glycyrrhizae (*Gan Cao*), Folium Lophatheri Gracilis (*Dan Zhu Ye*), Folium Eriobotryae Japonicae (*Pi Pa Ye*)

50. *Chuan Shan Jia San* (Squama Manitis Powder): Squama Manitis Pentadactylis (*Chuan Shan Jia*), Carapax Amydae Sinensis (*Bie Jia*), Radix Rubrus Paeoniae Lactiflorae (*Chi Shao Yao*), Radix Et Rhizoma Rhei (*Da Huang*), Lacca Sinica Exciccata (*Gan Qi*), Cortex Cinnamomi (*Rou Gui*), Radix Ligustici Wallichii (*Chuan Xiong*), Flos Daphnis Genkwae (*Yuan Hua*), Radix Angelicae Sinensis (*Dang Gui*), Secretio Moschi Moschiferi (*She Xiang*)

51. *Chuan Si Jun Zi Tang* (Dyspnea Four Gentlemen Decoction): Radix Panacis Ginseng (*Ren Shen*), Sclerotium Poriae Cocos (*Fu Ling*), Rhizoma Atractylodis Macrocephalae (*Bai Zhu*), mix-fried Radix Glycyrrhizae (*Zhi Gan Cao*), Radix Angelicae Sinensis (*Dang Gui*), Cortex Magnoliae Officinalis (*Hou Po*), Fructus Perillae Frutescentis (*Zi Su Zi*), Lignum Aquilariae Agallochae (*Chen Xiang*), Pericarpium Citri Reticulatae (*Chen Pi*), Radix Saussureae Seu Vladimiriae (*Mu Xiang*), Cortex Radicis Mori Albi (*Sang Bai Pi*), Fructus Amomi (*Sha Ren*)

52. *Chuan Xiong Cha Tiao San* (Ligusticum Wallichium & Tea Regulating Powder): Herba Cum Radice Asari (*Xi Xin*), Radix Ligustici Wallichii (*Chuan Xiong*), Radix Et Rhizoma Notopterygii (*Qiang Huo*), Radix Ledebouriellae Sesloidis (*Fang Feng*), Herba Schizonepetae Tenuifoliae (*Jing Jie*), Herba Menthae Haplocalycis (*Bo He*), Radix Angelicae Dahuricae (*Bai Zhi*), Radix Glycyrrhizae (*Gan Cao*)

53. *Ci Shi Liu Wei Wan* (Magnetite Six Flavors Pills): Magnetitum (*Ci Shi*), prepared Radix Rehmanniae (*Shu Di Huang*), Fructus Corni Officinalis (*Shan Zhu Yu*), Radix Dioscoreae Oppositae (*Shan Yao*), Rhizoma Alismatis (*Ze Xie*), Sclerotium Poriae Cocos (*Fu Ling*), Cortex Radicis Moutan (*Mu Dan Pi*)

54. *Ci Zhu Wan* (Magnetite & Cinnabar Pills): Magnetitum (*Ci Shi*), Cinnabar (*Zhu Sha*), Massa Medica Fermentata (*Shen Qu*)

55. *Cong Chi Jie Geng Tang* (Allium Fistulosum, Prepared Soybean & Platycodon Decoction): Bulbus Allii Fistulosi (*Cong Bai*), Semen

Praeparatum Sojae (*Dan Dou Chi*), Radix Platycodi Grandiflori (*Jie Geng*), Herba Menthae Haplocalycis (*Bo He*), Fructus Forsythiae Suspensae (*Lian Qiao*), Folium Lophatheri Gracilis (*Dan Zhu Ye*), Radix Glycyrrhizae (*Gan Cao*)

56. *Cong Chi Tang* (Allium Fistulosum & Prepared Soybeans Decoction [I]): Bulbus Allii Fistulosi (*Cong Bai*), Semen Praeparatum Sojae (*Dan Dou Chi*)

57. *Cong Chi Tang* (Allium Fistulosum & Prepared Soybeans Decoction [II]): Bulbus Allii Fistulosi (*Cong Bai*), Semen Praeparatum Sojae (*Dan Dou Chi*), Herba Ephedrae (*Ma Huang*), Radix Puerariae (*Ge Gen*)

58. *Cong Rong Run Chang Tang* (Cistanches Moisten the Intestines Decoction): Herba Cistanchis (*Rou Cong Rong*), Radix Angelicae Sinensis (*Dang Gui*), uncooked Radix Rehmanniae (*Sheng Di Huang*), Radix Albus Paeoniae Lactiflorae (*Bai Shao Yao*), Semen Cannabis Sativae (*Huo Ma Ren*)

59. *Da Bu Yin Wan* (Great Supplement Yin Pills): Prepared Radix Rehmanniae (*Shu Di Huang*), Rhizoma Anemarrhenae (*Zhi Mu*), Cortex Phellodendri (*Huang Bai*), Plastrum Testudinis (*Gui Ban*), Pig Spinal Marrow (*Zhu Ji Sui*)

60. *Da Chai Hu Tang* (Major Bupleurum Decoction): Radix Bupleuri (*Chai Hu*), Rhizoma Pinelliae Ternatae (*Ban Xia*), Radix Scutellariae Baicalensis (*Huang Qin*), Radix Et Rhizoma Rhei (*Da Huang*), Fructus Immaturus Citri Seu Ponciri (*Zhi Shi*), uncooked Rhizoma Zingiberis (*Sheng Jiang*), Radix Albus Paeoniae Lactiflorae (*Bai Shao Yao*), Fructus Zizyphi Jujubae (*Da Zao*)

61. *Da Cheng Qi Tang* (Major Support the Qi Decoction): Radix Et Rhizoma Rhei (*Da Huang*), Mirabilitum (*Mang Xiao*), Cortex Magnoliae Officinalis (*Hou Po*), Fructus Immaturus Citri Seu Ponciri (*Zhi Shi*)

62. *Da An Wan* (Great Quieting Pills): Massa Medica Fermentata (*Shen Qu*), Rhizoma Atractylodis Macrocephalae (*Bai Zhu*), Sclerotium Poriae Cocos (*Fu Ling*), Fructus Crataegi (*Shan Zha*), Semen Raphani Sativi (*Lai Fu Zi*), Pericarpium Citri Reticulatae (*Chen Pi*), Rhizoma Pinelliae Ternatae (*Ban Xia*), Fructus Forsythiae Suspensae (*Lian Qiao*)

62a. *Da Ding Feng Zhu* (Great Stabilize Wind Pearls): Concha Ostreae (*Mu Li*), Plastrum Testudinis (*Gui Ban*), Carapax Amydae Sinensis (*Bie Jia*), Fructus Schizandrae Chinensis (*Wu Wei Zi*), uncooked Radix Rehmanniae (*Sheng Di Huang*), Tuber Ophiopogonis Japonicae (*Mai Men Dong*), Radix Albus Paeoniae Lactiflorae (*Bai Shao Yao*), Semen Cannabis Sativae (*Huo Ma Ren*), Gelatinum Corii Asini (*E Jiao*), mix-fried Radix Glycyrrhizae (*Zhi Gan Cao*), Egg Yolk (*Ji Zi Huang*)

63. *Da Huang Fu Zi Tang* (Rhubarb & Aconite Decoction): Radix Lateralis Praeparatus Aconiti Carmichaeli (*Fu Zi*), Herba Cum Radice Asari (*Xi Xin*), Radix Et Rhizoma Rhei (*Da Huang*)

64. *Da Huang Mu Dan Pi Tang* (Rhubarb & Moutan Decoction): Radix Et Rhizoma Rhei (*Da Huang*), Cortex Radicis Moutan (*Mu Dan Pi*), Semen Pruni Persicae (*Tao Ren*), Mirabilitum (*Mang Xiao*), Semen Benincasae Hispidae (*Dong Gua Ren*)

65. *Da Huang Zhe Chong Wan* (Rhubarb & Eupolyphaga Pills): Radix Et Rhizoma Rhei (*Da Huang*), Eupolyphaga Seu Opisthoplatiae (*Zhe Chong*), Radix Scutellariae Baicalensis (*Huang Qin*), Semen Pruni Persicae (*Tao Ren*), Semen Pruni Armeniacae (*Xing Ren*), Radix Albus Paeoniae Lactiflorae (*Bai Shao Yao*), uncooked Radix Rehmanniae (*Sheng Di Huang*), Lacca Sinica Exciccata (*Gan Qi*), Tabanus (*Meng Chong*), Hirudo (*Shui Zhi*), Radix Glycyrrhizae (*Gan Cao*), Holotrichia Diomphala (*Qi Cao*)

66. *Da Jian Zhong Tang* (Major Fortify the Center Decoction): Pericarpium Zanthoxyli Bungeani (*Hua Jiao*), dry Rhizoma Zingiberis (*Gan Jiang*), Radix Panacis Ginseng (*Ren Shen*), Saccharum Granorum (*Yi Tang*)

67. *Da Tao Hua Tang* (Major Hallyositum Decoction): Hallyositum Rubrum (*Chi Shi Zhi*), Radix Panacis Ginseng (*Ren Shen*), Rhizoma Atractylodis Macrocephalae (*Bai Zhu*), dry Rhizoma Zingiberis (*Gan Jiang*), Radix Lateralis Praeparatus Aconiti Carmichaeli (*Fu Zi*), Radix Angelicae Sinensis (*Dang Gui*), Radix Albus Paeoniae Lactiflorae (*Bai Shao Yao*), Os Draconis (*Long Gu*), Concha Ostreae (*Mu Li*), mix-fried Glycyrrhizae (*Zhi Gan Cao*)

68. *Da Xian Xiong Tang* (Great Fell [*i.e.,* Drain] the Chest Decoction): Radix Et Rhizoma Rhei (*Da Huang*), Mirabilitum (*Mang Xiao*), Radix Euphorbiae Kansui (*Gan Sui*)

69. *Da Xian Xiong Wan* (Great Fell [*i.e.,* Drain] the Chest Pills): Radix Euphorbiae Kansui (*Gan Sui*), Semen Lepidii (*Ting Li Zi*), Radix Et Rhizoma Rhei (*Da Huang*), Semen Pruni Armeniacae (*Xing Ren*), Mirabilitum (*Mang Xiao*)

70. *Da Zao Wan* (Great Creation Pills): Placenta Hominis (*Zi He Che*), Plastrum Testudinis (*Gui Ban*), Cortex Phellodendri (*Huang Bai*), Cortex Eucommiae Ulmoidis (*Du Zhong*), Radix Achyranthis Bidentatae (*Huai Niu Xi*), Tuber Ophiopogonis Japonicae (*Mai Men Dong*), Tuber Asparagi Cochinensis (*Tian Men Dong*), uncooked Radix Rehmanniae (*Sheng Di Huang*), Radix Panacis Ginseng (*Ren Shen*)

71. *Dai Ge San* (Indigo & Clam Shell Powder): Pulvis Indigonis (*Qing Dai*), Concha Cyclinae (*Hai Ge Ke*)

72. *Dan Shen Yin* (Salvia Drink): Radix Salviae Miltiorrhizae (*Dan Shen*), Lignum Santali Albi (*Tan Xiang*), Fructus Amomi (*Sha Ren*)

73. *Dang Gui Bu Xue Tang* (*Dang Gui* Supplement the Blood Decoction): Radix Angelicae Sinensis (*Dang Gui*), Radix Astragali Membranacei (*Huang Qi*)

74. *Dang Gui Jian Zhong Tang* (*Dang Gui* Fortify the Center Decoction): Saccharum Granorum (*Yi Tang*), Ramulus Cinnamomi (*Gui Zhi*), Radix Albus Paeoniae Lactiflorae (*Bai Shao Yao*), mix-fried Radix Glycyrrhizae (*Zhi Gan Cao*), uncooked Rhizoma Zingiberis (*Sheng Jiang*), Fructus Zizyphi Jujubae (*Da Zao*), Radix Angelicae Sinensis (*Dang Gui*)

75. *Dang Gui Liu Huang Tang* (*Dang Gui* Six Yellows Decoction): Radix Angelicae Sinensis (*Dang Gui*), uncooked Radix Rehmanniae (*Sheng Di Huang*), prepared Radix Rehmanniae (*Shu Di Huang*), Radix Astragali Membranacei (*Huang Qi*), Rhizoma Coptidis Chinensis (*Huang Lian*), Cortex Phellodendri (*Huang Bai*), Radix Scutellariae Baicalensis (*Huang Qin*)

76. *Dang Gui San* (*Dang Gui* Powder [I]): Radix Angelicae Sinensis (*Dang Gui*), Rhizoma Atractylodis Macrocephalae (*Bai Zhu*), Radix Scutellariae Baicalensis (*Huang Qin*), Radix Albus Paeoniae Lactiflorae (*Bai Shao Yao*), Radix Ligustici Wallichii (*Chuan Xiong*)

77. *Dang Gui San* (*Dang Gui* Powder [II]): Radix Angelicae Sinensis (*Dang Gui*), carbonized Folium Et Petiolus Trachycarpi (*Zong Lu Tan*), Os Draconis (*Long Gu*), Rhizoma Cyperi Rotundi (*Xiang Fu*)

78. *Dang Gui Sheng Jiang Yang Rou Tang* (*Dang Gui*, Fresh Ginger & Mutton Decoction): Radix Angelicae Sinensis (*Dang Gui*), uncooked Rhizoma Zingiberis (*Sheng Jiang*), Mutton (*Yang Rou*)

79. *Dang Gui Si Ni Tang* (*Dang Gui* Four Counterflows Decoction): Ramulus Cinnamomi (*Gui Zhi*), Radix Angelicae Sinensis (*Dang Gui*), Herba Cum Radice Asari (*Xi Xin*), Radix Albus

Paeoniae Lactiflorae (*Bai Shao Yao*), Caulis Akebiae Mutong (*Mu Tong*), Fructus Zizyphi Jujubae (*Da Zao*), uncooked Rhizoma Zingiberis (*Sheng Jiang*)

80. *Dao Qi Tang* (Abduct the Qi Decoction):
Fructus Foeniculi Vulgaris (*Xiao Hui Xiang*), Fructus Evodiae Rutecarpae (*Wu Zhu Yu*), Radix Saussureae Seu Vladimiriae (*Mu Xiang*), Fructus Meliae Toosendan (*Chuan Lian Zi*)

81. *Dao Tan Tang* (Abduct Phlegm Decoction):
Rhizoma Pinelliae Ternatae (*Ban Xia*), Exocarpium Citri Rubri (*Ju Hong*), Fructus Immaturus Citri Seu Ponciri (*Zhi Shi*), Sclerotium Poriae Cocos (*Fu Ling*), Rhizoma Arisaematis (*Tian Nan Xing*), mix-fried Radix Glycyrrhizae (*Zhi Gan Cao*), uncooked Rhizoma Zingiberis (*Sheng Jiang*)

82. *Di Dang Tang* (Resistance Decoction):
Radix Et Rhizoma Rhei (*Da Huang*), Hirudo (*Shui Zhi*), Tabanus (*Meng Chong*), Semen Pruni Persicae (*Tao Ren*)

83. *Di Huang Jiu* (Rehmannia Wine):
Succus Rehmanniae (*Di Huang Zhi*), Succus Leonuri Heterophylli (*Yi Mu Cao Zhi*), Rice Wine (*Huang Jiu*)

84. *Di Huang Yin* (Rehmannia Drink):
Succus Rehmanniae (*Di Huang Zhi*), Gelatinum Cornu Cervi (*Lu Jiao Jiao*), Infant's Urine (*Tong Bian*)

85. *Di Tan Tang* (Scour Phlegm Decoction):
Bile[-processed] Rhizoma Arisaematis (*Dan Nan Xing*), Rhizoma Acori Graminei (*Shi Chang Pu*), Fructus Immaturus Citri Seu Ponciri (*Zhi Shi*), Exocarpium Citri Rubri (*Ju Hong*), Rhizoma Pinelliae Ternatae (*Ban Xia*), Sclerotium Poriae Cocos (*Fu Ling*), Caulis In Taeniis Bambusae (*Zhu Ru*), Radix Panacis Ginseng (*Ren Shen*), Radix Glycyrrhizae (*Gan Cao*)

86. *Ding Ming San* (Determine Destiny Powder):
Agkistrodon Seu Bungarus (*Bai Hua She*), Zaocys Dhummades (*Wu Shao She*), Scolopendra Subspinipes (*Wu Gong*), Rhizoma Gastrodiae Elatae (*Tian Ma*), Rhizoma Arisaematis (*Tian Nan Xing*)

87. *Ding Xian Wan* (Stabilize Epilepsy Pills):
Rhizoma Gastrodiae Elatae (*Tian Ma*), Buthus Martensi (*Quan Xie*), Bombyx Batryticatus (*Jiang Can*), Succus Bambusae (*Zhu Li*), bile[-processed] Rhizoma Arisaematis (*Dan Nan Xing*), Medulla Junci Effusi (*Deng Xin Cao*), Rhizoma Acori Graminei (*Shi Chang Pu*), Succinum (*Hu Po*), Rhizoma Pinelliae Ternatae (*Ban Xia*), Sclerotium Poriae Cocos (*Fu Ling*), Tuber Ophiopogonis Japonicae (*Mai Men Dong*), Pericarpium Citri Reticulatae (*Chen Pi*), Bulbus Fritillariae Cirrhosae (*Chuan Bei Mu*), Radix Salviae Miltiorrhizae (*Dan Shen*), Sclerotium Pararadicis Poriae Cocos (*Fu Shen*), Cinnabar (*Zhu Sha*), Radix Polygalae Tenuifoliae (*Yuan Zhi*), Radix Glycyrrhizae (*Gan Cao*)

88. *Du Huo Ji Sheng Tang* (*Du Huo* & Loranthus Decoction):
Radix Angelicae Pubescentis (*Du Huo*), Ramus Loranthi Seu Visci (*Sang Ji Sheng*), Radix Gentianae Macrophyllae (*Qin Jiao*), Radix Ledebouriellae Sesloidis (*Fang Feng*), Herba Cum Radice Asari (*Xi Xin*), Radix Angelicae Sinensis (*Dang Gui*), Radix Albus Paeoniae Lactiflorae (*Bai Shao Yao*), Radix Ligustici Wallichii (*Chuan Xiong*), prepared Radix Rehmanniae (*Shu Di Huang*), Cortex Eucommiae Ulmoidis (*Du Zhong*), Radix Achyranthis Bidentatae (*Huai Niu Xi*), Radix Panacis Ginseng (*Ren Shen*), Sclerotium Poriae Cocos (*Fu Ling*), mix-fried Radix Glycyrrhizae (*Zhi Gan Cao*), Cortex Cinnamomi (*Rou Gui*)

89. *Du Qi Wan* (Capital Qi Pills):
Prepared Radix Rehmanniae (*Shu Di Huang*), Fructus Corni Officinalis (*Shan Zhu Yu*), Radix Dioscoreae Oppositae (*Shan Yao*), Rhizoma Alismatis (*Ze Xie*), Sclerotium Poriae Cocos (*Fu Ling*), Cortex Radicis Moutan (*Mu Dan Pi*), Fructus Schizandrae Chinensis (*Wu Wei Zi*)

90. *E Jiao Ji Zi Huang Tang* (Donkey Skin Glue

& Egg Yolk Decoction): Gelatinum Corii Asini (*E Jiao*), Egg Yolk (*Ji Zi Huang*), Radix Albus Paeoniae Lactiflorae (*Bai Shao Yao*), uncooked Radix Rehmanniae (*Sheng Di Huang*), Ramulus Uncariae Cum Uncis (*Gou Teng*), Caulis Trachelospermi (*Luo Shi Teng*), Concha Ostreae (*Mu Li*), Concha Haliotidis (*Shi Jue Ming*), Sclerotium Pararadicis Poriae Cocos (*Fu Shen*), mix-fried Radix Glycyrrhizae (*Zhi Gan Cao*)

91. *E Jiao Zhi Ke Wan* (Donkey Skin Glue & Citrus Pills): Gelatinum Corii Asini (*E Jiao*), Fructus Citri Seu Ponciri (*Zhi Ke*), Talcum (*Hua Shi*)

92. *E Leng Zhu Yu Tang* (Zedoaria & Sparganium Dispel Stasis Decoction): Rhizoma Curcumae Zedoariae (*E Zhu*), Rhizoma Sparganii (*Sang Leng*), Flos Carthami Tinctorii (*Hong Hua*), Radix Salviae Miltiorrhizae (*Dan Shen*), Carapax Amydae Sinensis (*Bie Jia*), Squama Manitis Pentadactylis (*Chuan Shan Jia*), Radix Codonopsis Pilosulae (*Dang Shen*), Radix Astragali Membranacei (*Huang Qi*), Radix Angelicae Sinensis (*Dang Gui*), Pericarpium Citri Reticulatae (*Chen Pi*)

93. *E Zhu San* (Zedoaria Powder): Rhizoma Curcumae Zedoariae (*E Zhu*), Radix Angelicae Sinensis (*Dang Gui*), Radix Albus Paeoniae Lactiflorae (*Bai Shao Yao*), Radix Ligustici Wallichii (*Chuan Xiong*), Radix Angelicae Dahuricae (*Bai Zhi*), prepared Radix Rehmanniae (*Shu Di Huang*)

94. *E Zhu Wan* (Zedoaria Pills): Rhizoma Curcumae Zedoariae (*E Zhu*), Flos Caryophylli (*Ding Xiang*), Pericarpium Viridis Citri Reticulatae (*Qing Pi*), Fructus Hordei Vulgaris (*Mai Ya*), Rhizoma Sparganii (*San Leng*), Semen Arecae Catechu (*Bing Lang*), Rhizoma Cyperi Rotundi (*Xiang Fu*), Semen Pharbitidis (*Qian Niu Zi*), Fructus Cubebae (*Bi Cheng Qie*)

95. *Er Chen Tang* (Two Aged [Ingredients] Decoction): Rhizoma Pinelliae Ternatae (*Ban Xia*), Pericarpium Citri Reticulatae (*Chen Pi*), Sclerotium Poriae Cocos (*Fu Ling*), mix-fried Radix Glycyrrhizae (*Zhi Gan Cao*), uncooked Rhizoma Zingiberis (*Sheng Jiang*), Fructus Pruni Mume (*Wu Mei*)

96. *Er Huang Wan* (Two Yellows Pills): Uncooked Radix Rehmanniae (*Sheng Di Huang*), prepared Radix Rehmanniae (*Shu Di Huang*)

97. *Er Jia Fu Mai Tang* (Two Carapaces Restore the Pulse Decoction): Mix-fried Radix Glycyrrhizae (*Zhi Gan Cao*), uncooked Radix Rehmanniae (*Sheng Di Huang*), Radix Albus Paeoniae Lactiflorae (*Bai Shao Yao*), Tuber Ophiopogonis Japonicae (*Mai Men Dong*), Gelatinum Corii Asini (*E Jiao*), Concha Ostreae (*Mu Li*), Carapax Amydae Sinensis (*Bie Jia*), Semen Cannabis Sativae (*Huo Ma Ren*)

98. *Er Long Zuo Ci Wan* (Deafness Left [Kidney] Good Pills): Prepared Radix Rehmanniae (*Shu Di Huang*), Radix Dioscoreae Oppositae (*Shan Yao*), Fructus Corni Officinalis (*Shan Zhu Yu*), Cortex Radicis Moutan (*Mu Dan Pi*), Rhizoma Alismatis (*Ze Xie*), Sclerotium Poriae Cocos (*Fu Ling*), Radix Bupleuri (*Chai Hu*), Magnetitum (*Ci Shi*)

99. *Er Mu San* (Two Mu Powder): Bulbus Fritillariae Cirrhosae (*Chuan Bei Mu*), Rhizoma Anemarrhenae (*Zhi Mu*)

100. *Er Xian Tang* (Two Immortals Decoction): Rhizoma Curculiginis Orchioidis (*Xian Mao*), Herba Epimedii (*Yin Yang Huo*), Radix Morindae Officinalis (*Ba Ji Tian*), Radix Angelicae Sinensis (*Dang Gui*), Rhizoma Anemarrhenae (*Zhi Mu*), Cortex Phellodendri (*Huang Bai*)

101. *Er Zhi Wan* (Two Ultimates Pills): Herba Ecliptae Prostratae (*Han Lian Cao*), Fructus Ligustri Lucidi (*Nu Zhen Zi*)

102. *Fa Sheng San* (Emit the Voice Powder): Pericarpium Trichosanthis Kirlowii (*Gua Lou Pi*),

Radix Glycyrrhizae (*Gan Cao*), Bombyx Batryticatus (*Jiang Can*)

103. *Fang Feng Chong He Tang* (Ledebouriella Harmonious Flow Decoction): Radix Ledebouriellae Sesloidis (*Fang Feng*), Radix Angelicae Dahuricae (*Bai Zhi*), Radix Ligustici Wallichii (*Chuan Xiong*), Rhizoma Atractylodis Macrocephalae (*Bai Zhu*), uncooked Radix Rehmanniae (*Sheng Di Huang*), Radix Et Rhizoma Notopterygii (*Qiang Huo*), Radix Scutellariae Baicalensis (*Huang Qin*), Radix Glycyrrhizae (*Gan Cao*)

103a. *Fang Feng Tang* (Ledebouriella Decoction): Radix Ledebouriellae Sesloidis (*Fang Feng*), Radix Angelicae Pubescentis (*Du Huo*), Radix Gentianae Macrophyllae (*Qin Jiao*), Ramulus Cinnamomi (*Gui Zhi*), Radix Albus Paeoniae Lactiflorae (*Bai Shao Yao*), Radix Angelicae Sinensis (*Dang Gui*), Semen Pruni Armeniacae (*Xing Ren*), Sclerotium Poriae Cocos (*Fu Ling*), Radix Scutellariae Baicalensis (*Huang Qin*), Radix Glycyrrhizae (*Gan Cao*), uncooked Rhizoma Zingiberis (*Sheng Jiang*)

104. *Fang Ji Huang Qi Tang* (Stephania & Astragalus Decoction): Radix Stephaniae Tetrandrae (*Fang Ji*), Radix Astragali Membranacei (*Huang Qi*), Rhizoma Atractylodis Macrocephalae (*Bai Zhu*), mix-fried Radix Glycyrrhizae (*Zhi Gan Cao*), uncooked Rhizoma Zingiberis (*Sheng Jiang*), Fructus Zizyphi Jujubae (*Da Zao*)

105. *Fen Qing Wan* (Separate the Clear Pills): Sclerotium Poriae Cocos (*Fu Ling*), Semen Euryalis Ferocis (*Qian Shi*)

106. *Fu Yuan Huo Xue Tang* (Restore the Source & Quicken the Blood Decoction): Radix Et Rhizoma Rhei (*Da Huang*), Flos Carthami Tinctorii (*Hong Hua*), Semen Pruni Persicae (*Tao Ren*), Radix Angelicae Sinensis (*Dang Gui*), Squama Manitis Pentadactylis (*Chuan Shan Jia*), Radix Bupleuri (*Chai Hu*), Radix Trichosanthis Kirlowii (*Tian Hua Fen*), Radix Glycyrrhizae (*Gan Cao*)

107. *Fu Zi Li Zhong Wan* (Aconite Rectify the Center Pills): Radix Lateralis Praeparatus Aconiti Carmichaeli (*Fu Zi*), dry Rhizoma Zingiberis (*Gan Jiang*), Radix Panacis Ginseng (*Ren Shen*), Rhizoma Atractylodis Macrocephalae (*Bai Zhu*), mix-fried Radix Glycyrrhizae (*Zhi Gan Cao*)

108. *Gan Cao Fu Zi Tang* (Licorice & Aconite Decoction): Mix-fried Radix Glycyrrhizae (*Zhi Gan Cao*), Radix Lateralis Praeparatus Aconiti Carmichaeli (*Fu Zi*), Rhizoma Atractylodis Macrocephalae (*Bai Zhu*), Ramulus Cinnamomi (*Gui Zhi*)

109. *Gan Cao Xie Xin Tang* (Licorice Drain the Heart Decoction): Mix-fried Radix Glycyrrhizae (*Zhi Gan Cao*), Rhizoma Pinelliae Ternatae (*Ban Xia*), dry Rhizoma Zingiberis (*Gan Jiang*), Rhizoma Coptidis Chinensis (*Huang Lian*), Radix Scutellariae Baicalensis (*Huang Qin*), Radix Panacis Ginseng (*Ren Shen*), Fructus Zizyphi Jujubae (*Da Zao*)

110. *Gan Mao Re Ke Fang* (Common Cold Hot Cough Formula): Radix Peucedani (*Qian Hu*), Fructus Arctii Lappae (*Niu Bang Zi*), Folium Mori Albi (*Sang Ye*), Radix Platycodi Grandiflori (*Jie Geng*), Herba Menthae Haplocalycis (*Bo He*), Herba Schizonepetae Tenuifoliae (*Jing Jie*), Flos Chrysanthemi Indici (*Ye Ju Hua*), Semen Pruni Armeniacae (*Xing Ren*), Radix Glycyrrhizae (*Gan Cao*)

111. *Gan Sui Tong Jie Tang* (Euphorbia Kansui Free the Bound Decoction): Radix Euphorbiae Kansui (*Gan Sui*), Radix Et Rhizoma Rhei (*Da Huang*), Cortex Magnoliae Officinalis (*Hou Po*), Radix Saussureae Seu Vladimiriae (*Mu Xiang*)

112. *Ge Gen Qin Lian Tang* (Pueraria, Scutellaria & Coptis Decoction): Radix Puerariae (*Ge Gen*), Rhizoma Coptidis Chinensis (*Huang Lian*), Radix Scutellariae Baicalensis (*Huang Qin*), Radix Glycyrrhizae (*Gan Cao*)

113. *Ge Gen Tang* (Pueraria Decoction):
Herba Ephedrae (*Ma Huang*), Radix Puerariae (*Ge Gen*), Ramulus Cinnamomi (*Gui Zhi*), Radix Albus Paeoniae Lactiflorae (*Bai Shao Yao*), uncooked Rhizoma Zingiberis (*Sheng Jiang*), mix-fried Radix Glycyrrhizae (*Zhi Gan Cao*), Fructus Zizyphi Jujubae (*Da Zao*)

114. *Ge Xia Zhu Yu Tang* (Below the Diaphragm Dispel Stasis Decoction): Semen Pruni Persicae (*Tao Ren*), Flos Carthami Tinctorii (*Hong Hua*), Feces Trogopterori Seu Pteromi (*Wu Ling Zhi*), Radix Angelicae Sinensis (*Dang Gui*), Radix Ligustici Wallichii (*Chuan Xiong*), Radix Rubrus Paeoniae Lactiflorae (*Chi Shao Yao*), Cortex Radicis Moutan (*Mu Dan Pi*), Rhizoma Corydalis Yanhusuo (*Yan Hu Suo*), Fructus Citri Seu Ponciri (*Zhi Ke*), Radix Linderae Strychnifoliae (*Wu Yao*), Rhizoma Cyperi Rotundi (*Xiang Fu*), Radix Glycyrrhizae (*Gan Cao*)

115. *Gou Ji Yin* (Cibotium Drink): Rhizoma Cibotii Barmetz (*Gou Ji*), Radix Cyathulae (*Chuan Niu Xi*), Caulis Piperis (*Hai Feng Teng*), Fructus Chaenomelis Lagenariae (*Mu Gua*), Ramulus Mori Albi (*Sang Zhi*), Cortex Eucommiae Ulmoidis (*Du Zhong*), Radix Gentianae Macrophyllae (*Qin Jiao*), Ramulus Cinnamomi (*Gui Zhi*), prepared Radix Rehmanniae (*Shu Di Huang*), Radix Angelicae Sinensis (*Dang Gui*), Os Tigridis (*Hu Gu*) [substitute Pig Bone]

116. *Gou Qi Wan* (Lycium Pills): Fructus Lycii Chinensis (*Gou Qi Zi*), Rhizoma Polygonati (*Huang Jing*)

117. *Gu Chong Tang* (Secure the *Chong* Decoction): Os Draconis (*Long Gu*), Concha Ostreae (*Mu Li*), carbonized Folium Et Petiolus Trachycarpi (*Zong Lu Tan*), Os Sepiae Seu Sepiellae (*Hai Piao Xiao*), Radix Albus Paeoniae Lactiflorae (*Bai Shao Yao*), Rhizoma Atractylodis Macrocephalae (*Bai Zhu*), Radix Astragali Membranacei (*Huang Qi*), Fructus Corni Officinalis (*Shan Zhu Yu*), Radix Rubiae Cordifoliae (*Qian Cao Gen*), Galla Rhi Chinensis (*Wu Bei Zi*)

118. *Gu Jing Wan* (Secure the Menses Pills): Radix Scutellariae Baicalensis (*Huang Qin*), Cortex Phellodendri (*Huang Bai*), Cortex Ailanthi Altissimi (*Chun Gen Pi*), Radix Albus Paeoniae Lactiflorae (*Bai Shao Yao*), Plastrum Testudinis (*Gui Ban*), Rhizoma Cyperi Rotundi (*Xiang Fu*)

119. *Gua Lou Jian* (Trichosanthes Decoction): Pericarpium Trichosanthis Kirlowii (*Gua Lou Pi*), Radix Glycyrrhizae (*Gan Cao*), Honey (*Feng Mi*)

120. *Gua Lou Xie Bai Ban Xia Tang* (Trichosanthes, Allium Macrostemi & Pinellia Decoction): Fructus Trichosanthis Kirlowii (*Gua Lou*), Bulbus Allii Macrostemi (*Xie Bai*), Rhizoma Pinelliae Ternatae (*Ban Xia*), White Alcohol (*Bai Jiu*)

121. *Gui Pi Tang* (Return the Spleen Decoction): Rhizoma Atractylodis Macrocephalae (*Bai Zhu*), Sclerotium Poriae Cocos (*Fu Ling*), Radix Astragali Membranacei (*Huang Qi*), Radix Panacis Ginseng (*Ren Shen*), mix-fried Radix Glycyrrhizae (*Zhi Gan Cao*), Radix Angelicae Sinensis (*Dang Gui*), Radix Saussureae Seu Vladimiriae (*Mu Xiang*), Radix Polygalae Tenuifoliae (*Yuan Zhi*), Arillus Euphoriae Longanae (*Long Yan Rou*), Semen Zizyphi Spinosae (*Suan Zao Ren*)

122. *Gui Shao Di Huang Wan* (Dang Gui, Peony & Rehmannia Pills): Radix Angelicae Sinensis (*Dang Gui*), Radix Albus Paeoniae Lactiflorae (*Bai Shao Yao*), prepared Radix Rehmanniae (*Shu Di Huang*), Fructus Corni Officinalis (*Shan Zhu Yu*), Radix Dioscoreae Oppositae (*Shan Yao*), Cortex Radicis Moutan (*Mu Dan Pi*), Rhizoma Alismatis (*Ze Xie*), Sclerotium Poriae Cocos (*Fu Ling*)

123. *Gui Zhi Fu Ling Wan* (Cinnamon Twig & Poria Pills): Ramulus Cinnamomi (*Gui Zhi*), Cortex Radicis Moutan (*Mu Dan Pi*), Semen Pruni Persicae (*Tao Ren*), Radix Albus Paeoniae Lactiflorae (*Bai Shao Yao*), Sclerotium Poriae Cocos (*Fu Ling*)

124. *Gui Zhi Fu Zi Tang* (Cinnamon Twig & Aconite Decoction): Ramulus Cinnamomi (*Gui Zhi*), Radix Lateralis Praeparatus Aconiti Carmichaeli (*Fu Zi*), Radix Albus Paeoniae Lactiflorae (*Bai Shao Yao*), uncooked Rhizoma Zingiberis (*Sheng Jiang*), Fructus Zizyphi Jujubae (*Da Zao*), mix-fried Radix Glycyrrhizae (*Zhi Gan Cao*)

125. *Gui Zhi Gan Cao Tang* (Cinnamon Twig & Licorice Decoction): Ramulus Cinnamomi (*Gui Zhi*), mix-fried Radix Glycyrrhizae (*Zhi Gan Cao*)

126. *Gui Zhi Jia Hou Po Xing Ren Tang* (Cinnamon Twig Plus Magnolia & Armeniaca Decoction): Ramulus Cinnamomi (*Gui Zhi*), Radix Albus Paeoniae Lactiflorae (*Bai Shao Yao*), uncooked Rhizoma Zingiberis (*Sheng Jiang*), Cortex Magnoliae Officinalis (*Hou Po*), Semen Pruni Armeniacae (*Xing Ren*), mix-fried Radix Glycyrrhizae (*Zhi Gan Cao*), Fructus Zizyphi Jujubae (*Da Zao*)

127. *Gui Zhi Jia Long Gu Mu Li Tang* (Cinnamon Twig Plus Dragon Bone & Oyster Shell Decoction): Ramulus Cinnamomi (*Gui Zhi*), Radix Albus Paeoniae Lactiflorae (*Bai Shao Yao*), Os Draconis (*Long Gu*), Concha Ostreae (*Mu Li*), uncooked Rhizoma Zingiberis (*Sheng Jiang*), Fructus Zizyphi Jujubae (*Da Zao*), mix-fried Radix Glycyrrhizae (*Zhi Gan Cao*)

128. *Gui Zhi Shao Yao Zhi Mu Tang* (Cinnamon Twig Peony & Anemarrhena Decoction): Ramulus Cinnamomi (*Gui Zhi*), Radix Albus Paeoniae Lactiflorae (*Bai Shao Yao*), Rhizoma Anemarrhenae (*Zhi Mu*), Herba Ephedrae (*Ma Huang*), Rhizoma Atractylodis Macrocephalae (*Bai Zhu*), Radix Lateralis Praeparatus Aconiti Carmichaeli (*Fu Zi*), Radix Ledebouriellae Sesloidis (*Fang Feng*), uncooked Rhizoma Zingiberis (*Sheng Jiang*), mix-fried Radix Glycyrrhizae (*Zhi Gan Cao*)

129. *Gui Zhi Tang* (Cinnamon Twig Decoction): Ramulus Cinnamomi (*Gui Zhi*), Radix Albus Paeoniae Lactiflorae (*Bai Shao Yao*), uncooked Rhizoma Zingiberis (*Sheng Jiang*), Fructus Zizyphi Jujubae (*Da Zao*), mix-fried Radix Glycyrrhizae (*Zhi Gan Cao*)

130. *Hai Ge Tang* (Concha Cyclinae Decoction): Concha Cyclinae (*Hai Ge Ke*), Caulis Akebiae Mutong (*Mu Tong*), Sclerotium Polypori Umbellati (*Zhu Ling*), Rhizoma Alismatis (*Ze Xie*), Talcum (*Hua Shi*), Semen Benincasae Hispidae (*Dong Gua Ren*), Cortex Radicis Mori Albi (*Sang Bai Pi*), Medulla Junci Effusi (*Deng Xin Cao*)

131. *Hai Ge Wan* (Concha Cyclinae Pills): Concha Cyclinae (*Hai Ge Ke*), Semen Trichosanthis Kirlowii (*Gua Lou Ren*)

132. *He Li Le Wan* (Terminalia Pills): Fructus Terminaliae Chebulae (*He Zi*), Semen Pruni Armeniacae (*Xing Ren*), Bulbus Fritillariae Thunbergii (*Zhe Bei Mu*), Semen Trichosanthis Kirlowii (*Gua Lou Ren*), Pulvis Indigonis (*Qing Dai*), Rhizoma Cyperi Rotundi (*Xiang Fu*)

133. *He Shou Wu Tang* (Polygonum Multiflorum Decoction): Radix Polygoni Multiflori (*He Shou Wu*), Flos Lonicerae Japonicae (*Jin Yin Hua*), Fructus Forsythiae Suspensae (*Lian Qiao*), Cortex Radicis Dictamni (*Bai Xian Pi*), Radix Sophorae Flavescentis (*Ku Shen*), Rhizoma Atractylodis (*Cang Zhu*), Herba Schizonepetae Tenuifoliae (*Jing Jie*), Radix Ledebouriellae Sesloidis (*Fang Feng*), Caulis Akebiae Mutong (*Mu Tong*), Radix Glycyrrhizae (*Gan Cao*)

134. *He Zi Pi San* (Terminalia Powder): Fructus Terminaliae Chebulae (*He Zi*), dry Rhizoma Zingiberis (*Gan Jiang*), Pericarpium Citri Reticulatae (*Chen Pi*), Pericarpium Papaveris Somniferi (*Ying Su Ke*)

135. *He Zi Qing Yin Tang* (Terminalia Clear the Voice Decoction): Fructus Terminaliae Chebulae (*He Zi*), Radix Platycodi Grandiflori (*Jie Geng*), Radix Glycyrrhizae (*Gan Cao*)

136. *He Zi San* (Terminalia Powder): Fructus Terminaliae Chebulae (*He Zi*), Rhizoma Coptidis Chinensis (*Huang Lian*), Radix Saussureae Seu Vladimiriae (*Mu Xiang*), Radix Glycyrrhizae (*Gan Cao*)

137. *Hou Po Ma Huang Tang* (Magnolia & Ephedra Decoction): Herba Ephedrae (*Ma Huang*), Cortex Magnoliae Officinalis (*Hou Po*), Herba Cum Radice Asari (*Xi Xin*), dry Rhizoma Zingiberis (*Gan Jiang*), Semen Pruni Armeniacae (*Xing Ren*), Rhizoma Pinelliae Ternatae (*Ban Xia*), Gypsum Fibrosum (*Shi Gao*), Fructus Levis Tritici Aestivi (*Fu Xiao Mai*), Fructus Schizandrae Chinensis (*Wu Wei Zi*)

138. *Hou Po San Wu Tang* (Magnolia Three Materials Decoction): Cortex Magnoliae Officinalis (*Hou Po*), Fructus Citri Seu Ponciri (*Zhi Ke*), Radix Et Rhizoma Rhei (*Da Huang*)

139. *Hou Po Sheng Jiang Ban Xia Gan Cao Ren Shen Tang* (Magnolia, Fresh Ginger, Pinellia, Licorice & Ginseng Decoction): Cortex Magnoliae Officinalis (*Hou Po*), uncooked Rhizoma Zingiberis (*Sheng Jiang*), Rhizoma Pinelliae Ternatae (*Ban Xia*), mix-fried Radix Glycyrrhizae (*Zhi Gan Cao*), Radix Panacis Ginseng (*Ren Shen*)

140. *Hou Po Wen Zhong Tang* (Magnolia Warm the Center Decoction): Cortex Magnoliae Officinalis (*Hou Po*), Pericarpium Citri Reticulatae (*Chen Pi*), mix-fried Radix Glycyrrhizae (*Zhi Gan Cao*), Sclerotium Poriae Cocos (*Fu Ling*), Semen Alpiniae Katsumadai (*Cao Dou Kou*), Radix Saussureae Seu Vladimiriae (*Mu Xiang*), dry Rhizoma Zingiberis (*Gan Jiang*), uncooked Rhizoma Zingiberis (*Sheng Jiang*)

141. *Hu Lu Ba San* (Fenugreek Powder): Semen Trigonellae Foeni-graeci (*Hu Lu Ba*), Rhizoma Sparganii (*San Leng*), dry Rhizoma Zingiberis (*Gan Jiang*), Fructus Evodiae Rutecarpae (*Wu Zhu Yu*), Radix Et Rhizoma Ligustici Chinensis (*Gao Ben*)

142. *Hu Lu Ba Wan* (Fenugreek Pills [I]): Semen Trigonellae Foeni-graeci (*Hu Lu Ba*), Radix Lateralis Praeparatus Aconiti Carmichaeli (*Fu Zi*), Sulfur (*Liu Huang*)

143. *Hu Lu Ba Wan* (Fenugreek Pills [II]): Semen Trigonellae Foeni-graeci (*Hu Lu Ba*), Fructus Feoniculi Vulgaris (*Xiao Hui Xiang*), Radix Morindae Officinalis (*Ba Ji Tian*), Radix Aconiti Carmichaeli (*Chuan Wu Tou*), Fructus Meliae Toosendan (*Chuan Lian Zi*), Fructus Evodiae Rutecarpae (*Wu Zhu Yu*)

144. *Hu Qian Wan* (Hidden Tiger Pills): Radix Angelicae Sinensis (*Dang Gui*), Radix Achyranthis Bidentatae (*Huai Niu Xi*), Cortex Phellodendri (*Huang Bai*), Plastrum Testudinis (*Gui Ban*), Rhizoma Anemarrhenae (*Zhi Mu*), prepared Radix Rehmanniae (*Shu Di Huang*), Pericarpium Citri Reticulatae (*Chen Pi*), Herba Cynomorii Sangarici (*Suo Yang*), Os Tigridis (*Hu Gu*) [substitute Pig Bone], dry Rhizoma Zingiberis (*Gan Jiang*), Mutton (*Yang Rou*)

145. *Hu Wei Cheng Qi Tang* (Protect the Stomach & Support the Qi Decoction): Rhizoma Anemarrhenae (*Zhi Mu*), Radix Et Rhizoma Rhei (*Da Huang*), Radix Scrophulariae Ningpoensis (*Xuan Shen*), Tuber Ophiopogonis Japonicae (*Mai Men Dong*), uncooked Radix Rehmanniae (*Sheng Di Huang*), Cortex Radicis Moutan (*Mu Dan Pi*)

146. *Hua Ban Tang* (Transform Macules Decoction): Gypsum Fibrosum (*Shi Gao*), Cornu Rhinocerotis (*Xi Jiao*) [substitute Cornu Bubali (*Shui Niu Jiao*)], uncooked Radix Rehmanniae (*Sheng Di Huang*), Rhizoma Anemarrhenae (*Zhi Mu*), Radix Scrophulariae Ningpoensis (*Xuan*

Shen), mix-fried Radix Glycyrrhizae (*Zhi Gan Cao*), Semen Oryzae Sativae (*Geng Mi*)

147. *Hua Chong Wan* (Transform Parasites Pills): Semen Arecae Catechu (*Bing Lang*), Omphalia (*Lei Wan*), Cortex Radicis Meliae Azerdach (*Ku Lian Pi*), Fructus Quisqualis Indicae (*Shi Jun Zi*), Alumen (*Bai Fan*), Pasta Ulmi (*Wu Yi*)

148. *Hua Jian Wan* (Transform the Hard Pills): Concha Ostreae (*Mu Li*), Concha Cyclinae (*Hai Ge Ke*), Herba Sargassii (*Hai Zao*), Thallus Algae (*Kun Bu*), Bulbus Fritillariae Thunbergii (*Zhe Bei Mu*), Spica Prunellae Vulgaris (*Xia Ku Cao*), Radix Angelicae Sinensis (*Dang Gui*), Radix Ligustici Wallichii (*Chuan Xiong*), Ramulus Cinnamomi (*Gui Zhi*), Herba Cum Radice Asari (*Xi Xin*), Radix Angelicae Dahuricae (*Bai Zhi*), Herba Agastachis Seu Pogostemi (*Huo Xiang*), Tuber Cremastrae Seu Plieonis (*Shang Ci Gu*)

149. *Huai Hua San* (Flos Sophorae Powder): Flos Immaturus Sophorae Japonicae (*Huai Hua*), Cacumen Biotae Orientalis (*Ce Bai Ye*), Herba Schizonepetae Tenuifoliae (*Jing Jie*), Radix Platycodi Grandiflori (*Jie Geng*)

150. *Huai Jiao Wan* (Fructus Sophorae Pills): Fructus Sophorae Japonicae (*Huai Jiao*), Radix Sanguisorbae (*Di Yu*), Radix Angelicae Sinensis (*Dang Gui*), Radix Ledebouriellae Sesloidis (*Fang Feng*), Radix Scutellariae Baicalensis (*Huang Qin*), Fructus Citri Seu Ponciri (*Zhi Ke*)

151. *Huang Lian E Jiao Tang* (Coptis & Donkey Skin Glue Decoction): Rhizoma Coptidis Chinensis (*Huang Lian*), Gelatinum Corii Asini (*E Jiao*), Radix Albus Paeoniae Lactiflorae (*Bai Shao Yao*), Radix Scutellariae Baicalensis (*Huang Qin*), Egg Yolk (*Ji Zi Huang*)

152. *Huang Lian Jie Du Tang* (Coptis Resolve Toxins Decoction): Radix Scutellariae Baicalensis (*Huang Qin*), Rhizoma Coptidis Chinensis (*Huang Lian*), Cortex Phellodendri (*Huang Bai*), Fructus Gardeniae Jasminoidis (*Shan Zhi Zi*)

153. *Huang Lian Xiang Ru Yin* (Coptis & Elsholtzia Drink): Rhizoma Coptidis Chinensis (*Huang Lian*), Herba Elsholtziae (*Xiang Ru*), Cortex Magnoliae Officinalis (*Hou Po*), Semen Dolichoris Lablab (*Bai Bian Dou*)

154. *Huang Lian Zhu Ru Ju Pi Ban Xia Tang* (Coptis, Caulis In Taeniis Bambusae, Orange Peel & Pinellia Decoction): Rhizoma Coptidis Chinensis (*Huang Lian*), Caulis In Taeniis Bambusae (*Zhu Ru*), Pericarpium Citri Reticulatae (*Chen Pi*), Rhizoma Pinelliae Ternatae (*Ban Xia*)

155. *Huang Long Tang* (Yellow Dragon Decoction): Radix Et Rhizoma Rhei (*Da Huang*), Mirabilitum (*Mang Xiao*), Radix Angelicae Sinensis (*Dang Gui*), Radix Panacis Ginseng (*Ren Shen*), Fructus Immaturus Citri Seu Ponciri (*Zhi Shi*), Cortex Magnoliae Officinalis (*Hou Po*), Radix Platycodi Grandiflori (*Jie Geng*), uncooked Rhizoma Zingiberis (*Sheng Jiang*), Fructus Zizyphi Jujubae (*Da Zao*), mix-fried Radix Glycyrrhizae (*Zhi Gan Cao*)

156. *Huang Qi Gui Zhi Wu Wu Tang* (Astragalus & Cinnamon Twig Five Materials Decoction): Radix Astragali Membranacei (*Huang Qi*), Ramulus Cinnamomi (*Gui Zhi*), Radix Albus Paeoniae Lactiflorae (*Bai Shao Yao*), uncooked Rhizoma Zingiberis (*Sheng Jiang*), Fructus Zizyphi Jujubae (*Da Zao*)

157. *Huang Qi Jian Zhong Tang* (Astragalus Fortify the Center Decoction): Radix Astragali Membranacei (*Huang Qi*), Saccharum Granorum (*Yi Tang*), Ramulus Cinnamomi (*Gui Zhi*), Radix Albus Paeoniae Lactiflorae (*Bai Shao Yao*), uncooked Rhizoma Zingiberis (*Sheng Jiang*), Fructus Zizyphi Jujubae (*Da Zao*), mix-fried Radix Glycyrrhizae (*Zhi Gan Cao*)

158. *Huang Qi Tang* (Astragalus Decoction): Radix Astragali Membranacei (*Huang Qi*), Semen Cannabis Sativae (*Huo Ma Ren*), Honey (*Feng Mi*), Pericarpium Citri Reticulatae (*Chen Pi*)

159. *Huang Qin Hua Shi Tang* (Scutellaria & Talcum Decoction): Radix Scutellariae Baicalensis (*Huang Qin*), Talcum (*Hua Shi*), Medulla Tetrapanacis Papyriferi (*Tong Cao*), Fructus Cardamomi (*Bai Dou Kou*), Pericarpium Arecae Catechu (*Da Fu Pi*), Sclerotium Polypori Umbellati (*Zhu Ling*), Cortex Sclerotii Poriae Cocos (*Fu Ling Pi*)

160. *Huang Qin Tang* (Scutellaria Decoction): Radix Scutellariae Baicalensis (*Huang Qin*), Radix Albus Paeoniae Lactiflorae (*Bai Shao Yao*), Radix Glycyrrhizae (*Gan Cao*), Fructus Zizyphi Jujubae (*Da Zao*)

161. *Huang Qin Xie Fei Tang* (Scutellaria Drain the Lungs Decoction): Radix Scutellariae Baicalensis (*Huang Qin*), Radix Et Rhizoma Rhei (*Da Huang*), Fructus Forsythiae Suspensae (*Lian Qiao*), Fructus Gardeniae Jasminoidis (*Shan Zhi Zi*), Semen Pruni Armeniacae (*Xing Ren*), Fructus Immaturus Citri Seu Ponciri (*Zhi Shi*), Radix Platycodi Grandiflori (*Jie Geng*), Herba Menthae Haplocalycis (*Bo He*), Radix Glycyrrhizae (*Gan Cao*)

162. *Huo Luo Xiao Ling Dan* (Quicken the Network Vessels Fantastically Effective Elixir): Radix Salviae Miltiorrhizae (*Dan Shen*), Resina Olibani (*Ru Xiang*), Resina Myrrhae (*Mo Yao*), Radix Angelicae Sinensis (*Dang Gui*)

163. *Huo Xiang Ban Xia Tang* (Agastaches & Pinellia Decoction): Herba Agastachis Seu Pogostemi (*Huo Xiang*), Flos Caryophylli (*Ding Xiang*), Rhizoma Pinelliae Ternatae (*Ban Xia*), uncooked Rhizoma Zingiberis (*Sheng Jiang*)

164. *Ji Chi Tang* (Chicken Gizzard Membrane Decoction): Endothelium Corneum Gigeriae Galli (*Ji Nei Jin*), Rhizoma Atractylodis Macrocephalae (*Bai Zhu*), Radix Albus Paeoniae Lactiflorae (*Bai Shao Yao*), Radix Bupleuri (*Chai Hu*), Pericarpium Citri Reticulatae (*Chen Pi*), uncooked Rhizoma Zingiberis (*Sheng Jiang*)

165. *Ji Chuan Jian* (Benefit the River [Flow] Decoction): Herba Cistanchis (*Rou Cong Rong*), Radix Achyranthis Bidentatae (*Huai Niu Xi*), Radix Angelicae Sinensis (*Dang Gui*), Rhizoma Cimicifugae (*Sheng Ma*), Fructus Citri Seu Ponciri (*Zhi Ke*), Rhizoma Alismatis (*Ze Xie*)

166. *Ji Jiao Li Huang Wan* (Stephania, Zanthoxylum, Lepidium & Rhubarb Pills): Radix Stephaniae Tetrandrae (*Fang Ji*), Semen Zanthoxyli Bungeani (*Jiao Mu*), Semen Lepidii (*Ting Li Zi*), Radix Et Rhizoma Rhei (*Da Huang*)

167. *Ji Ming San* (Cock Crow Powder): Semen Arecae Catechu (*Bing Lang*), Fructus Chaenomelis Lagenariae (*Mu Gua*), Fructus Evodiae Rutecarpae (*Wu Zhu Yu*), Folium Perillae Frutescentis (*Zi Su Ye*), Pericarpium Citri Reticulatae (*Chen Pi*), Radix Platycodi Grandiflori (*Jie Geng*), uncooked Rhizoma Zingiberis (*Sheng Jiang*)

168. *Jia Jian Jing Fang Bai Du San* (Additions & Subtractions Schizonepeta & Ledebouriella Resolve Toxins Powder): Herba Schizonepetae Tenuifoliae (*Jing Jie*), Radix Ledebouriellae Sesloidis (*Fang Feng*), Fructus Arctii Lappae (*Niu Bang Zi*), Flos Lonicerae Japonicae (*Jin Yin Hua*), Fructus Forsythiae Suspensae (*Lian Qiao*), Herba Menthae Haplocalycis (*Bo He*), Herba Lophatheri Gracilis (*Dan Zhu Ye*), Radix Platycodi Grandiflori (*Jie Geng*), Semen Praeparatum Sojae (*Dan Dou Chi*), Fructificatio Lasiosphaerae (*Ma Bo*), Periostracum Cicadae (*Chan Tui*), Bombyx Batryticatus (*Jiang Can*), Rhizoma Belamcandae (*She Gan*)

169. *Jia Jian Lou Rui Tang* (Additions & Subtractions Polygonatum Decoction): Rhizoma Polygonati Odorati (*Yu Zhu*), Bulbus Allii Fistulosi (*Cong Bai*), Radix Platycodi Grandiflori (*Jie Geng*), Radix Cynanchi Atrati (*Bai Wei*), Herba Menthae Haplocalycis (*Bo He*), Semen Praeparatum Sojae (*Dan Dou Chi*), Radix Glycyrrhizae (*Gan Cao*), Fructus Zizyphi Jujubae (*Da Zao*)

170. *Jia Wei Qing Wei San* (Added Flavors Clear the Stomach Powder): Cortex Radicis Moutan (*Mu Dan Pi*), uncooked Radix Rehmanniae (*Sheng Di*), Radix Angelicae Sinensis (*Dang Gui*), Rhizoma Coptidis Chinensis (*Huang Lian*), Rhizoma Cimicifugae (*Sheng Ma*), Radix Achyranthis Bidentatae (*Huai Niu Xi*), Radix Glycyrrhizae (*Gan Cao*)

171. *Jian Pi Wan* (Fortify the Spleen Pills): Rhizoma Atractylodis Macrocephalae (*Bai Zhu*), Sclerotium Poriae Cocos (*Fu Ling*), Radix Panacis Ginseng (*Ren Shen*), Radix Dioscoreae Oppositae (*Shan Yao*), mix-fried Radix Glycyrrhizae (*Zhi Gan Cao*), Fructus Germinatus Hordei Vulgaris (*Mai Ya*), Massa Medica Fermentata (*Shen Qu*), Fructus Crataegi (*Shan Zha*), Pericarpium Citri Reticulatae (*Chen Pi*), Semen Myristicae Fragrantis (*Rou Dou Kou*), Fructus Amomi (*Sha Ren*), Radix Saussureae Seu Vladimiriae (*Mu Xiang*), Rhizoma Coptidis Chinensis (*Huang Lian*)

172. *Jiang Gui Wan* (Ginger & Cinnamon Pills): Uncooked Rhizoma Zingiberis (*Sheng Jiang*), Cortex Cinnamomi (*Rou Gui*), Rhizoma Arisaematis (*Tian Nan Xing*)

173. *Jiao Ai Tang* (Donkey Skin Glue & Artemisia Argyium Decoction): Folium Artemisiae Argyii (*Ai Ye*), Gelatinum Corii Asini (*E Jiao*), mix-fried Radix Glycyrrhizae (*Zhi Gan Cao*), Radix Ligustici Wallichii (*Chuan Xiong*), Radix Angelicae Sinensis (*Dang Gui*), Radix Albus Paeoniae Lactiflorae (*Bai Shao Yao*), uncooked Radix Rehmanniae (*Sheng Di Huang*)

174. *Jiao Tai Wan* (Supreme Communication Pills): Rhizoma Coptidis Chinensis (*Huang Lian*), Cortex Cinnamomi (*Rou Gui*)

175. *Jiao Zhu Wan* (Zanthoxylum & Atractylodes Pills): Rhizoma Atractylodis (*Cang Zhu*), Pericarpium Zanthoxyli Bungeani (*Hua Jiao*)

176. *Jie Geng Tang* (Platycodon Decoction): Radix Glycyrrhizae (*Gan Cao*), Radix Platycodi Grandiflori (*Jie Geng*)

177. *Jie Gu San* (Knit Bone Powder): Resina Olibani (*Ru Xiang*), Resina Myrrhae (*Mo Yao*), Pyritum (*Zi Ran Tong*), Eupolyphaga Seu Opisthoplatiae (*Zhe Chong*), Sanguis Draconis (*Xue Jie*), Radix Dipsaci (*Xu Duan*), Radix Angelicae Sinensis (*Dang Gui*), Rhizoma Drynariae (*Gu Sui Bu*), Flos Carthami Tinctorii (*Hong Hua*), Radix Saussureae Seu Vladimiriae (*Mu Xiang*)

178. *Jie Nue Qi Bao Yin* (Resolve *Nue* Seven Treasures Drink): Radix Dichroae Febrifugae (*Chang Shan*), Semen Arecae Catechu (*Bing Lang*), Cortex Magnoliae Officinalis (*Hou Po*), Pericarpium Viridis Citri Reticulatae (*Qing Pi*), Pericarpium Citri Reticulatae (*Chen Pi*), mix-fried Radix Glycyrrhizae (*Zhi Gan Cao*), Fructus Amomi Tsao-ko (*Cao Guo*)

179. *Jin Fei Cao San* (Inula Powder): Flos Inulae (*Xuan Fu Hua*), Herba Ephedrae (*Ma Huang*), Herba Schizonepetae Tenuifoliae (*Jing Jie*), Rhizoma Pinelliae Ternatae (*Ban Xia*), Radix Rubrus Paeoniae Lactiflorae (*Chi Shao Yao*), Radix Peucedani (*Qian Hu*), Radix Glycyrrhizae (*Gan Cao*)

180. *Jin Jian Yi Yi Ren Tang* (Golden Mirror Coix Decoction): Semen Coicis Lachryma-jobi (*Yi Yi Ren*), Cortex Radicis Moutan (*Mu Dan Pi*), Semen Pruni Persicae (*Tao Ren*), Radix Rubrus Paeoniae Lactiflorae (*Chi Shao Yao*), Pericarpium Trichosanthis Kirlowii (*Gua Lou Pi*)

181. *Jin Ling Zi San* (Melia Powder): Rhizoma Corydalis Yanhusuo (*Yan Hu Suo*), Fructus Meliae Toosendan (*Chuan Lian Zi*)

182. *Jin Suo Gu Jing Wan* (Golden Lock Secure the Essence Pills): Semen Astragali (*Sha Yuan Zi*), Semen Euryalis Ferocis (*Qian Shi*), Stamen Nelumbinis Nuciferae (*Lian Xu*), Os Draconis (*Long Gu*), Concha Ostreae (*Mu Li*), Semen Nelumbinis Nuciferae (*Lian Zi*)

183. *Jing Fang Bai Du San* **(Schizonepeta &
Ledebouriella Vanquish Toxins Powder):**
Herba Menthae Haplocalycis (*Bo He*), Herba
Schizonepetae Tenuifoliae (*Jing Jie*), Radix
Ledebouriellae Sesloidis (*Fang Feng*), Radix Et
Rhizoma Notopterygii (*Qiang Huo*), Radix
Angelicae Pubescentis (*Du Huo*), Sclerotium
Poriae Cocos (*Fu Ling*), Fructus Citri Seu Ponciri
(*Zhi Ke*), Radix Platycodi Grandiflori (*Jie Geng*),
Radix Bupleuri (*Chai Hu*), Radix Peucedani
(*Qian Hu*), Radix Glycyrrhizae (*Gan Cao*), un-
cooked Rhizoma Zingiberis (*Sheng Jiang*)

184. *Jing Jie Tang* **(Schizonepeta Decoction):**
Herba Schizonepetae Tenuifoliae (*Jing Jie*), Ra-
dix Platycodi Grandiflori (*Jie Geng*), Radix
Glycyrrhizae (*Gan Cao*)

185. *Jiu Wei Qiang Huo Tang* **(Nine Flavors
Notopterygium Decoction):** Radix Et Rhizoma
Notopterygii (*Qiang Huo*), Radix Scutellariae
Baicalensis (*Huang Qin*), Radix Ledebouriellae
Sesloidis (*Fang Feng*), Radix Angelicae Dahu-
ricae (*Bai Zhi*), Herba Cum Radice Asari (*Xi
Xin*), Rhizoma Atractylodis (*Cang Zhu*), Radix
Ligustici Wallichii (*Chuan Xiong*), uncooked
Radix Rehmanniae (*Sheng Di Huang*), Radix
Glycyrrhizae (*Gan Cao*)

186. *Jiu Xian San* **(Nine Immortals Powder):**
Radix Panacis Ginseng (*Ren Shen*), Flos Tussil-
aginis Farfarae (*Kuan Dong Hua*), Radix Platy-
codi Grandiflori (*Jie Geng*), Cortex Radicis Mori
Albi (*Sang Bai Pi*), Fructus Schizandrae Chinen-
sis (*Wu Wei Zi*), Gelatinum Corii Asini (*E Jiao*),
Bulbus Fritillariae Cirrhosae (*Chuan Bei Mu*),
Fructus Pruni Mume (*Wu Mei*), Pericarpium
Papaveris Somniferi (*Ying Su Ke*)

187. *Jiu Yi Dan* **(Nine [to] One Powder):** Gyp-
sum Fibrosum (*Shi Gao*), Upbearing Medicinal
(*Sheng Yao, i.e.,* a combination of Alumen [*Ming
Fan*], Mercury [*Shui Yin*], and Niter [*Xiao Shi*])

188. *Ju Hua Cha Tiao San* **(Chrysanthemum &
Tea Regulating Powder):** Flos Chrysanthemi
Morifolii (*Ju Hua*), Radix Ligustici Wallichii

(*Chuan Xiong*), Herba Schizonepetae Tenuifoliae
(*Jing Jie*), Herba Cum Radice Asari (*Xi Xin*),
Radix Glycyrrhizae (*Gan Cao*), Radix Lede-
bouriellae Sesloidis (*Fang Feng*), Radix Angel-
icae Dahuricae (*Bai Zhi*), Herba Menthae Haplo-
calycis (*Bo He*), Radix Et Rhizoma Notopterygii
(*Qiang Huo*), Bombyx Batryticatus (*Jiang Can*),
Periostracum Cicadae (*Chan Tui*)

189. *Ju Hua San* **(Chrysanthemum Powder):**
Flos Chrysanthemi Morifolii (*Ju Hua*), Fructus
Viticis (*Man Jing Zi*), Radix Et Rhizoma Noto-
pterygii (*Qiang Huo*), Radix Ledebouriellae Ses-
loidis (*Fang Feng*), Flos Inulae (*Xuan Fu Hua*),
Gypsum Fibrosum (*Shi Gao*), Fructus Citri Seu
Ponciri (*Zhi Ke*), Radix Glycyrrhizae (*Gan Cao*),
uncooked Rhizoma Zingiberis (*Sheng Jiang*)

190. *Ju Pi Tang* **(Orange Peel Decoction):**
Pericarpium Citri Reticulatae (*Chen Pi*), uncooked Rhizoma Zingiberis (*Sheng Jiang*)

191. *Ju Pi Zhu Ru Tang* **(Orange Peel & Caulis
Bambusae Decoction):** Pericarpium Citri Reticulatae (*Chen Pi*), Radix Panacis Ginseng (*Ren
Shen*), Caulis In Taeniis Bambusae (*Zhu Ru*),
uncooked Rhizoma Zingiberis (*Sheng Jiang*),
mix-fried Radix Glycyrrhizae (*Zhi Gan Cao*),
Fructus Zizyphi Jujubae (*Da Zao*)

192. *Juan Bi Tang* **(Alleviate** *Bi* **Decoction):**
Radix Ledebouriellae Sesloidis (*Fang Feng*),
Rhizoma Curcumae (*Jiang Huang*), Radix Angel-
icae Sinensis (*Dang Gui*), Radix Astragali Mem-
branacei (*Huang Qi*), Radix Et Rhizoma Noto-
pterygii (*Qiang Huo*), Radix Rubrus Paeoniae
Lactiflorae (*Chi Shao Yao*), Radix Glycyrrhizae
(*Gan Cao*)

193. *Jue Ming Zi San* **(Cassia Seed Powder):**
Semen Cassiae Torae (*Jue Ming Zi*), Flos Chry-
santhemi Morifolii (*Ju Hua*), Herba Equiseti Hie-
malis (*Mu Zei*), Radix Scutellariae Baicalensis
(*Huang Qin*), Gypsum Fibrosum (*Shi Gao*), Ra-
dix Rubrus Paeoniae Lactiflorae (*Chi Shao Yao*),
Radix Ligustici Wallichii (*Chuan Xiong*), Radix
Et Rhizoma Notopterygii (*Qiang Huo*), Fructus

Viticis (*Man Jing Zi*), Concha Haliotidis (*Shi Jue Ming*), Radix Glycyrrhizae (*Gan Cao*)

194. *Ke Xue Fang* (Coughing Blood Formula): Pumice (*Hai Fu Shi*), Pulvis Indigonis (*Qing Dai*), Semen Trichosanthis Kirlowii (*Gua Lou Ren*), Fructus Gardeniae Jasminoidis (*Shan Zhi Zi*), Fructus Terminaliae Chebulae (*He Zi*)

195. *Kong Xian Dan* (Control Drool Elixir): Radix Euphorbiae Kansui (*Gan Sui*), Radix Euphorbiae Pekinensis (*Jing Da Ji*), Semen Sinapis Albae (*Bai Jie Zi*)

195a. *Kuan Dong Hua Tang* (Tussilago Decoction): Flos Tussilaginis Farfare (*Kuan Dong Hua*), Bulbus Fritillariae Thunbergii (*Zhe Bei Mu*), Cortex Radicis Mori (*Sang Bai Pi*), Rhizoma Anemarrhenae (*Zhi Mu*), Semen Pruni Armeniacae (*Xing Ren*), Radix Glycyrrhizae (*Gan Cao*), Fructus Schizandrae Chinensis (*Wu Wei Zi*)

196. *Li Zhong Wan* (Rectify the Center Pills): Radix Panacis Ginseng (*Ren Shen*), Rhizoma Atractylodis Macrocephalae (*Bai Zhu*), dry Rhizoma Zingiberis (*Gan Jiang*), mix-fried Radix Glycyrrhizae (*Zhi Gan Cao*)

197. *Liang Fu Wan* (Alpinia Officinarus & Cyperus Pills): Rhizoma Cyperi Rotundi (*Xiang Fu*), Rhizoma Alpiniae Officinari (*Gao Liang Jiang*)

198. *Liang Xue Tang* (Cool the Blood Decoction): Fructus Gardeniae Jasminoidis (*Shan Zhi Zi*), Rhizoma Anemarrhenae (*Zhi Mu*), Rhizoma Imperatae Cylindricae (*Bai Mao Gen*), Cacumen Biotae Orientalis (*Ce Bai Ye*), Rhizoma Bletillae Striatae (*Bai Ji*), Nodus Nelumbinis Nuciferae (*Ou Jie*)

199. *Liang Yi Tang* (Two Principles Decoction): Prepared Radix Rehmanniae (*Shu Di*), Radix Codonopsis Pilosulae (*Dang Shen*)

200. *Ling Gan Wu Wei Jiang Xin Tang* (Poria, Licorice, Schizandra, Ginger & Asarum Decoction): Sclerotium Poriae Cocos (*Fu Ling*), mix-fried Radix Glycyrrhizae (*Zhi Gan Cao*), Fructus Schizandrae Chinensis (*Wu Wei Zi*), dry Rhizoma Zingiberis (*Gan Jiang*), Herba Cum Radice Asari (*Xi Xin*)

201. *Ling Gui Zhu Gan Tang* (Poria, Cinnamon, Atractylodes & Licorice Decoction): Ramulus Cinnamomi (*Gui Zhi*), Sclerotium Poriae Cocos (*Fu Ling*), Rhizoma Atractylodis Macrocephalae (*Bai Zhu*), mix-fried Radix Glycyrrhizae (*Zhi Gan Cao*)

202. *Liu An Jian* (Six Quiets Decoction): Rhizoma Pinelliae Ternatae (*Ban Xia*), Pericarpium Citri Reticulatae (*Chen Pi*), Sclerotium Poriae Cocos (*Fu Ling*), Semen Pruni Armeniacae (*Xing Ren*), Semen Sinapis Albae (*Bai Jie Zi*), mix-fried Radix Glycyrrhizae (*Zhi Gan Cao*), uncooked Rhizoma Zingiberis (*Sheng Jiang*)

203. *Liu Jun Zi Tang* (Six Gentlemen Decoction): Radix Panacis Ginseng (*Ren Shen*), Sclerotium Poriae Cocos (*Fu Ling*), Rhizoma Atractylodis Macrocephalae (*Bai Zhu*), mix-fried Radix Glycyrrhizae (*Zhi Gan Cao*), Pericarpium Citri Reticulatae (*Chen Pi*), Rhizoma Pinelliae Ternatae (*Ban Xia*)

204. *Liu Wei Di Huang Wan* (Six Flavors Rehmannia Pills): Prepared Radix Rehmanniae (*Shu Di Huang*), Fructus Corni Officinalis (*Shan Zhu Yu*), Radix Dioscoreae Oppositae (*Shan Yao*), Sclerotium Poriae Cocos (*Fu Ling*), Rhizoma Alismatis (*Ze Xie*), Cortex Radicis Moutan (*Mu Dan Pi*)

205. *Long Chi San* (Dragon Tooth Powder): Dens Draconis (*Long Chi*), Ramulus Uncariae Cum Uncis (*Gou Teng*), Periostracum Cicadae (*Chan Tui*), Sclerotium Poriae Cocos (*Fu Ling*), Radix Glycyrrhizae (*Gan Cao*), Frustra Ferri (*Tie Luo*), Cinnabar (*Zhu Sha*), Radix Et Rhizoma Rhei (*Da Huang*), Minium (*Huang Dan*)

206. Long Chi Wan (Dragon Tooth Pills): Dens Draconis (*Long Chi*), Sclerotium Pararadicis Poriae Cocos (*Fu Shen*), Frustra Ferri (*Tie Luo*), Calcitum (*Han Shui Shi*)

207. Long Gu San (Dragon Bone Powder): Os Draconis (*Long Gu*), Fructus Terminaliae Chebulae (*He Zi*), Hallyositum Rubrum (*Chi Shi Zhi*), Pericarpium Papaveris Somniferi (*Ying Su Ke*), Quercus Infectoria (*Mo Shi Zi*)

208. Lu Jiao Jiao Fang (Deer Antler Glue Formula): Gelatinum Cornu Cervi (*Lu Jiao Jiao*), Succus Rehmanniae (*Di Huang Zhi*)

209. Lu Jiao Jiao San (Deer Antler Glue Powder): Gelatinum Cornu Cervi (*Lu Jiao Jiao*), Fructus Rubi (*Fu Pen Zi*), Semen Plantaginis (*Che Qian Zi*)

210. Lu Jiao Jiao Wan (Deer Antler Glue Pills): Gelatinum Cornu Cervi (*Lu Jiao Jiao*), prepared Radix Rehmanniae (*Shu Di Huang*), Crinis Carbonisatus (*Xue Yu Tan*)

211. Lu Jiao Wan (Deer Antler Pills): Cornu Cervi (*Lu Jiao*), Radix Achyranthis Bidentatae (*Huai Niu Xi*)

212. Ma Dou Ling Tang (Aristolochia Decoction): Fructus Aristolochiae (*Ma Dou Ling*), Semen Lepidii (*Ting Li Zi*), Rhizoma Pinelliae Ternatae (*Ban Xia*), Cortex Radicis Mori Albi (*Sang Bai Pi*), Radix Glycyrrhizae (*Gan Cao*), uncooked Rhizoma Zingiberis (*Sheng Jiang*)

213. Ma Huang Fu Zi Xi Xin Tang (Ephedra, Aconite & Asarum Decoction): Herba Ephedrae (*Ma Huang*), Radix Lateralis Praeparatus Aconiti Carmichaeli (*Fu Zi*), Herba Cum Radice Asari (*Xi Xin*)

214. Ma Huang Lian Qiao Chi Xiao Dou Tang (Ephedra, Forsythia & Aduki Bean Decoction): Herba Ephedrae (*Ma Huang*), Fructus Forsythiae Suspensae (*Lian Qiao*), Semen Pruni Armeniacae (*Xing Ren*), Semen Phaseoli Calcarati (*Chi Xiao Dou*), Fructus Zizyphi Jujubae (*Da Zao*), uncooked Rhizoma Zingiberis (*Sheng Jiang*), Radix Glycyrrhizae (*Gan Cao*), Cortex Caltalpae Ovatae (*Zi Bai Pi*)

215. Ma Huang Tang (Ephedra Decoction): Herba Ephedrae (*Ma Huang*), Ramulus Cinnamomi (*Gui Zhi*), Semen Pruni Armeniacae (*Xing Ren*), mix-fried Radix Glycyrrhizae (*Zhi Gan Cao*)

216. Ma Xing Shi Gan Tang (Ephedra, Armeniaca, Gypsum & Licorice Decoction): Herba Ephedrae (*Ma Huang*), Semen Pruni Armeniacae (*Xing Ren*), Gypsum Fibrosum (*Shi Gao*), Radix Glycyrrhizae (*Gan Cao*)

217. Ma Xing Yi Gan Tang (Ephedra, Armeniaca, Coix & Licorice Decoction): Herba Ephedrae (*Ma Huang*), Semen Pruni Armeniacae (*Xing Ren*), Semen Coicis Lachryma-jobi (*Yi Yi Ren*), mix-fried Radix Glycyrrhizae (*Zhi Gan Cao*)

218. Ma Zi Ren Wan (Cannabis Seed Pills): Semen Cannabis Sativae (*Huo Ma Ren*), Semen Pruni Armeniacae (*Xing Ren*), Fructus Immaturus Citri Seu Ponciri (*Zhi Shi*), Radix Et Rhizoma Rhei (*Da Huang*), Cortex Magnoliae Officinalis (*Hou Po*), Radix Albus Paeoniae Lactiflorae (*Bai Shao Yao*)

219. Mai Men Dong Tang (Ophiopogon Decoction): Tuber Ophiopogonis Japonicae (*Mai Men Dong*), Herba Artemisiae Apiaceae (*Qing Hao*), Radix Glycyrrhizae (*Gan Cao*), Radix Platycodi Grandiflori (*Jie Geng*)

220. Mi Yuan Jian (Secret Source Decoction): Radix Dioscoreae Oppositae (*Shan Yao*), Fructus Schizandrae Chinensis (*Wu Wei Zi*), Semen Euryalis Ferocis (*Qian Shi*), Fructus Rosae Laevigatae (*Jin Ying Zi*), Radix Panacis Ginseng (*Ren Shen*), Rhizoma Atractylodis Macrocephalae (*Bai Zhu*), Sclerotium Poriae Cocos (*Fu Ling*), Semen Zizyphi Spinosae (*Suan Zao Ren*), Radix Polygalae

Tenuifoliae (*Yuan Zhi*), mix-fried Radix Glycyrrhizae (*Zhi Gan Cao*)

221. *Mu Dan Pi San* (Moutan Powder): Cortex Radicis Moutan (*Mu Dan Pi*), Radix Rubrus Paeoniae Lactiflorae (*Chi Shao Yao*), uncooked Radix Rehmanniae (*Sheng Di Huang*), Radix Angelicae Sinensis (*Dang Gui*), Semen Pruni Persicae (*Tao Ren*), Radix Ligustici Wallichii (*Chuan Xiong*), Resina Olibani (*Ru Xiang*), Resina Myrrhae (*Mo Yao*), Rhizoma Drynariae (*Gu Sui Bu*), Radix Dipsaci (*Xu Duan*)

222. *Mu Gua San* (Chaenomeles Powder): Fructus Chaenomelis Lagenariae (*Mu Gua*), Pericarpium Papaveris Somniferi (*Ying Su Ke*), Semen Plantaginis (*Che Qian Zi*)

223. *Mu Gua Tang* (Chaenomeles Decoction): Fructus Chaenomelis Lagenariae (*Mu Gua*), Fructus Foeniculi Vulgaris (*Xiao Hui Xiang*), Fructus Evodiae Rutecarpae (*Wu Zhu Yu*), Caulis Perillae Frutescentis (*Zi Su Geng*), uncooked Rhizoma Zingiberis (*Sheng Jiang*), mix-fried Radix Glycyrrhizae (*Zhi Gan Cao*)

224. *Mu Li San* (Oyster Shell Powder): Radix Astragali Membranacei (*Huang Qi*), Semen Levis Tritici Aestivi (*Fu Xiao Mai*), Concha Ostreae (*Mu Li*), Radix Ephedrae (*Ma Huang Gen*)

225. *Mu Xiang Bing Lang Wan* (Saussurea & Areca Pills): Radix Saussureae Seu Vladimiriae (*Mu Xiang*), Semen Arecae Catechu (*Bing Lang*), Rhizoma Coptidis Chinensis (*Huang Lian*), Radix Et Rhizoma Rhei (*Da Huang*), Pericarpium Viridis Citri Reticulatae (*Qing Pi*), Rhizoma Curcumae Zedoariae (*E Zhu*), Semen Pharbitidis (*Qian Niu Zi*), Pericarpium Citri Reticulatae (*Chen Pi*), Rhizoma Cyperi Rotundi (*Xiang Fu*), Cortex Phellodendri (*Huang Bai*)

226. *Mu Xiang San* (Saussurea Powder): Radix Saussureae Seu Vladimiriae (*Mu Xiang*), Rhizoma Coptidis Chinensis (*Huang Lian*), uncooked Rhizoma Zingiberis (*Sheng Jiang*), Pericarpium Papaveris Somniferi (*Ying Su Ke*)

227. *Mu Xiang Tiao Qi San* (Saussurea Regulate the Qi Powder): Radix Saussureae Seu Vladimiriae (*Mu Xiang*), Fructus Amomi (*Sha Ren*), Fructus Cardamomi (*Bai Dou Kou*), Flos Caryophylli (*Ding Xiang*), Lignum Santali Albi (*Tan Xiang*), Herba Agastachis Seu Pogostemi (*Huo Xiang*), mix-fried Radix Glycyrrhizae (*Zhi Gan Cao*)

228. *Niu Xi San* (Cyathula Powder): Radix Cyathulae (*Chuan Niu Xi*), Radix Angelicae Sinensis (*Dang Gui*), Cortex Cinnamomi (*Rou Gui*), Radix Rubrus Paeoniae Lactiflorae (*Chi Shao Yao*), Semen Pruni Persicae (*Tao Ren*), Rhizoma Corydalis Yanhusuo (*Yan Hu Suo*), Cortex Radicis Moutan (*Mu Dan Pi*), Radix Saussureae Seu Vladimiriae (*Mu Xiang*)

229. *Niu Xi Tang* (Cyathula Decoction): Radix Cyathulae (*Chuan Niu Xi*), Radix Angelicae Sinensis (*Dang Gui*), Herba Dianthi (*Qu Mai*), Caulis Akebiae Mutong (*Mu Tong*), Talcum (*Hua Shi*), Semen Benincasae Hispidae (*Dong Gua Ren*)

230. *Ping Bu Zhen Xin Dan* (Equally Supplementing & Settling the Heart Elixir): Sclerotium Poriae Cocos (*Fu Ling*), Radix Polygalae Tenuifoliae (*Yuan Zhi*), Radix Panacis Ginseng (*Ren Shen*), Dens Draconis (*Long Chi*), Semen Zizyphi Spinosae (*Suan Zao Ren*), Fructus Schizandrae Chinensis (*Wu Wei Zi*), Tuber Asparagi Cochinensis (*Tian Men Dong*), Tuber Ophiopogonis Japonicae (*Mai Men Dong*), prepared Radix Rehmanniae (*Shu Di Huang*), Radix Dioscoreae Oppositae (*Shan Yao*), Cortex Cinnamomi (*Rou Gui*), Cinnabar (*Zhu Sha*), Sclerotium Pararadicis Poriae Cocos (*Fu Shen*), Semen Plantaginis (*Che Qian Zi*)

231. *Ping Wei San* (Level the Stomach Powder): Rhizoma Atractylodis (*Cang Zhu*), Cortex Magnoliae Officinalis (*Hou Po*), Pericarpium Citri Reticulatae (*Chen Pi*), uncooked Rhizoma Zingiberis (*Sheng Jiang*), Fructus Zizyphi Jujubae (*Da Zao*), mix-fried Radix Glycyrrhizae (*Zhi Gan Cao*)

232. *Pu Huang San* (Pollen Typhae Powder): Pollen Typhae (*Pu Huang*), Semen Malvae Seu Abutilonis (*Dong Kui Zi*), uncooked Radix Rehmanniae (*Sheng Di Huang*

233. *Pu Huang Wan* (Pollen Typhae Pills): Pollen Typhae (*Pu Huang*), Folium Artemisiae Argyii (*Ai Ye*), Os Draconis (*Long Gu*)

234. *Pu Ji Xiao Du Yin* (Universal Benefit Disperse Toxins Drink): Fructus Arctii Lappae (*Niu Bang Zi*), Fructificatio Lasiosphaerae (*Ma Bo*), Radix Isatidis Seu Baphicacanthi (*Ban Lan Gen*), Radix Astragali Membranacei (*Huang Qi*), Rhizoma Coptidis Chinensis (*Huang Lian*), Fructus Forsythiae Suspensae (*Lian Qiao*), Herba Menthae Haplocalycis (*Bo He*), Radix Scrophulariae Ningpoensis (*Xuan Shen*), Bombyx Batryticatus (*Jiang Can*), Radix Platycodi Grandiflori (*Jie Geng*), Radix Glycyrrhizae (*Gan Cao*), Pericarpium Citri Reticulatae (*Chen Pi*), Rhizoma Cimicifugae (*Sheng Ma*), Radix Bupleuri (*Chai Hu*)

235. *Qi Bao Mei Ran Dan* (Seven Treasures Beautiful Beard Elixir): Radix Polygoni Multiflori (*He Shou Wu*), Sclerotium Poriae Cocos (*Fu Ling*), Radix Achyranthis Bidentatae (*Huai Niu Xi*), Radix Angelicae Sinensis (*Dang Gui*), Fructus Lycii Chinensis (*Gou Qi Zi*), Semen Cuscutae (*Tu Si Zi*), Fructus Psoraleae Corylifoliae (*Bu Gu Zhi*)

236. *Qi Li San* (Seven Li Powder): Sanguis Draconis (*Xue Jie*), Resina Olibani (*Ru Xiang*), Resina Myrrhae (*Mo Yao*), Secretio Moschi Moschiferi (*She Xiang*), Flos Carthami Tinctorii (*Hong Hua*), Borneol (*Bing Pian*), Acacia Catechu (*Er Cha*), Cinnabar (*Zhu Sha*)

237. *Qi Wei Bai Zhu San* (Seven Flavors Atractylodes Powder): Radix Panacis Ginseng (*Ren Shen*), Sclerotium Poriae Cocos (*Fu Ling*), Rhizoma Atractylodis Macrocephalae (*Bai Zhu*), Radix Puerariae (*Ge Gen*), Radix Saussureae Seu Vladimiriae (*Mu Xiang*), Herba Agastachis Seu Pogostemi (*Huo Xiang*), Radix Glycyrrhizae (*Gan Cao*)

238. *Qi Wei Tiao Qi Tang* (Seven Flavors Regulate the Qi Decoction): Pericarpium Viridis Citri Reticulatae (*Qing Pi*), Rhizoma Cyperi Rotundi (*Xiang Fu*), Radix Saussureae Seu Vladimiriae (*Mu Xiang*), Herba Agastachis Seu Pogostemi (*Huo Xiang*), Radix Linderae Strychnifoliae (*Wu Yao*), Fructus Amomi (*Sha Ren*), mix-fried Radix Glycyrrhizae (*Zhi Gan Cao*)

239. *Qian Bei Xing Gua Tang* (Peucedanum, Fritillaria, Armeniaca & Benincasa Decoction): Radix Peucedani (*Qian Hu*), Bulbus Fritillariae Thunbergii (*Zhe Bei Mu*), Semen Pruni Armeniacae (*Xing Ren*), Semen Benincasae Hispidae (*Dong Gua Ren*)

240. *Qian Gen San* (Rubia Root Powder): Radix Rubiae Cordifoliae (*Qian Cao Gen*), Radix Scutellariae Baicalensis (*Huang Qin*), Gelatinum Corii Asini (*E Jiao*), Cacumen Biotae Orientalis (*Ce Bai Ye*), uncooked Radix Rehmanniae (*Sheng Di Huang*), Radix Glycyrrhizae (*Gan Cao*)

241. *Qian Gen Tang* (Rubia Root Decoction): Radix Rubiae Cordifoliae (*Qian Cao Gen*), Rhizoma Coptidis Chinensis (*Huang Lian*), Cortex Phellodendri (*Huang Bai*), Radix Sanguisorbae (*Di Yu*), Hallyositum Rubrum (*Chi Shi Zhi*), Gelatinum Corii Asini (*E Jiao*)

242. *Qian Hu San* (Peucedanum Powder): Radix Peucedani (*Qian Hu*), Cortex Radicis Mori Albi (*Sang Bai Pi*), Semen Pruni Armeniacae (*Xing Ren*), Bulbus Fritillariae Thunbergii (*Zhe Bei Mu*), Tuber Ophiopogonis Japonicae (*Mai Men Dong*)

243. *Qian Jin San* (Thousand [Ounces of] Gold Powder): Bile[-processed] Rhizoma Arisaematis (*Dan Nan Xing*), Rhizoma Coptidis Chinensis (*Huang Lian*), Calculus Bovis (*Niu Huang*), Buthus Martensi (*Quan Xie*), Rhizoma Gastrodiae Elatae (*Tian Ma*), Borneol (*Bing Pian*), Cinnabar (*Zhu Sha*)

244. *Qian Niu San* (Morning Glory Powder): Semen Pharbitidis (*Qian Niu Zi*), Semen Arecae Catechu (*Bing Lang*), Radix Et Rhizoma Rhei (*Da Huang*), Realgar (*Xiong Huang*)

245. *Qian Niu Zi San* (Morning Glory Seed Powder): Semen Pharbitidis (*Qian Niu Zi*), Caulis Akebiae Mutong (*Mu Tong*), Rhizoma Atractylodis Macrocephalae (*Bai Zhu*), Cortex Radicis Mori Albi (*Sang Bai Pi*), Radix Saussureae Seu Vladimiriae (*Mu Xiang*), Cortex Cinnamomi (*Rou Gui*), Pericarpium Citri Reticulatae (*Chen Pi*)

246. *Qian Zheng San* (Lead to Righteousness Powder): Rhizoma Typhonii (*Bai Fu Zi*), Bombyx Batryticatus (*Jiang Can*), Buthus Martensi (*Quan Xie*)

247. *Qiang Huo Sheng Shi Tang* (Notopterygium Overcome Dampness Decoction): Radix Et Rhizoma Notopterygii (*Qiang Huo*), Radix Ledebouriellae Sesloidis (*Fang Feng*), Radix Angelicae Pubescentis (*Du Huo*), Radix Et Rhizoma Ligustici Chinensis (*Gao Ben*), Radix Ligustici Wallichii (*Chuan Xiong*), Fructus Viticis (*Man Jing Zi*), Radix Glycyrrhizae (*Gan Cao*)

248. *Qin Jiao Tian Ma Tang* (Gentiana Macrophylla & Gastrodia Decoction): Radix Gentianae Macrophyllae (*Qin Jiao*), Rhizoma Gastrodiae Elatae (*Tian Ma*), Radix Et Rhizoma Notopterygii (*Qiang Huo*), Pericarpium Citri Reticulatae (*Chen Pi*), Radix Angelicae Sinensis (*Dang Gui*), Radix Ligustici Wallichii (*Chuan Xiong*), mix-fried Radix Glycyrrhizae (*Zhi Gan Cao*), Ramulus Mori Albi (*Sang Zhi*), uncooked Rhizoma Zingiberis (*Sheng Jiang*)

249. *Qin Lian Si Wu Tang* (Scutellaria & Coptis Four Materials Decoction): Uncooked Radix Rehmanniae (*Sheng Di Huang*), Radix Albus Paeoniae Lactiflorae (*Bai Shao Yao*), Radix Angelicae Sinensis (*Dang Gui*), Radix Ligustici Wallichii (*Chuan Xiong*), Radix Scutellariae Baicalensis (*Huang Qin*), Rhizoma Coptidis Chinensis (*Huang Lian*)

250. *Qing Dai Tang* (Clear Abnormal Vaginal Discharge Decoction): Concha Ostreae (*Mu Li*), Os Draconis (*Long Gu*), Radix Dioscoreae Oppositae (*Shan Yao*), Os Sepiae Seu Sepiellae (*Hai Piao Xiao*), Radix Rubiae Cordifoliae (*Qian Cao Gen*)

251. *Qing Gu San* (Clear the Bones Powder): Radix Stellariae (*Yin Chai Hu*), Cortex Radicis Lycii (*Di Gu Pi*), Radix Gentianae Macrophyllae (*Qin Jiao*), Rhizoma Picrorrhizae (*Hu Huang Lian*), Carapax Amydae Sinensis (*Bie Jia*), Rhizoma Anemarrhenae (*Zhi Mu*), Herba Artemisiae Apiaceae (*Qing Hao*), Radix Glycyrrhizae (*Gan Cao*)

252. *Qing Hao Bie Jia Tang* (Artemisia Apiacea & Carapax Amydae Decoction): Herba Artemisiae Apiaceae (*Qing Hao*), Carapax Amydae Sinensis (*Bie Jia*), Cortex Radicis Moutan (*Mu Dan Pi*), uncooked Radix Rehmanniae (*Sheng Di Huang*), Rhizoma Anemarrhenae (*Zhi Mu*)

253. *Qing Pi Tang* (Clear the Spleen Decoction): Radix Bupleuri (*Chai Hu*), Pericarpium Viridis Citri Reticulatae (*Qing Pi*), Rhizoma Pinelliae Ternatae (*Ban Xia*), Radix Scutellariae Baicalensis (*Huang Qin*), Cortex Magnoliae Officinalis (*Hou Po*), Rhizoma Atractylodis Macrocephalae (*Bai Zhu*), Sclerotium Poriae Cocos (*Fu Ling*), Fructus Amomi Tsao-ko (*Cao Guo*), Radix Glycyrrhizae (*Gan Cao*)

253a. *Qing Pi Wan* (Green Orange Peel Pills): Pericarpium Viridis Citri Reticulatae (*Qing Pi*), Massa Medica Fermentata (*Shen Qu*), Fructus Germinatus Hordei Vulgaris (*Mai Ya*), Fructus Crataegi (*Shan Zha*), Fructus Amomi Tsao-ko (*Cao Guo*)

254. *Qing Qi Hua Tan Wan* (Clear the Qi & Transform Phlegm Pills): Bile[-processed] Rhizoma Arisaematis (*Dan Nan Xing*), Semen Trichosanthis Kirlowii (*Gua Lou Ren*), Rhizoma Pinelliae Ternatae (*Ban Xia*), Pericarpium Citri Reticulatae (*Chen Pi*), Semen Pruni Armeniacae

(*Xing Ren*), Fructus Immaturus Citri Seu Ponciri (*Zhi Shi*), Radix Scutellariae Baicalensis (*Huang Qin*), Sclerotium Poriae Cocos (*Fu Ling*)

255. *Qing Shi Hua Tan Tang* (Clear Dampness & Transform Phlegm Decoction): Rhizoma Arisaematis (*Tian Nan Xing*), Sclerotium Poriae Cocos (*Fu Ling*), Rhizoma Pinelliae Ternatae (*Ban Xia*), Semen Sinapis Albae (*Bai Jie Zi*), Radix Et Rhizoma Notopterygii (*Qiang Huo*), Radix Scutellariae Baicalensis (*Huang Qin*), dry Rhizoma Zingiberis (*Gan Jiang*), Pericarpium Citri Reticulatae (*Chen Pi*), Rhizoma Atractylodis (*Cang Zhu*), Radix Angelicae Dahuricae (*Bai Zhi*), uncooked Rhizoma Zingiberis (*Sheng Jiang*), Radix Glycyrrhizae (*Gan Cao*)

256. *Qing Wei San* (Clear the Stomach Powder): Cortex Radicis Moutan (*Mu Dan Pi*), Rhizoma Cimicifugae (*Sheng Ma*), Rhizoma Coptidis Chinensis (*Huang Lian*), uncooked Radix Rehmanniae (*Sheng Di Huang*), Radix Angelicae Sinensis (*Dang Gui*)

257. *Qing Wen Bai Du San* (Clear Warmth & Vanquish Toxins Powder): Gypsum Fibrosum (*Shi Gao*), Rhizoma Coptidis Chinensis (*Huang Lian*), uncooked Radix Rehmanniae (*Sheng Di Huang*), Cornu Rhinocerotis (*Xi Jiao*) [substitute Cornu Bubali, *Shui Niu Jiao*], Radix Scutellariae Baicalensis (*Huang Qin*), Fructus Gardeniae Jasminoidis (*Shan Zhi Zi*), Radix Platycodi Grandiflori (*Jie Geng*), Rhizoma Anemarrhenae (*Zhi Mu*), Radix Rubrus Paeoniae Lactiflorae (*Chi Shao Yao*), Radix Scrophulariae Ningpoensis (*Xuan Shen*), Fructus Forsythiae Suspensae (*Lian Qiao*), Radix Glycyrrhizae (*Gan Cao*), Cortex Radicis Moutan (*Mu Dan Pi*), Folium Lophatheri Gracilis (*Dan Zhu Ye*)

258. *Qing Yan Tang* (Clear the Throat Decoction): Fructus Viticis (*Man Jing Zi*), Radix Glycyrrhizae (*Gan Cao*), Radix Platycodi Grandiflori (*Jie Geng*), Bombyx Batryticatus (*Jiang Can*), Herba Schizonepetae Tenuifoliae (*Jing Jie*), Radix Ledebouriellae Seslodis (*Fang Feng*), Semen Pruni Armeniacae (*Xing Ren*),

Fructus Citri Seu Ponciri (*Zhi Ke*), Herba Menthae Haplocalycis (*Bo He*), Radix Peucedani (*Qian Hu*), Herba Spirodelae Seu Lemnae (*Fu Ping*), Fructus Canarii Albi (*Gan Lan*)

259. *Qing Ying Tang* (Clear the Constructive Decoction): Cornu Rhinocerotis (*Xi Jiao*) [substitute Cornu Bubali, *Shui Niu Jiao*], uncooked Radix Rehmanniae (*Sheng Di Huang*), Radix Scrophulariae Ningpoensis (*Xuan Shen*), Folium Lophatheri Gracilis (*Dan Zhu Ye*), Flos Lonicerae Japonicae (*Jin Yin Hua*), Fructus Forsythiae Suspensae (*Lian Qiao*), Rhizoma Coptidis Chinensis (*Huang Lian*), Radix Salviae Miltiorrhizae (*Dan Shen*), Tuber Ophiopogonis Japonicae (*Mai Men Dong*)

260. *Qing Zao Jiu Fei Tang* (Clear Dryness & Rescue the Lungs Decoction): Folium Mori Albi (*Sang Ye*), Gypsum Fibrosum (*Shi Gao*), Radix Panacis Ginseng (*Ren Shen*), Radix Glycyrrhizae (*Gan Cao*), Semen Sesami Indici (*Hei Zhi Ma*), Gelatinum Corii Asini (*E Jiao*), Tuber Ophiopogonis Japonicae (*Mai Men Dong*), Semen Pruni Armeniacae (*Xing Ren*), Folium Eriobotryae Japonicae (*Pi Pa Ye*)

261. *Qing Zhen Tang* (Clear Tremors Decoction): Rhizoma Cimicifugae (*Sheng Ma*), Rhizoma Atractylodis (*Cang Zhu*), Folium Nelumbinis Nuciferae (*He Ye*), Fructus Viticis (*Man Jing Zi*)

262. *Qu Feng Gao* (Expel Wind Paste): Agkistrodon Seu Bungarus (*Bai Hua She*), Rhizoma Gastrodiae Elatae (*Tian Ma*), Herba Schizonepetae Tenuifoliae (*Jing Jie*), Herba Menthae Haplocalycis (*Bo He*), Radix Ledebouriellae Sesloidis (*Fang Feng*)

263. *Qu Mai Tang* (Dianthus Decoction): Herba Dianthi (*Qu Mai*), Talcum (*Hua Shi*), Rhizoma Imperatae Cylindricae (*Bai Mao Gen*), Semen Malvae Seu Abutilonis (*Dong Kui Zi*), Folium Lophatheri Gracilis (*Dan Zhu Ye*), Radix Scutellariae Baicalensis (*Huang Qin*), Semen Benincasae Hispidae (*Dong Gua Ren*)

264. *Qu Mai Zhi Zhu Wan* (Massa Medica Fermentata, Sprouted Barley, Citrus & Atractylodes Pills): Massa Medica Fermentata (*Shen Qu*), Rhizoma Atractylodis Macrocephalae (*Bai Zhu*), Fructus Germinatus Hordei Vulgaris (*Mai Ya*), Fructus Immaturus Citri Seu Ponciri (*Zhi Shi*)

265. *Qu Tan Yin Zi* (Dispel Phlegm Drink): Fructus Amomi Tsao-ko (*Cao Guo*), Rhizoma Arisaematis (*Tian Nan Xing*), Rhizoma Pinelliae Ternatae (*Ban Xia*), Sclerotium Poriae Cocos (*Fu Ling*), Pericarpium Viridis Citri Reticulatae (*Qing Pi*), Pericarpium Citri Reticulatae (*Chen Pi*)

266. *Rou Cong Rong Wan* (Cistanches Pills): Herba Cistanchis (*Rou Cong Rong*), Radix Dipsaci (*Xu Duan*), Cortex Eucommiae Ulmoidis (*Du Zhong*), Semen Cuscutae (*Tu Si Zi*), Fructus Schizandrae Chinensis (*Wu Wei Zi*), Radix Polygalae Tenuifoliae (*Yuan Zhi*), Fructus Cnidii Monnieri (*She Chuang Zi*)

267. *Ru Shen Tang* (Like Magic Decoction): Rhizoma Imperatae Cylindricae (*Bai Mao Gen*), Cortex Radicis Mori Albi (*Sang Bai Pi*)

268. *Ru Zhi Xia Xing Fang* (Breast Milk Descend & Move Formula): Radix Angelicae Sinensis (*Dang Gui*), Radix Ligustici Wallichii (*Chuan Xiong*), Squama Manitis Pentadactylis (*Chuan Shan Jia*), Radix Dipsaci (*Xu Duan*), Radix Trichosanthis Kirlowii (*Tian Hua Fen*), Herba Ephedrae (*Ma Huang*)

269. *Run Chang Wan* (Moisten the Intestines Pills): Semen Pruni Armeniacae (*Xing Ren*), Semen Pruni Persicae (*Tao Ren*), Semen Cannabis Sativae (*Huo Ma Ren*), Radix Angelicae Sinensis (*Dang Gui*), uncooked Radix Rehmanniae (*Sheng Di Huang*), Fructus Citri Seu Ponciri (*Zhi Ke*)

270. *Run Zao Tang* (Moisten Dryness Decoction): Semen Pruni Persicae (*Tao Ren*), Semen Cannabis Sativae (*Huo Ma Ren*), Radix Angelicae Sinensis (*Dang Gui*), uncooked Radix Rehmanniae (*Sheng Di Huang*), Rhizoma Cimicifugae (*Sheng Ma*), Radix Et Rhizoma Rhei (*Da Huang*), Flos Carthami Tinctorii (*Hong Hua*), prepared Radix Rehmanniae (*Shu Di Huang*), Radix Glycyrrhizae (*Gan Cao*)

271. *San Ao Tang* (Three [Ingredients] Unbinding Decoction): Herba Ephedrae (*Ma Huang*), Semen Pruni Armeniacae (*Xing Ren*), Radix Glycyrrhizae (*Gan Cao*)

272. *San Leng Wan* (Sparganium Pills): Rhizoma Sparganii (*San Leng*), Rhizoma Curcumae Zedoariae (*E Zhu*), Radix Ligustici Wallichii (*Chuan Xiong*), Cortex Radicis Moutan (*Mu Dan Pi*), Radix Cyathulae (*Chuan Niu Xi*), Radix Et Rhizoma Rhei (*Da Huang*), Rhizoma Corydalis Yanhusuo (*Yan Hu Suo*)

273. *San Miao Wan* (Three Marvels Pills): Cortex Phellodendri (*Huang Bai*), Rhizoma Atractylodis (*Cang Zhu*), Radix Achyranthis Bidentatae (*Huai Niu Xi*)

273a. *San Shi San* (Three Stones Powder): Gypsum Fibrosum (*Shi Gao*), Smithsonitum (*Lu Gan Shi*), Hallyositum Rubrum (*Chi Shi Zhi*)

274. *San Zi Yang Xin Tang* (Three Seeds Nourish the Aged Decoction): Semen Raphani Sativi (*Lai Fu Zi*), Semen Sinapis Albae (*Bai Jie Zi*), Fructus Perillae Frutescentis (*Zi Su Zi*)

275. *Sang Bai Pi Tang* (Cortex Mori Decoction): Cortex Radicis Mori Albi (*Sang Bai Pi*), Herba Ephedrae (*Ma Huang*), Ramulus Cinnamomi (*Gui Zhi*), Semen Pruni Armeniacae (*Xing Ren*), Herba Cum Radice Asari (*Xi Xin*), dry Rhizoma Zingiberis (*Gan Jiang*)

276. *Sang Ju Yin* (Morus & Chrysanthemum Drink): Flos Chrysanthemi Morifolii (*Ju Hua*), Folium Mori Albi (*Sang Ye*), Semen Pruni Armeniacae (*Xing Ren*), Herba Menthae Haplocalycis (*Bo He*), Fructus Forsythiae Suspensae (*Lian Qiao*), Radix Platycodi Grandiflori (*Jie Geng*), Radix Glycyrrhizae (*Gan Cao*), Rhizoma Phragmitis Communis (*Lu Gen*)

277. _Sang Ma Wan_ (Morus & Sesame Pills): Semen Sesami Indici (_Hei Zhi Ma_), Folium Mori Albi (_Sang Ye_), Honey (_Feng Mi_)

278. _Sang Piao Xiao San_ (Mantis Egg Case Powder): Ootheca Mantidis (_Sang Piao Xiao_), Os Draconis (_Long Gu_), Plastrum Testudinis (_Gui Ban_), Radix Panacis Ginseng (_Ren Shen_), Radix Polygalae Tenuifoliae (_Yuan Zhi_), Sclerotium Pararadicis Poriae Cocos (_Fu Shen_), Rhizoma Acori Graminei (_Shi Chang Pu_), Radix Angelicae Sinensis (_Dang Gui_)

279. _Sang Xing Tang_ (Morus & Armeniaca Decoction): Folium Mori Albi (_Sang Ye_), Semen Pruni Armeniacae (_Xing Ren_), Radix Glehniae Littoralis (_Bei Sha Shen_), Bulbus Fritillariae Thunbergii (_Zhe Bei Mu_), Semen Praeparatum Sojae (_Dan Dou Chi_), Fructus Gardeniae Jasminoidis (_Shan Zhi Zi_), Pericarpium Pyri (_Li Pi_)

280. _Sang Zhi Tang_ (Morus Twig Decoction): Radix Stephaniae Tetrandrae (_Fang Ji_), Ramulus Mori Albi (_Sang Zhi_), Fasciculus Vascularis Luffae (_Si Gua Luo_), Radix Cyathulae (_Chuan Niu Xi_)

281. _Shan Yao Xiao Ke Yin_ (Dioscorea Wasting Thirst Drink): Radix Dioscoreae Oppositae (_Shan Yao_), Radix Astragali Membranacei (_Huang Qi_), Radix Trichosanthis Kirlowii (_Tian Hua Fen_), Tuber Ophiopogonis Japonicae (_Mai Men Dong_), uncooked Radix Rehmanniae (_Sheng Di Huang_)

282. _Shan Yu Wan_ (Dioscorea Pills): Radix Dioscoreae Oppositae (_Shan Yao_), Rhizoma Atractylodis Macrocephalae (_Bai Zhu_), Radix Panacis Ginseng (_Ren Shen_)

283. _Shang Dang Shen Tang_ (Superior Codonopsis Decoction): Radix Codonopsis Pilosulae (_Dang Shen_), Radix Glehniae Littoralis (_Bei Sha Shen_), Cortex Cinnamomi (_Rou Gui_)

284. _Shao Yao Gan Cao Tang_ (Peony & Licorice Decoction): Radix Albus Paeoniae Lactiflorae (_Bai Shao Yao_), mix-fried Radix Glycyrrhizae (_Zhi Gan Cao_)

285. _Shao Yao Tang_ (Peony Decoction): Radix Albus Paeoniae Lactiflorae (_Bai Shao Yao_), Radix Scutellariae Baicalensis (_Huang Qin_), Rhizoma Coptidis Chinensis (_Huang Lian_), Radix Saussureae Seu Vladimiriae (_Mu Xiang_), Radix Angelicae Sinensis (_Dang Gui_), Semen Arecae Catechu (_Bing Lang_), Cortex Cinnamomi (_Rou Gui_), Radix Et Rhizoma Rhei (_Da Huang_), Radix Glycyrrhizae (_Gan Cao_)

286. _She Dan Chen Pi Mo_ (Snake Gall & Orange Peel Powder): Fel Agkistrodonis (_She Dan_), Pericarpium Citri Reticulatae (_Chen Pi_), Lumbricus (_Di Long_), Cinnabar (_Zhu Sha_), Bombyx Batryticatus (_Jiang Can_), Succinum (_Hu Po_)

287. _She Gan Ma Huang Tang_ (Belamcanda & Ephedra Decoction): Rhizoma Belamcandae (_She Gan_), Herba Ephedrae (_Ma Huang_), uncooked Rhizoma Zingiberis (_Sheng Jiang_), Herba Cum Radice Asari (_Xi Xin_), Radix Asteris Tatarici (_Zi Wan_), Flos Tussilaginis Farfarae (_Kuan Dong Hua_), Fructus Schizandrae Chinensis (_Wu Wei Zi_), Fructus Zizyphi Jujubae (_Da Zao_), Rhizoma Pinelliae Ternatae (_Ban Xia_)

288. _Shen Ling Bai Zhu San_ (Ginseng, Poria & Atractylodes Powder): Radix Panacis Ginseng (_Ren Shen_), Sclerotium Poriae Cocos (_Fu Ling_), Rhizoma Atractylodis Macrocephalae (_Bai Zhu_), Radix Dioscoreae Oppositae (_Shan Yao_), Semen Coicis Lachryma-jobi (_Yi Yi Ren_), Semen Dolichoris Lablab (_Bai Bian Dou_), Semen Nelumbinis Nuciferae (_Lian Zi_), mix-fried Radix Glycyrrhizae (_Zhi Gan Cao_), Radix Platycodi Grandiflori (_Jie Geng_), Fructus Amomi (_Sha Ren_)

289. _Shen Qi Bai Zhu Tang_ (Codonopsis, Astragalus & Atractylodes Decoction): Radix Codonopsis Pilosulae (_Dang Shen_), Radix Astragali Membranacei (_Huang Qi_), Rhizoma

Atractylodis Macrocephalae (*Bai Zhu*), Rhizoma Cimicifugae (*Sheng Ma*), Radix Bupleuri (*Chai Hu*)

290. *Shen Qi Tang* (Ginseng & Astragalus Decoction): Radix Panacis Ginseng (*Ren Shen*), Radix Astragali Membranacei (*Huang Qi*)

291. *Shen Qi Wan* (Kidney Qi Pills): Prepared Radix Rehmanniae (*Shu Di Huang*), Radix Dioscoreae Oppositae (*Shan Yao*), Fructus Corni Officinalis (*Shan Zhu Yu*), Rhizoma Alismatis (*Ze Xie*), Sclerotium Poriae Cocos (*Fu Ling*), Cortex Radicis Moutan (*Mu Dan Pi*), Radix Lateralis Praeparatus Aconiti Carmichaeli (*Fu Zi*), Ramulus Cinnamomi (*Gui Zhi*)

292. *Shen Zhu San* (Ginseng & Atractylodes Powder): Radix Panacis Ginseng (*Ren Shen*), Rhizoma Atractylodis Macrocephalae (*Bai Zhu*), Sclerotium Poriae Cocos (*Fu Ling*), Fructus Amomi (*Sha Ren*), mix-fried Radix Glycyrrhizae (*Zhi Gan Cao*), Semen Coicis Lachryma-jobi (*Yi Yi Ren*), Semen Nelumbinis Nuciferae (*Lian Zi*), Massa Medica Fermentata (*Shen Qu*), Fructus Crataegi (*Shan Zha*), Semen Myristicae Fragrantis (*Rou Dou Kou*), Fructus Terminaliae Chebulae (*He Zi*), Pericarpium Citri Reticulatae (*Chen Pi*), Radix Saussureae Seu Vladimiriae (*Mu Xiang*)

293. *Shen Zhu San* (Magic Atractylodes Powder): Rhizoma Atractylodis (*Cang Zhu*), Radix Et Rhizoma Ligustici Chinensis (*Gao Ben*), Radix Angelicae Dahuricae (*Bai Zhi*), Herba Cum Radice Asari (*Xi Xin*), Radix Et Rhizoma Notopterygii (*Qiang Huo*), Radix Ligustici Wallichii (*Chuan Xiong*), mix-fried Radix Glycyrrhizae (*Zhi Gan Cao*), Bulbus Allii Fistulosi (*Cong Bai*), uncooked Rhizoma Zingiberis (*Sheng Jiang*)

294. *Sheng Hua Tang* (Engender & Transform Decoction): Blast-fried Rhizoma Zingiberis (*Pao Jiang*), Radix Angelicae Sinensis (*Dang Gui*), Radix Ligustici Wallichii (*Chuan Xiong*), Semen Pruni Persicae (*Tao Ren*), mix-fried Radix Glycyrrhizae (*Zhi Gan Cao*)

295. *Sheng Ji Ze Xie Tang* (*Sheng Ji* Alisma Decoction): Rhizoma Alismatis (*Ze Xie*), Cortex Cinnamomi (*Rou Gui*), Rhizoma Atractylodis Macrocephalae (*Bai Zhu*), Sclerotium Poriae Cocos (*Fu Ling*), Radix Achyranthis Bidentatae (*Huai Niu Xi*), dry Rhizoma Zingiberis (*Gan Jiang*), Cortex Eucommiae Ulmoidis (*Du Zhong*), mix-fried Radix Glycyrrhizae (*Zhi Gan Cao*)

296. *Sheng Jiang Ban Xia Tang* (Fresh Ginger & Pinellia Decoction): Uncooked Rhizoma Zingiberis (*Sheng Jiang*), Rhizoma Pinelliae Ternatae (*Ban Xia*)

297. *Sheng Ma Ge Gen Tang* (Cimicifuga & Pueraria Decoction): Rhizoma Cimicifugae (*Sheng Ma*), Radix Puerariae (*Ge Gen*), mix-fried Radix Glycyrrhizae (*Zhi Gan Cao*), Radix Albus Paeoniae Lactiflorae (*Bai Shao Yao*)

298. *Sheng Mai San* (Engender the Pulse Powder): Radix Panacis Ginseng (*Ren Shen*), Fructus Schizandrae Chinensis (*Wu Wei Zi*), Tuber Ophiopogonis Japonicae (*Mai Men Dong*)

299. *Shi Hui San* (Ten Ashes Powder): Cacumen Biotae Orientalis (*Ce Bai Ye*), Cortex Radicis Moutan (*Mu Dan Pi*), Rhizoma Imperatae Cylindricae (*Bai Mao Gen*), Herba Cirsii Japonici (*Da Ji*), Herba Cephalanoploris Segeti (*Xiao Ji*), Radix Rubiae Cordifoliae (*Qian Cao Gen*), Radix Et Rhizoma Rhei (*Da Huang*), Fructus Gardeniae Jasminoidis (*Shan Zhi Zi*), carbonized Folium Et Petiolus Trachycarpi (*Zong Lu Tan*), Folium Nelumbinis Nuciferae (*He Ye*)

300. *Shi Jue Ming San* (Concha Haliotidis Powder): Concha Haliotidis (*Shi Jue Ming*), Fructus Lycii Chinensis (*Gou Qi Zi*), Herba Equiseti Hiemalis (*Mu Zei*), Herba Schizonepetae Tenuifoliae (*Jing Jie*), Folium Mori Albi (*Sang Ye*), Radix Glycyrrhizae (*Gan Cao*), Rhizoma Atractylodis (*Cang Zhu*), Flos Chrysanthemi Morifolii (*Ju Hua*), Herba Inulae Britannicae (*Jin Fei Cao*), Exuviae Serpentis (*She Tui*)

301. *Shi Xiao San* (Sudden Smile Powder):

Pollen Typhae (*Pu Huang*), Feces Trogopterori Seu Pteromi (*Wu Ling Zhi*)

302. *Shi Zao Tang* (Ten Dates Decoction): Radix Euphorbiae Kansui (*Gan Sui*), Flos Daphnis Genkwae (*Yuan Hua*), Radix Euphorbiae Pekinensis (*Jing Da Ji*), Fructus Zizyphi Jujubae (*Da Zao*)

303. *Shu Xue San* (Course the Blood Powder): Nodus Nelumbinis Nuciferae (*Ou Jie*), Cacumen Biotae Orientalis (*Ce Bai Ye*), Rhizoma Imperatae Cylindricae (*Bai Mao Gen*), Gelatinum Corii Asini (*E Jiao*)

304. *Shu Yu Wan* (Dioscorea Pills): Radix Dioscoreae Oppositae (*Shan Yao*), Tuber Ophiopogonis Japonicae (*Mai Men Dong*), Semen Pruni Armeniacae (*Xing Ren*), Radix Platycodi Grandiflori (*Jie Geng*), Gelatinum Corii Asini (*E Jiao*), uncooked Radix Rehmanniae (*Sheng Di Huang*), Rhizoma Bletillae Striatae (*Bai Ji*), Radix Angelicae Sinensis (*Dang Gui*), Radix Albus Paeoniae Lactiflorae (*Bai Shao Yao*), Radix Panacis Ginseng (*Ren Shen*), Radix Glycyrrhizae (*Gan Cao*), Sclerotium Poriae Cocos (*Fu Ling*), Radix Bupleuri (*Chai Hu*), Radix Ligustici Wallichii (*Chuan Xiong*), Ramulus Cinnamomi (*Gui Zhi*), dry Rhizoma Zingiberis (*Gan Jiang*), Radix Ledebouriellae Sesloidis (*Fang Feng*), Fructus Zizyphi Jujubae (*Da Zao*), Massa Medica Fermentata (*Shen Qu*), Semen Germinatum Glycinis (*Da Dou Huang Juan*), Rhizoma Atractylodis Macrocephalae (*Bai Zhu*)

305. *Shu Zao Yin Zi* (Coursing & Chiselling Drink): Cortex Sclerotii Poriae Cocos (*Fu Ling Pi*), Pericarpium Arecae Catechu (*Da Fu Pi*), Cortex Rhizomatis Zingiberis (*Sheng Jiang Pi*), Semen Phaseoli Calcarati (*Chi Xiao Dou*), Rhizoma Alismatis (*Ze Xie*), Caulis Akebiae Mutong (*Mu Tong*), Semen Zanthoxyli Bungeani (*Jiao Mu*), Semen Arecae Catechu (*Bing Lang*), Radix Gentianae Macrophyllae (*Qin Jiao*), Radix Et Rhizoma Notopterygii (*Qiang Huo*), Radix Phytolaccae (*Shang Lu*)

306. *Shuang He San* (Two Lotuses Powder): Nodus Nelumbinis Nuciferae (*Ou Jie*), Folium Nelumbinis Nuciferae (*He Ye*)

307. *Shuang Sang Tang* (Two Moruses Decoction): Folium Mori Albi (*Sang Ye*), Ramulus Mori Albi (*Sang Zhi*), Semen Leonuri Heterophylli (*Chong Wei Zi*)

308. *Shui Tu Er Xian Dan* (Water & Earth Two Immortals Elixir): Fructus Rosae Laevigatae (*Jin Ying Zi*), Semen Euryalis Ferocis (*Qian Shi*)

309. *Si Hai Shu Yu Wan* (Four Seas Soothe Depression Pills): Concha Cyclinae (*Hai Ge Ke*), Herba Sargassii (*Hai Zao*), Herba Zosterae Marinae (*Hai Dai*), Thallus Algae (*Kun Bu*), Radix Aristolochiae (*Qing Mu Xiang*), Os Sepiae Seu Sepiellae (*Hai Piao Xiao*), Pericarpium Citri Reticulatae (*Chen Pi*)

310. *Si Jun Zi Tang* (Four Gentlemen Decoction): Radix Panacis Ginseng (*Ren Shen*), Sclerotium Poriae Cocos (*Fu Ling*), Rhizoma Atractylodis Macrocephalae (*Bai Zhu*), mix-fried Radix Glycyrrhizae (*Zhi Gan Cao*)

311. *Si Mo Yin Zi* (Four Grindings Drink): Semen Arecae Catechu (*Bing Lang*), Radix Linderae Strychnifoliae (*Wu Yao*), Lignum Aquilariae Agallochae (*Chen Xiang*), Radix Panacis Ginseng (*Ren Shen*)

312. *Si Ni Tang* (Four Counterflows Decoction): Radix Lateralis Praeparatus Aconiti Carmichaeli (*Fu Zi*), dry Rhizoma Zingiberis (*Gan Jiang*), mix-fried Radix Glycyrrhizae (*Zhi Gan Cao*)

313. *Si Shen Wan* (Four Spirits Pills): Fructus Psoraleae Corylifoliae (*Bu Gu Zhi*), Semen Myristicae Fragrantis (*Rou Dou Kou*), Fructus Evodiae Rutecarpae (*Wu Zhu Yu*), Fructus Schizandrae Chinensis (*Wu Wei Zi*)

314. *Si Sheng Wan* (Four Uncooked [Ingredients] Pills): Uncooked Rhizoma Imperatae Cylindricae (*Sheng Bai Mao Gen*), uncooked Radix Rehmanniae (*Sheng Di Huang*), uncooked Folium Nelumbinis Nuciferae (*Sheng He Ye*), uncooked Folium Artemisiae Argyii (*Ai Ye*)

315. *Si Wu Tang* (Four Materials Decoction): Prepared Radix Rehmanniae (*Shu Di Huang*), Radix Albus Paeoniae Lactiflorae (*Bai Shao Yao*), Radix Angelicae Sinensis (*Dang Gui*), Radix Ligustici Wallichii (*Chuan Xiong*)

316. *Su Zi Jiang Qi Tang* (Perilla Seed Downbear Qi Decoction): Fructus Perillae Frutescentis (*Zi Su Zi*), Cortex Magnoliae Officinalis (*Hou Po*), Radix Peucedani (*Qian Hu*), Radix Angelicae Sinensis (*Dang Gui*), Rhizoma Pinelliae Ternatae (*Ban Xia*), Folium Perillae Frutescentis (*Zi Su Ye*), Pericarpium Citri Reticulatae (*Chen Pi*), Cortex Cinnamomi (*Rou Gui*), uncooked Rhizoma Zingiberis (*Sheng Jiang*), mix-fried Radix Glycyrrhizae (*Zhi Gan Cao*), Fructus Zizyphi Jujubae (*Da Zao*)

317. *Suan Zao Ren Tang* (Zizyphus Spinosa Decoction): Semen Zizyphi Spinosae (*Suan Zao Ren*), Sclerotium Poriae Cocos (*Fu Ling*), Radix Glycyrrhizae (*Gan Cao*), Radix Ligustici Wallichii (*Chuan Xiong*), Rhizoma Anemarrhenae (*Zhi Mu*)

318. *Sui Xin Dan* (Follow [Your] Heart Elixir): Radix Euphorbiae Kansui (*Gan Sui*), Cinnabar (*Zhu Sha*), Lapis Micae Seu Chloriti (*Meng Shi*)

319. *Suo Quan Wan* (Shut the Spring Pills): Radix Dioscoreae Oppositae (*Shan Yao*), Fructus Alpiniae Oxyphyllae (*Yi Zhi Ren*), Radix Linderae Strychnifoliae (*Wu Yao*)

320. *Tao He Cheng Qi Tang* (Persica Seed Support the Qi Decoction): Semen Pruni Persicae (*Tao Ren*), Ramulus Cinnamomi (*Gui Zhi*), Radix Et Rhizoma Rhei (*Da Huang*), Mirabilitum (*Mang Xiao*), mix-fried Radix Glycyrrhizae (*Zhi Gan Cao*)

321. *Tao Hong Si Wu Tang* (Persica & Carthamus Four Materials Decoction): Semen Pruni Persicae (*Tao Ren*), Flos Carthami Tinctorii (*Hong Hua*), Radix Angelicae Sinensis (*Dang Gui*), Radix Ligustici Wallichii (*Chuan Xiong*), Radix Albus Paeoniae Lactiflorae (*Bai Shao Yao*), prepared Radix Rehmanniae (*Shu Di Huang*)

322. *Tao Hua Tang* (Hallyositum Decoction): Dry Rhizoma Zingiberis (*Gan Jiang*), Hallyositum Rubrum (*Chi Shi Zhi*), Semen Oryzae Sativae (*Geng Mi*)

323. *Tian Ma Gou Teng Yin* (Gastrodia & Uncaria Drink): Rhizoma Gastrodiae Elatae (*Tian Ma*), Ramulus Uncariae Cum Uncis (*Gou Teng*), Cortex Eucommiae Ulmoidis (*Du Zhong*), Radix Achyranthis Bidentatae (*Huai Niu Xi*), Concha Haliotidis (*Shi Jue Ming*), Ramus Loranthi Seu Visci (*Sang Ji Sheng*), Fructus Gardeniae Jasminoidis (*Shan Zhi Zi*), Radix Scutellariae Baicalensis (*Huang Qin*), Herba Leonuri Heterophylli (*Yi Mu Cao*), Caulis Polygoni Multiflori (*Ye Jiao Teng*), Sclerotium Pararadicis Poriae Cocos (*Fu Shen*)

324. *Tian Ma Wan* (Gastrodia Pills): Rhizoma Gastrodiae Elatae (*Tian Ma*), Radix Angelicae Pubescentis (*Du Huo*), Radix Lateralis Praeparatus Aconiti Carmichaeli (*Fu Zi*), Herba Ephedrae (*Ma Huang*), Cortex Cinnamomi (*Rou Gui*), Zaocys Dhummades (*Wu Shao She*), Radix Panacis Ginseng (*Ren Shen*), Radix Ledebouriellae Sesloidis (*Fang Feng*), Herba Cum Radice Asari (*Xi Xin*), Lumbricus (*Di Long*), Radix Angelicae Sinensis (*Dang Gui*), Rhizoma Atractylodis Macrocephalae (*Bai Zhu*), Cornu Antelopis (*Ling Yang Jiao*), Buthus Martensi (*Quan Xie*), Radix Cyathulae (*Chuan Niu Xi*), Radix Ligustici Wallichii (*Chuan Xiong*), Sclerotium Pararadicis Poriae Cocos (*Fu Shen*), Semen Coicis Lachryma-jobi (*Yi Yi Ren*), Rhizoma Arisaematis (*Tian Nan Xing*), Bombyx Batryticatus (*Jiang Can*), Calculus Bovis (*Niu Huang*), Borneol (*Bing Pian*), Secretio Moschi Moschiferi (*She Xiang*), Cinnabar (*Zhu Sha*)

325. Tian Tai Wu Yao San (Tian Tai Lindera Powder): Radix Linderae Strychnifoliae (*Wu Yao*), Radix Saussureae Seu Vladimiriae (*Mu Xiang*), Fructus Foeniculi Vulgaris (*Xiao Hui Xiang*), Pericarpium Viridis Citri Reticulatae (*Qing Pi*), Semen Arecae Catechu (*Bing Lang*), Rhizoma Alpiniae Officinari (*Gao Liang Jiang*), Fructus Meliae Toosendan (*Chuan Lian Zi*), Semen Crotoni Tiglii (*Ba Dou*)

326. Tian Wang Bu Xin Dan (Heavenly Emperor Supplement the Heart Elixir): Radix Panacis Ginseng (*Ren Shen*), Radix Scrophulariae Ningpoensis (*Xuan Shen*), Radix Salviae Miltiorrhizae (*Dan Shen*), Sclerotium Poriae Cocos (*Fu Ling*), Fructus Schizandrae Chinensis (*Wu Wei Zi*), Radix Polygalae Tenuifoliae (*Yuan Zhi*), Radix Platycodi Grandiflori (*Jie Geng*), Radix Angelicae Sinensis (*Dang Gui*), Tuber Ophiopogonis Japonicae (*Mai Men Dong*), Tuber Asparagi Cochinensis (*Tian Men Dong*), Semen Biotae Orientalis (*Bai Zi Ren*), Semen Zizyphi Spinosae (*Suan Zao Ren*), uncooked Radix Rehmanniae (*Sheng Di Huang*), Cinnabar (*Zhu Sha*)

327. Tiao Wei Cheng Qi Tang (Regulate the Stomach & Support the Qi Decoction): Radix Et Rhizoma Rhei (*Da Huang*), Mirabilitum (*Mang Xiao*), Radix Glycyrrhizae (*Gan Cao*)

327a. Ting Li Zi Da Zao Xie Fei Tang (Lepidium & Red Dates Drain the Lungs Decoction): Semen Lepidii (*Ting Li Zi*), Fructus Zizyphi Jujubae (*Da Zao*)

328. Ting Li Zi San (Lepidium Powder): Semen Lepidii (*Ting Li Zi*), Cortex Sclerotii Poriae Cocos (*Fu Ling Pi*), Cortex Radix Mori Albi (*Sang Bai Pi*), Rhizoma Atractylodis Macrocephalae (*Bai Zhu*), Semen Pruni (*Yu Li Ren*)

329. Tong Guan San (Open the Gate Powder): Bombyx Batryticatus (*Jiang Can*), Secretio Moschi Moschiferi (*She Xiang*), Radix Et Rhizoma Notopterygii (*Qiang Huo*), uncooked Rhizoma Zingiberis Juice (*Sheng Jiang Zhi*)

330. Tong Guan Wan (Open the Gate Pills): Cortex Phellodendri (*Huang Bai*), Rhizoma Anemarrhenae (*Zhi Mu*), Cortex Cinnamomi (*Rou Gui*)

331. Tong Luo Zhi Tong Tang (Open the Network Vessels & Stop Pain Decoction): Fasciculus Vascularis Luffae (*Si Gua Luo*), Fasciculus Vascularis Citri Reticulatae (*Ju Luo*), Fructus Citri Seu Ponciri (*Zhi Ke*), Radix Bupleuri (*Chai Hu*), Radix Albus Paeoniae Lactiflorae (*Bai Shao Yao*), Resina Olibani (*Ru Xiang*), Resina Myrrhae (*Mo Yao*), Herba Epimedii (*Yin Yang Huo*)

332. Tong Ru Tang (Open the Breast Decoction): Semen Vaccariae Segetalis (*Wang Bu Liu Xing*), Squama Manitis Pentadactylis (*Chuan Shan Jia*), Medulla Tetrapanacis Papyriferi (*Tong Cao*), Radix Astragali Membranacei (*Huang Qi*), Fructus Liquidambaris Taiwaniae (*Lu Lu Tong*)

333. Tong Xie Yao Fang (Painful Diarrhea Essential Formula): Rhizoma Atractylodis Macrocephalae (*Bai Zhu*), Pericarpium Citri Reticulatae (*Chen Pi*), Radix Albus Paeoniae Lactiflorae (*Bai Shao Yao*), Radix Ledebouriellae Sesloidis (*Fang Feng*)

334. Tou Nong San (Outthrust Pus Powder): Radix Astragali Membranacei (*Huang Qi*), Squama Manitis Pentadactylis (*Chuan Shan Jia*), Radix Angelicae Sinensis (*Dang Gui*), Fructus Gleditschiae Chinensis (*Zao Jiao*), Radix Ligustici Wallichii (*Chuan Xiong*)

335. Wan Dai Tang (End Abnormal Vaginal Discharge Decoction): Radix Dioscoreae Oppositae (*Shan Yao*), Rhizoma Atractylodis Macrocephalae (*Bai Zhu*), Rhizoma Atractylodis (*Cang Zhu*), Semen Plantaginis (*Che Qian Zi*), Radix Panacis Ginseng (*Ren Shen*), Pericarpium Citri Reticulatae (*Chen Pi*), Radix Bupleuri (*Chai Hu*),

Herba Schizonepetae Tenuifoliae (*Jing Jie*), Radix Albus Paeoniae Lactiflorae (*Bai Shao Yao*), Radix Glycyrrhizae (*Gan Cao*)

336. *Wan Ying Wan* (Ten Thousand Responses Pills): Radix Et Rhizoma Rhei (*Da Huang*), Semen Pharbitidis (*Qian Niu Zi*), Fructus Gleditschiae Chinensis (*Zao Jiao*), Cortex Radicis Meliae Azerdach (*Ku Lian Pi*), Lignum Aquilariae Agallochae (*Chen Xiang*), Radix Saussureae Seu Vladimiriae (*Mu Xiang*), Omphalia (*Lei Wan*)

337. *Wu Bei San* (Sepia & Fritillaria Powder): Os Sepiae Seu Sepiellae (*Hai Piao Xiao*), Bulbus Fritillariae Thunbergii (*Zhe Bei Mu*), Radix Glycyrrhizae (*Gan Cao*)

338. *Wei Jing Tang* (Phragmites Decoction): Rhizoma Phragmitis Communis (*Lu Gen*), Semen Benincasae Hispidae (*Dong Gua Ren*), Semen Pruni Persicae (*Tao Ren*), Semen Coicis Lachryma-jobi (*Yi Yi Ren*)

339. *Wei Rui Tang* (Solomon Seal Decoction): Rhizoma Polygonati Odorati (*Yu Zhu*), Herba Ephedrae (*Ma Huang*), Radix Cynanchi Atrati (*Bai Wei*), Radix Angelicae Pubescentis (*Du Huo*), Semen Pruni Armeniacae (*Xing Ren*), Radix Ligustici Wallichii (*Chuan Xiong*), Radix Glycyrrhizae (*Gan Cao*), Radix Aristolochiae (*Qing Mu Xiang*), Gypsum Fibrosum (*Shi Gao*)

340. *Wen Dan Tang* (Warm the Gallbladder Decoction): Caulis In Taeniis Bambusae (*Zhu Ru*), Rhizoma Pinelliae Ternatae (*Ban Xia*), Fructus Immaturus Citri Seu Ponciri (*Zhi Shi*), Pericarpium Citri Reticulatae (*Chen Pi*), Sclerotium Poriae Cocos (*Fu Ling*), uncooked Rhizoma Zingiberis (*Sheng Jiang*), Radix Glycyrrhizae (*Gan Cao*), Fructus Zizyphi Jujubae (*Da Zao*)

341. *Wen Jing Tang* (Warm the Channels [or Menses] Decoction): Ramulus Cinnamomi (*Gui Zhi*), Fructus Evodiae Rutecarpae (*Wu Zhu Yu*), Radix Ligustici Wallichii (*Chuan Xiong*), Radix Angelicae Sinensis (*Dang Gui*), Radix Albus Paeoniae Lactiflorae (*Bai Shao Yao*), Tuber Ophiopogonis Japonicae (*Mai Men Dong*), Radix Panacis Ginseng (*Ren Shen*), Cortex Radicis Moutan (*Mu Dan Pi*), Gelatinum Corii Asini (*E Jiao*), Rhizoma Pinelliae Ternatae (*Ban Xia*), Radix Glycyrrhizae (*Gan Cao*), uncooked Rhizoma Zingiberis (*Sheng Jiang*)

342. *Wen Pi Tang* (Warm the Spleen Decoction): Radix Lateralis Praeparatus Aconiti Carmichaeli (*Fu Zi*), dry Rhizoma Zingiberis (*Gan Jiang*), Radix Panacis Ginseng (*Ren Shen*), Radix Et Rhizoma Rhei (*Da Huang*), mix-fried Radix Glycyrrhizae (*Zhi Gan Cao*)

343. *Wu Ao Tang* (Five [Ingredients] Unbinding Decoction): Herba Ephedrae (*Ma Huang*), Semen Pruni Armeniacae (*Xing Ren*), Herba Schizonepetae Tenuifoliae (*Jing Jie*), Radix Platycodi Grandiflori (*Jie Geng*), Radix Glycyrrhizae (*Gan Cao*)

344. *Wu Fa Wan* (Blacken the Hair Pills): Radix Polygoni Multiflori (*He Shou Wu*), Cacumen Biotae Orientalis (*Ce Bai Ye*), Fructus Ligustri Lucidi (*Nu Zhen Zi*), uncooked Radix Rehmanniae (*Sheng Di Huang*), Semen Sesami Indici (*Hei Zhi Ma*), prepared Radix Rehmanniae (*Shu Di Huang*), Radix Angelicae Sinensis (*Dang Gui*)

345. *Wu Ji Wan* (Fifth & Sixth Heavenly Stems Pills): Fructus Evodiae Rutecarpae (*Wu Zhu Yu*), Rhizoma Coptidis Chinensis (*Huang Lian*), Radix Albus Paeoniae Lactiflorae (*Bai Shao Yao*)

346. *Wu Jia Pi San* (Acanthopanax Powder): Cortex Radicis Acanthopanacis (*Wu Jia Pi*), Fructus Chaenomelis Lagenariae (*Mu Gua*), Nodus Ligni Pini (*Song Jie*)

347. *Wu Jia Pi Wan* (Acanthopanax Pills): Cortex Radicis Acanthopanacis (*Wu Jia Pi*), Radix Dipsaci (*Xu Duan*), Cortex Eucommiae Ulmoidis (*Du Zhong*), Rhizoma Cibotii Barometz (*Gou Ji*), Radix Angelicae Pubescentis (*Du Huo*), Rhizoma Dioscoreae Hypoglaucae (*Bei Xie*), Fructus Terminaliae Chebulae (*He Zi*), Radix Albus Paeoniae Lactiflorae (*Bai Shao Yao*), Radix Ligustici Wallichii (*Chuan Xiong*)

348. *Wu Ling San* (Five [Ingredients] *Ling* Powder): Sclerotium Polypori Umbellati (*Zhu Ling*), Sclerotium Poriae Cocos (*Fu Ling*), Rhizoma Alismatis (*Ze Xie*), Rhizoma Atractylodis Macrocephalae (*Bai Zhu*), Ramulus Cinnamomi (*Gui Zhi*)

349. *Wu Long Dan* (Aconite & Borneol Elixir): Radix Aconiti Carmichaeli (*Chuan Wu Tou*), Borneol (*Bing Pian*), Feces Trogopterori Seu Pteromi (*Wu Ling Zhi*), Secretio Moschi Moschiferi (*She Xiang*)

350. *Wu Mei Wan* (Mume Pills): Fructus Pruni Mume (*Wu Mei*), Pericarpium Zanthoxyli Bungeani (*Hua Jiao*), Herba Cum Radice Asari (*Xi Xin*), dry Rhizoma Zingiberis (*Gan Jiang*), Rhizoma Coptidis Chinensis (*Huang Lian*), Radix Angelicae Sinensis (*Dang Gui*), Radix Lateralis Praeparatus Aconiti Carmichaeli (*Fu Zi*), Ramulus Cinnamomi (*Gui Zhi*), Radix Panacis Ginseng (*Ren Shen*), Cortex Phellodendri (*Huang Bai*)

351. *Wu Pi San* (Five Peels Powder): Cortex Radicis Mori Albi (*Sang Bai Pi*), Cortex Sclerotii Poriae Cocos (*Fu Ling Pi*), Pericarpium Arecae Catechu (*Da Fu Pi*), Cortex Rhizomatis Zingiberis (*Sheng Jiang Pi*), Pericarpium Citri Reticulatae (*Chen Pi*)

352. *Wu Pi Yin* (Five Peels Drink): Cortex Radicis Acanthopanacis (*Wu Jia Pi*), Pericarpium Citri Reticulatae (*Chen Pi*), Cortex Sclerotii Poriae Cocos (*Fu Ling Pi*), Cortex Rhizomatis Zingiberis (*Sheng Jiang Pi*), Pericarpium Arecae Catechu (*Da Fu Pi*)

353. *Wu Ren Wan* (Five Seeds Pills): Semen Pruni (*Yu Li Ren*), Semen Pruni Armeniacae (*Xing Ren*), Semen Pini (*Song Zi Ren*), Semen Biotae Orientalis (*Bai Zi Ren*), Semen Pruni Persicae (*Tao Ren*), Pericarpium Citri Reticulatae (*Chen Pi*)

354. *Wu Tou Chi Shi Zhi Wan* (Aconite & Hallyositum Pills): Pericarpium Zanthoxyli Bungeani (*Hua Jiao*), Radix Aconiti Carmichaeli (*Chuan Wu Tou*), Radix Lateralis Praeparatus Aconiti Carmichaeli (*Fu Zi*), dry Rhizoma Zingiberis (*Gan Jiang*), Hallyositum Rubrum (*Chi Shi Zhi*)

355. *Wu Tou Gui Zhi Tang* (Aconite & Cinnamon Twig Decoction): Radix Aconiti Carmichaeli (*Chuan Wu Tou*), Ramulus Cinnamomi (*Gui Zhi*), Radix Albus Paeoniae Lactiflorae (*Bai Shao Yao*), uncooked Rhizoma Zingiberis (*Sheng Jiang*), Fructus Zizyphi Jujubae (*Da Zao*), mix-fried Radix Glycyrrhizae (*Zhi Gan Cao*)

356. *Wu Tou Tang* (Aconite Decoction): Radix Aconiti Carmichaeli (*Chuan Wu Tou*), Radix Astragali Membranacei (*Huang Qi*), Herba Ephedrae (*Ma Huang*), Radix Albus Paeoniae Lactiflorae (*Bai Shao Yao*), mix-fried Radix Glycyrrhizae (*Zhi Gan Cao*), Honey (*Feng Mi*)

357. *Wu Wei Xi Xin Tang* (Schizandra & Asarum Decoction): Fructus Schizandrae Chinensis (*Wu Wei Zi*), Herba Cum Radice Asari (*Xi Xin*), dry Rhizoma Zingiberis (*Gan Jiang*), Sclerotium Poriae Cocos (*Fu Ling*), mix-fried Radix Glycyrrhizae (*Zhi Gan Cao*)

358. *Wu Wei Xiao Du Yin* (Five Flavors Disperse Toxins Drink): Flos Lonicerae Japonicae (*Jin Yin Hua*), Herba Violae Yedoensis (*Zi Hua Di Ding*), Herba Cum Radice Taraxaci Mongolici

(*Pu Gong Ying*), Flos Chrysanthemi Indici (*Ye Ju Hua*), Semen Semiaquilegiae (*Tian Kui Zi*)

359. *Wu Xiang San* (Five Fragrances Powder): Radix Aconiti Kusnezofii (*Cao Wu Tou*), Herba Cum Radice Asari (*Xi Xin*), Secretio Moschi Moschiferi (*She Xiang*), Folium Camilliae Sinensis (*Cha Ye*)

360. *Wu Zhu Wan* (Aconite & Atractylodes Pills): Radix Aconiti Carmichaeli (*Chuan Wu Tou*), Rhizoma Atractylodis (*Cang Zhu*), Pyritum (*Zi Ran Tong*), Feces Trogopterori Seu Pteromi (*Wu Ling Zhi*)

361. *Wu Zhu Yu Tang* (Evodia Decoction): Fructus Evodiae Rutecarpae (*Wu Zhu Yu*), uncooked Rhizoma Zingiberis (*Sheng Jiang*), Radix Panacis Ginseng (*Ren Shen*), Fructus Zizyphi Jujubae (*Da Zao*)

362. *Xi Jiao Di Huang Tang* (Rhinoceros Horn & Rehmannia Decoction): Cornu Rhinocerotis (*Xi Jiao*) [substitute Cornu Bubali, *Shui Niu Jiao*], uncooked Radix Rehmanniae (*Sheng Di Huang*), Cortex Radicis Moutan (*Mu Dan Pi*), Radix Rubrus Paeoniae Lactiflorae (*Chi Shao Yao*)

363. *Xia Yu Xue Tang* (Descend Static Blood Decoction): Semen Pruni Persicae (*Tao Ren*), Radix Et Rhizoma Rhei (*Da Huang*), Eupolyphaga Seu Opisthoplatia (*Zhe Chong*)

364. *Xian Fang Huo Ming Yin* (Immortal Formula for Saving Life Drink): Squama Manitis Pentadactylis (*Chuan Shan Jia*), Radix Trichosanthis Kirlowii (*Tian Hua Fen*), Radix Glycyrrhizae (*Gan Cao*), Resina Olibani (*Ru Xiang*), Radix Angelicae Dahuricae (*Bai Zhi*), Radix Rubrus Paeoniae Lactiflorae (*Chi Shao Yao*), Bulbus Fritillariae Thunbergii (*Zhe Bei Mu*), Radix Ledebouriellae Sesloidis (*Fang Feng*), Resina Myrrhae (*Mo Yao*), Spina Gleditschiae Chinensis (*Zao Jiao Ci*), Radix Angelicae Sinensis (*Dang*

Gui), Pericarpium Citri Reticulatae (*Chen Pi*), Flos Lonicerae Japonicae (*Jin Yin Hua*)

365. *Xian Ling Pi San* (Epimedium Powder): Herba Epimedii (*Yin Yang Huo*), Radix Clematidis Chinensis (*Wei Ling Xian*), Radix Ligustici Wallichii (*Chuan Xiong*), Ramulus Cinnamomi (*Gui Zhi*), Fructus Xanthii (*Cang Er Zi*)

366. *Xian Mao Wan* (Curculigo Pills): Rhizoma Curculiginis Orchiidis (*Xian Mao*), Rhizoma Atractylodis (*Cang Zhu*), Fructus Lycii Chinensis (*Gou Qi Zi*), Semen Plantaginis (*Che Qian Zi*), Sclerotium Poriae Cocos (*Fu Ling*), Fructus Foeniculi Vulgaris (*Xiao Hui Xiang*), Semen Biotae Orientalis (*Bai Zi Ren*), uncooked Radix Rehmanniae (*Sheng Di Huang*), prepared Radix Rehmanniae (*Shu Di Huang*)

367. *Xiang Lian Wan* (Saussurea & Coptis Pills): Rhizoma Coptidis Chinensis (*Huang Lian*), Radix Saussureae Seu Vladimiriae (*Mu Xiang*)

368. *Xiang Ru San* (Elsholtzia Powder): Herba Elsholtziae (*Xiang Ru*), Semen Dolichoris Lablab (*Bai Bian Dou*), Cortex Magnoliae Officinalis (*Hou Po*)

369. *Xiang Sha Er Chen Tang* (Saussurea & Amomum Two Aged [Ingredients] Decoction): Radix Saussureae Seu Vladimiriae (*Mu Xiang*), Fructus Amomi (*Sha Ren*), Pericarpium Citri Reticulatae (*Chen Pi*), Rhizoma Pinelliae Ternatae (*Ban Xia*), Sclerotium Poriae Cocos (*Fu Ling*), mix-fried Radix Glycyrrhizae (*Zhi Gan Cao*)

370. *Xiang Su San* (Cyperus & Perilla Powder): Rhizoma Cyperi Rotundi (*Xiang Fu*), Folium Perillae Frutescentis (*Zi Su Ye*), Pericarpium Citri Reticulatae (*Chen Pi*), mix-fried Radix Glycyrrhizae (*Zhi Gan Cao*), Rhizoma Atractylodis (*Cang Zhu*)

371. *Xiao Ban Xia Jia Fu Ling Tang* (Minor Pinellia Plus Poriae Decoction): Rhizoma Pinelliae Ternatae (*Ban Xia*), uncooked Rhizoma Zingiberis (*Sheng Jiang*), Sclerotium Poriae Cocos (*Fu Ling*)

372. *Xiao Ban Xia Tang* (Minor Pinellia Decoction): Rhizoma Pinelliae Ternatae (*Ban Xia*), uncooked Rhizoma Zingiberis (*Sheng Jiang*)

373. *Xiao Bao He Wan* (Minor Protect Harmony Pills): Fructus Crataegi (*Shan Zha*), Massa Medica Fermentata (*Shen Qu*), Rhizoma Atractylodis Macrocephalae (*Bai Zhu*), Sclerotium Poriae Cocos (*Fu Ling*), Radix Albus Paeoniae Lactiflorae (*Bai Shao Yao*), Pericarpium Citri Reticulatae (*Chen Pi*)

374. *Xiao Chai Hu Tang* (Minor Bupleurum Decoction): Radix Bupleuri (*Chai Hu*), Radix Scutellariae Baicalensis (*Huang Qin*), Radix Codonopsis Pilosulae (*Dang Shen*), Rhizoma Pinelliae Ternatae (*Ban Xia*), mix-fried Radix Glycyrrhizae (*Zhi Gan Cao*), Fructus Zizyphi Jujubae (*Da Zao*), uncooked Rhizoma Zingiberis (*Sheng Jiang*)

375. *Xiao Huo Luo Dan* (Minor Quicken the Network Vessels Elixir): Radix Aconiti Carmichaeli (*Chuan Wu Tou*), Radix Aconiti Kusnezofii (*Cao Wu Tou*), Resina Myrrhae (*Mo Yao*), Resina Olibani (*Ru Xiang*), Lumbricus (*Di Long*), Rhizoma Arisaematis (*Tian Nan Xing*)

376. *Xiao Jian Zhong Tang* (Minor Fortify the Center Decoction): Saccharum Granorum (*Yi Tang*), Ramulus Cinnamomi (*Gui Zhi*), Radix Albus Paeoniae Lactiflorae (*Bai Shao Yao*), uncooked Rhizoma Zingiberis (*Sheng Jiang*), Fructus Zizyphi Jujubae (*Da Zao*), mix-fried Radix Glycyrrhizae (*Zhi Gan Cao*)

377. *Xiao Qing Long Tang* (Minor Blue Dragon Decoction): Herba Ephedrae (*Ma Huang*), Herba Cum Radice Asari (*Xi Xin*), dry Rhizoma Zingiberis (*Gan Jiang*), Ramulus Cinnamomi (*Gui Zhi*), Rhizoma Pinelliae Ternatae (*Ban Xia*), Fructus Schizandrae Chinensis (*Wu Wei Zi*), Radix Albus Paeoniae Lactiflorae (*Bai Shao Yao*), mix-fried Radix Glycyrrhizae (*Zhi Gan Cao*)

378. *Xiao Ru Tang* (Disperse the Breasts Decoction): Radix Salviae Miltiorrhizae (*Dan Shen*), Resina Olibani (*Ru Xiang*), Resina Myrrhae (*Mo Yao*), Fructus Forsythiae Suspensae (*Lian Qiao*), Flos Lonicerae Japonicae (*Jin Yin Hua*), Squama Manitis Pentadactylis (*Chuan Shan Jia*), Rhizoma Anemarrhenae (*Zhi Mu*), Fructus Trichosanthis Kirlowii (*Gua Lou*)

379. *Xiao Xian Xiong Tang* (Minor Fell [*i.e.*, Drain] the Chest Decoction): Rhizoma Coptidis Chinensis (*Huang Lian*), Rhizoma Pinelliae Ternatae (*Ban Xia*), Fructus Trichosanthis Kirlowii (*Gua Lou*)

380. *Xiao Yao San* (Rambling Powder): Radix Bupleuri (*Chai Hu*), Radix Albus Paeoniae Lactiflorae (*Bai Shao Yao*), Radix Angelicae Sinensis (*Dang Gui*), Sclerotium Poriae Cocos (*Fu Ling*), Rhizoma Atractylodis Macrocephalae (*Bai Zhu*), mix-fried Radix Glycyrrhizae (*Zhi Gan Cao*), Herba Menthae Haplocalycis (*Bo He*), uncooked Rhizoma Zingiberis (*Sheng Jiang*)

381. *Xie Bai San* (Drain the White Powder): Cortex Radicis Mori Albi (*Sang Bai Pi*), Cortex Radicis Lycii (*Di Gu Pi*), Radix Glycyrrhizae (*Gan Cao*), Semen Oryzae Sativae (*Geng Mi*)

382. *Xie Xin Tang* (Drain the Heart Decoction): Rhizoma Coptidis Chinensis (*Huang Lian*), Radix Scutellariae Baicalensis (*Huang Qin*), Radix Et Rhizoma Rhei (*Da Huang*)

383. *Xin Yi San* (Flos Magnoliae Powder): Flos Magnoliae Liliflorae (*Xin Yi Hua*), Herba Cum Radice Asari (*Xi Xin*), Radix Et Rhizoma Ligustici Chinensis (*Gao Ben*), Radix Angelicae Dahuricae (*Bai Zhi*), Radix Ligustici Wallichii (*Chuan Xiong*), Radix Ledebouriellae Sesloidis (*Fang Feng*), Caulis Akebiae Mutong (*Mu Tong*), Rhizoma Cimicifugae (*Sheng Ma*), Radix Glycyrrhizae (*Gan Cao*)

384. *Xing Su San* (Armeniaca & Perilla Powder): Semen Pruni Armeniacae (*Xing Ren*), Folium Perillae Frutescentis (*Zi Su Ye*), Radix Peucedani (*Qian Hu*), Rhizoma Pinelliae Ternatae (*Ban Xia*), Sclerotium Poriae Cocos (*Fu Ling*), mix-fried Radix Glycyrrhizae (*Zhi Gan Cao*), Radix Platycodi Grandiflori (*Jie Geng*), Fructus Citri Seu Ponciri (*Zhi Ke*), Pericarpium Citri Reticulatae (*Chen Pi*), uncooked Rhizoma Zingiberis (*Sheng Jiang*), Fructus Zizyphi Jujubae (*Da Zao*)

385. *Xing Xiao Wan* (Move & Disperse Pills): Resina Olibani (*Ru Xiang*), Resina Myrrhae (*Mo Yao*), Secretio Moschi Moschiferi (*She Xiang*), Realgar (*Xiong Huang*)

386. *Xu Duan Wan* (Dipsacus Pills): Radix Dipsaci (*Xu Duan*), Radix Ledebouriellae Sesloidis (*Fang Feng*), Radix Achyranthis Bidentatae (*Huai Niu Xi*), Radix Aconiti Carmichaeli (*Chuan Wu Tou*), Rhizoma Dioscoreae Hypoglaucae (*Bei Xie*)

387. *Xuan Du Jie Biao Tang* (Diffuse Toxins & Resolve the Exterior Decoction): Rhizoma Cimicifugae (*Sheng Ma*), Radix Puerariae (*Ge Gen*), Herba Schizonepetae Tenuifoliae (*Jing Jie*), Radix Ledebouriellae Sesloidis (*Fang Feng*), Herba Menthae Haplocalycis (*Bo He*), Fructus Forsythiae Suspensae (*Lian Qiao*), Radix Peucedani (*Qian Hu*), Semen Pruni Armeniacae (*Xing Ren*), Radix Platycodi Grandiflori (*Jie Geng*), Fructus Citri Seu Ponciri (*Zhi Ke*), Fructus Arctii Lappae (*Niu Bang Zi*), Folium Lophatheri Gracilis (*Dan Zhu Ye*), Caulis Akebiae Mutong (*Mu Tong*), Radix Glycyrrhizae (*Gan Cao*)

388. *Xuan Fu Dai Zhe Tang* (Inula & Hematite Decoction): Flos Inulae (*Xuan Fu Hua*), Haematitum (*Dai Zhe Shi*), Radix Panacis Ginseng (*Ren Shen*), uncooked Rhizoma Zingiberis (*Sheng Jiang*), Radix Glycyrrhizae (*Gan Cao*), Rhizoma Pinelliae Ternatae (*Ban Xia*), Fructus Zizyphi Jujubae (*Da Zao*)

389. *Xuan Fu Hua Tang* (Inula Decoction): Flos Inulae (*Xuan Fu Hua*), Bulbus Allii Fistulosi (*Cong Bai*), Radix Rubiae Cordifoliae (*Qian Cao Gen*)

390. *Xuan Fu Tang* (Corydalis & Aconite Decoction): Rhizoma Corydalis Yanhusuo (*Yan Hu Suo*), Radix Lateralis Praeparatus Aconiti Carmichaeli (*Fu Zi*), Radix Saussureae Seu Vladimiriae (*Mu Xiang*)

391. *Xuan Mai Gan Jie Tang* (Scrophularia, Ophiopogon, Licorice & Platycodon Decoction): Radix Scrophulariae Ningpoensis (*Xuan Shen*), Tuber Ophiopogonis Japonicae (*Mai Men Dong*), Radix Glycyrrhizae (*Gan Cao*), Radix Platycodi Grandiflori (*Jie Geng*)

392. *Xuan Qi San* (Diffuse the Qi Powder): Medulla Junci Effusi (*Deng Xin Cao*), Caulis Akebiae Mutong (*Mu Tong*), Fructus Gardeniae Jasminoidis (*Shan Zhi Zi*), Semen Malvae Seu Abutilonis (*Dong Kui Zi*), Talcum (*Hua Shi*), Radix Glycyrrhizae (*Gan Cao Shao*)

393. *Xue Fu Zhu Yu Tang* (Blood Mansion Dispel Stasis Decoction): Radix Angelicae Sinensis (*Dang Gui*), Radix Ligustici Wallichii (*Chuan Xiong*), uncooked Radix Rehmanniae (*Sheng Di Huang*), Semen Pruni Persicae (*Tao Ren*), Flos Carthami Tinctorii (*Hong Hua*), Radix Bupleuri (*Chai Hu*), Fructus Citri Seu Ponciri (*Zhi Ke*), Radix Rubrus Paeoniae Lactiflorae (*Chi Shao Yao*), Radix Cyathulae (*Chuan Niu Xi*), Radix Platycodi Grandiflori (*Jie Geng*), Radix Glycyrrhizae (*Gan Cao*)

394. Yang Gan Wan (Nourish the Liver Pills): Radix Angelicae Sinensis (*Dang Gui*), Radix Albus Paeoniae Lactiflorae (*Bai Shao Yao*), prepared Radix Rehmanniae (*Shu Di Huang*), Radix Ligustici Wallichii (*Chuan Xiong*), Radix Ledebouriellae Sesloidis (*Fang Feng*), Semen Plantaginis (*Che Qian Zi*), Fructus Prinsepiae (*Rui Ren*), Fructus Broussonetiae (*Chu Shi*)

395. Yang He Tang (Harmonize Yang Decoction): Gelatinum Cornu Cervi (*Lu Jiao Jiao*), Cortex Cinnamomi (*Rou Gui*), prepared Radix Rehmanniae (*Shu Di Huang*), blast-fried Rhizoma Zingiberis (*Pao Jiang*), Herba Ephedrae (*Ma Huang*), Semen Sinapis Albae (*Bai Jie Zi*), Radix Glycyrrhizae (*Gan Cao*)

396. Yang Huo San Zi Tang (Epimedium Three Seeds Decoction): Herba Epimedii (*Yin Yang Huo*), Fructus Schizandrae Chinensis (*Wu Wei Zi*), Fructus Lycii Chinensis (*Gou Qi Zi*), Semen Astragali (*Sha Yuan Zi*), Fructus Corni Officinalis (*Shan Zhu Yu*)

397. Yang Xin Tang (Nourish the Heart Decoction): Semen Biotae Orientalis (*Bai Zi Ren*), Semen Zizyphi Spinosae (*Suan Zao Ren*), Radix Angelicae Sinensis (*Dang Gui*), Fructus Schizandrae Chinensis (*Wu Wei Zi*), Radix Polygalae Tenuifoliae (*Yuan Zhi*), Radix Ligustici Wallichii (*Chuan Xiong*), Radix Panacis Ginseng (*Ren Shen*), Sclerotium Poriae Cocos (*Fu Ling*), Sclerotium Pararadicis Poriae Cocos (*Fu Shen*), Radix Astragali Membranacei (*Huang Qi*), Cortex Cinnamomi (*Rou Gui*), mix-fried Radix Glycyrrhizae (*Zhi Gan Cao*), Rhizoma Pinelliae Fermentata (*Ban Xia Qu*)

398. Yi Fu San (One Administration Powder): Pericarpium Papaveris Somniferi (*Ying Su Ke*), Fructus Pruni Mume (*Wu Mei*), Rhizoma Pinelliae Ternatae (*Ban Xia*), Semen Pruni Armeniacae (*Xing Ren*), Folium Perillae Frutescentis (*Zi Su Ye*), Gelatinum Corii Asini (*E Jiao*), Radix

Glycyrrhizae (*Gan Cao*), uncooked Rhizoma Zingiberis (*Sheng Jiang*)

399. Yi Gong San (Extraordinary Merit Powder): Rhizoma Atractylodis Macrocephalae (*Bai Zhu*), Pericarpium Citri Reticulatae (*Chen Pi*), Radix Panacis Ginseng (*Ren Shen*), Sclerotium Poriae Cocos (*Fu Ling*), mix-fried Radix Glycyrrhizae (*Zhi Gan Cao*)

400. Yi Huang San (Change Yellow Powder): Semen Plantaginis (*Che Qian Zi*), Cortex Phellodendri (*Huang Bai*), Radix Dioscoreae Oppositae (*Shan Yao*), Semen Euryalis Ferocis (*Qian Shi*), Semen Ginkgonis Bilobae (*Bai Guo*)

401. Yi Mu Si Wu Tang (Leonurus Four Materials Decoction): Herba Leonuri Heterophylli (*Yi Mu Cao*), prepared Radix Rehmanniae (*Shu Di Huang*), Radix Angelicae Sinensis (*Dang Gui*), Radix Albus Paeoniae Lactiflorae (*Bai Shao Yao*), Radix Ligustici Wallichii (*Chuan Xiong*)

402. Yi Mu Wan (Leonurus Pills): Radix Ligustici Wallichii (*Chuan Xiong*), Radix Angelicae Sinensis (*Dang Gui*), Herba Leonuri Heterophylli (*Yi Mu Cao*), Radix Rubrus Paeoniae Lactiflorae (*Chi Shao Yao*), Radix Saussureae Seu Vladimiriae (*Mu Xiang*)

403. Yi Qi Cong Ming Tang (Boost the Qi & Increase Acuity Decoction): Radix Panacis Ginseng (*Ren Shen*), Radix Astragali Membranacei (*Huang Qi*), Fructus Viticis (*Man Jing Zi*), Radix Puerariae (*Ge Gen*), Rhizoma Cimicifugae (*Sheng Ma*), Cortex Phellodendri (*Huang Bai*), Radix Albus Paeoniae Lactiflorae (*Bai Shao Yao*), mix-fried Radix Glycyrrhizae (*Zhi Gan Cao*)

404. Yi Wei Tang (Boost the Stomach Decoction): Tuber Ophiopogonis Japonicae (*Mai Men Dong*), Radix Glehniae Littoralis (*Bei Sha Shen*), uncooked Radix Rehmanniae (*Sheng Di Huang*),

Rhizoma Polygonati Odorati (*Yu Zhu*), Crystallized Sugar (*Bing Tang*)

405. *Yi Yi Du Zhong Tang* (Coix & Eucommia Decoction): Semen Coicis Lachryma-jobi (*Yi Yi Ren*), Cortex Eucommiae Ulmoidis (*Du Zhong*), Rhizoma Smilacis Glabrae (*Tu Fu Ling*), Semen Cuscutae (*Tu Si Zi*), Rhizoma Cibotii Barometz (*Gou Ji*), Radix Astragali Membranacei (*Huang Qi*), Herba Houttuyniae Cordatae (*Yu Xing Cao*), Radix Codonopsis Lanceolatae (*Shan Hai Luo*)

406. *Yi Yi Ren Tang* (Coix Decoction): Semen Coicis Lachryma-jobi (*Yi Yi Ren*), Rhizoma Atractylodis (*Cang Zhu*), Ramulus Cinnamomi (*Gui Zhi*), Radix Albus Paeoniae Lactiflorae (*Bai Shao Yao*), Radix Angelicae Sinensis (*Dang Gui*), Herba Ephedrae (*Ma Huang*), Radix Ligustici Wallichii (*Chuan Xiong*), Radix Angelicae Pubescentis (*Du Huo*), Radix Et Rhizoma Notopterygii (*Qiang Huo*), Radix Ledebouriellae Sesloidis (*Fang Feng*), Radix Aconiti Carmichaeli (*Chuan Wu Tou*), mix-fried Radix Glycyrrhizae (*Zhi Gan Cao*), uncooked Rhizoma Zingiberis (*Sheng Jiang*)

407. *Yi Zhi Ren Tang* (Alpinia Oxyphylla Decoction): Fructus Alpiniae Oxyphyllae (*Yi Zhi Ren*), Radix Aconiti Carmichaeli (*Chuan Wu Tou*), Pericarpium Viridis Citri Reticulatae (*Qing Pi*), Fructus Foeniculi Vulgaris (*Xiao Hui Xiang*), dry Rhizoma Zingiberis (*Gan Jiang*), mix-fried Radix Glycyrrhizae (*Zhi Gan Cao*), uncooked Rhizoma Zingiberis (*Sheng Jiang*)

408. *Yi Zhi San* (Alpinia Oxyphylla Powder): Fructus Alpiniae Oxyphyllae (*Yi Zhi Ren*), Radix Aconiti Carmichaeli (*Chuan Wu Tou*), dry Rhizoma Zingiberis (*Gan Jiang*), Pericarpium Viridis Citri Reticulatae (*Qing Pi*)

409. *Yin Chen Hao Tang* (Artemisia Capillaris Decoction): Herba Artemisiae Capillaris (*Yin Chen Hao*), Radix Et Rhizoma Rhei (*Da Huang*),

Fructus Gardeniae Jasminoidis (*Shan Zhi Zi*)

410. *Yin Chen Wu Ling San* (Artemisia Capillaris Five [Ingredients] *Ling* Powder): Herba Artemisiae Capillaris (*Yin Chen Hao*), Rhizoma Alismatis (*Ze Xie*), Sclerotium Polypori Umbellati (*Zhu Ling*), Sclerotium Poriae Cocos (*Fu Ling*), Rhizoma Atractylodis Macrocephalae (*Bai Zhu*), Ramulus Cinnamomi (*Gui Zhi*)

411. *Yin Feng Tang* (Conduct Wind Decoction): Fluoritum (*Zi Shi Ying*), Quartz Album (*Bai Shi Ying*), Ramulus Cinnamomi (*Gui Zhi*), Radix Glycyrrhizae (*Gan Cao*), Os Draconis (*Long Gu*), Concha Ostreae (*Mu Li*), Hallyositum Rubrum (*Chi Shi Zhi*), Calcitum (*Han Shui Shi*), Gypsum Fibrosum (*Shi Gao*), dry Rhizoma Zingiberis (*Gan Jiang*), Radix Et Rhizoma Rhei (*Da Huang*), Talcum (*Hua Shi*)

412. *Yin Qiao San* (Lonicera & Forsythia Powder): Flos Lonicerae Japonicae (*Jin Yin Hua*), Fructus Forsythiae Suspensae (*Lian Qiao*), Herba Menthae Haplocalycis (*Bo He*), Semen Praeparatum Sojae (*Dan Dou Chi*), Radix Platycodi Grandiflori (*Jie Geng*), Herba Schizonepetae Tenuifoliae (*Jing Jie*), Rhizoma Phragmitis Communis (*Lu Gen*), Folium Lophatheri Gracilis (*Dan Zhu Ye*), Fructus Arctii Lappae (*Niu Bang Zi*), Radix Glycyrrhizae (*Gan Cao*)

413. *Yu Fen Wan* (Jade Powder Pills): Pericarpium Citri Reticulatae (*Chen Pi*), Rhizoma Pinelliae Ternatae (*Ban Xia*), Rhizoma Arisaematis (*Tian Nan Xing*)

414. *Yu Feng Dan* (Heal Wind Elixir): Zaocys Dhummades (*Wu Shao She*), Agkistrodon Seu Bungarus (*Bai Hua She*), Elaphe (*Jin Qian Bai Hua She*), Fructus Gleditschiae Chinensis (*Zao Jiao*), Radix Sophorae Flavescentis (*Ku Shen*)

415. *Yu Hu Wan* (Jade Vase Pills): Rhizoma Arisaematis (*Tian Nan Xing*), Rhizoma Gastrodiae Elatae (*Tian Ma*), Rhizoma Pinelliae Ternatae (*Ban Xia*)

416. *Yu Nu Jian* (Jade Maiden Decoction): Gypsum Fibrosum (*Shi Gao*), Rhizoma Anemarrhenae (*Zhi Mu*), prepared Radix Rehmanniae (*Shu Di Huang*), Tuber Ophiopogonis Japonicae (*Mai Men Dong*), Radix Achyranthis Bidentatae (*Huai Niu Xi*)

417. *Yu Ping Feng San* (Jade Windscreen Powder): Radix Astragali Membranacei (*Huang Qi*), Rhizoma Atractylodis Macrocephalae (*Bai Zhu*), Radix Ledebouriellae Sesloidis (*Fang Feng*)

418. *Yu Quan Wan* (Jade Spring Pills): Tuber Ophiopogonis Japonicae (*Mai Men Dong*), Radix Trichosanthis Kirlowii (*Tian Hua Fen*), Fructus Pruni Mume (*Wu Mei*), Radix Puerariae (*Ge Gen*), Radix Astragali Membranacei (*Huang Qi*), mix-fried Radix Glycyrrhizae (*Zhi Gan Cao*)

419. *Yu Ye Tang* (Jade Humors Decoction): Radix Dioscoreae Oppositae (*Shan Yao*), Cortex Phellodendri (*Huang Bai*), Fructus Schizandrae Chinensis (*Wu Wei Zi*), Rhizoma Anemarrhenae (*Zhi Mu*), Endothelium Corneum Gigeriae Galli (*Ji Nei Jin*), Radix Puerariae (*Ge Gen*), Radix Trichosanthis Kirlowii (*Tian Hua Fen*), Radix Astragali Membranacei (*Huang Qi*)

420. *Yu Zhen San* (True Jade Powder): Radix Ledebouriellae Sesloidis (*Fang Feng*), Rhizoma Arisaematis (*Tian Nan Xing*), Rhizoma Typhonii (*Bai Fu Zi*), Rhizoma Gastrodiae Elatae (*Tian Ma*), Radix Angelicae Dahuricae (*Bai Zhi*), Radix Et Rhizoma Notopterygii (*Qiang Huo*)

421. *Yu Zhu Mai Men Dong Tang* (Solomon Seal & Ophiopogon Decoction): Rhizoma Polygonati Odorati (*Yu Zhu*), Tuber Ophiopogonis Japonicae (*Mai Men Dong*), Radix Glehniae Littoralis (*Bei Sha Shen*), Radix Glycyrrhizae (*Gan Cao*)

422. *Yuan Zhi Tang* (Polygala Decoction): Radix Polygalae Tenuifoliae (*Yuan Zhi*), Semen Zizyphi Spinosae (*Suan Zao Ren*), Radix Angelicae Sinensis (*Dang Gui*), Radix Panacis Ginseng (*Ren Shen*), Radix Astragali Membranacei (*Huang Qi*), Tuber Ophiopogonis Japonicae (*Mai Men Dong*), Herba Dendrobii (*Shi Hu*), Sclerotium Pararadicis Poriae Cocos (*Fu Shen*), Radix Glycyrrhizae (*Gan Cao*)

423. *Yue Bi Tang* (Maidservant from Yue Decoction): Herba Ephedrae (*Ma Huang*), Gypsum Fibrosum (*Shi Gao*), uncooked Rhizoma Zingiberis (*Sheng Jiang*), Fructus Zizyphi Jujubae (*Da Zao*), mix-fried Radix Glycyrrhizae (*Zhi Gan Cao*)

424. *Yue Ju Wan* (Escape Restraint Pills): Rhizoma Atractylodis (*Cang Zhu*), Rhizoma Cyperi Rotundi (*Xiang Fu*), Massa Medica Fermentata (*Shen Qu*), Radix Ligustici Wallichii (*Chuan Xiong*), Fructus Gardeniae Jasminoidis (*Shan Zhi Zi*)

425. *Yun Qi San* (Move Qi Powder): Radix Saussureae Seu Vladimiriae (*Mu Xiang*), Pericarpium Viridis Citri Reticulatae (*Qing Pi*), Fructus Crataegi (*Shan Zha*)

426. *Ze Xie Tang* (Alisma Decoction): Rhizoma Alismatis (*Ze Xie*), Rhizoma Atractylodis Macrocephalae (*Bai Zhu*)

427. *Zeng Ye Tang* (Increase Humors Decoction): Radix Scrophulariae Ningpoensis (*Xuan Shen*), uncooked Radix Rehmanniae (*Sheng Di Huang*), Tuber Ophiopogonis Japonicae (*Mai Men Dong*)

428. *Zhen Gan Xi Feng Tang* (Settle the Liver & Extinguish Wind Decoction): Radix Achyranthis Bidentatae (*Huai Niu Xi*), Haemititum (*Dai Zhe Shi*), Concha Ostreae (*Mu Li*), Os Draconis (*Long Gu*), Plastrum Testudinis (*Gui Ban*),

Radix Albus Paeoniae Lactiflorae (*Bai Shao Yao*), Radix Scrophulariae Ningpoensis (*Xuan Shen*), Tuber Asparagi Cochinensis (*Tian Men Dong*), Fructus Meliae Toosendan (*Chuan Lian Zi*), Fructus Germinatus Hordei Vulgaris (*Mai Ya*), Herba Artemisiae Capillaris (*Yin Chen Hao*), Radix Glycyrrhizae (*Gan Cao*)

429. *Zhen Wu Tang* (True Warrior Decoction): Radix Lateralis Praeparatus Aconiti Carmichaeli (*Fu Zi*), Rhizoma Atractylodis Macrocephalae (*Bai Zhu*), Radix Albus Paeoniae Lactiflorae (*Bai Shao Yao*), uncooked Rhizoma Zingiberis (*Sheng Jiang*), Sclerotium Poriae Cocos (*Fu Ling*)

430. *Zhen Zhong Dan* (Pillow Elixir): Os Draconis (*Long Gu*), Radix Polygalae Tenuifoliae (*Yuan Zhi*), Rhizoma Acori Graminei (*Shi Chang Pu*), Plastrum Testudinis (*Gui Ban*)

431. *Zhi Bai Di Huang Wan* (Anemarrhena & Phellodendron Rehmannia Pills): Rhizoma Anemarrhenae (*Zhi Mu*), Cortex Phellodendri (*Huang Bai*), prepared Radix Rehmanniae (*Shu Di Huang*), Fructus Corni Officinalis (*Shan Zhu Yu*), Rhizoma Alismatis (*Ze Xie*), Sclerotium Poriae Cocos (*Fu Ling*), Radix Dioscoreae Oppositae (*Shan Yao*), Cortex Radicis Moutan (*Mu Dan Pi*)

432. *Zhi Gan Cao Tang* (Mix-fried Licorice Decoction): Mix-fried Radix Glycyrrhizae (*Zhi Gan Cao*), Radix Panacis Ginseng (*Ren Shen*), uncooked Radix Rehmanniae (*Sheng Di Huang*), Gelatinum Corii Asini (*E Jiao*), Ramulus Cinnamomi (*Gui Zhi*), Semen Cannabis Sativae (*Huo Ma Ren*), Fructus Zizyphi Jujubae (*Da Zao*), uncooked Rhizoma Zingiberis (*Sheng Jiang*), Tuber Ophiopogonis Japonicae (*Mai Men Dong*)

433. *Zhi Mu San* (Anemarrhena Powder): Rhizoma Anemarrhenae (*Zhi Mu*), Cortex Radicis Mori Albi (*Sang Bai Pi*), Radix Scutellariae Bai-

calensis (*Huang Qin*), Radix Peucedani (*Qian Hu*), Radix Glycyrrhizae (*Gan Cao*)

434. *Zhi Shi Dao Zhi Wan* (Immature Citrus Abduct Stagnation Pills): Fructus Immaturus Citri Seu Ponciri (*Zhi Shi*), Radix Et Rhizoma Rhei (*Da Huang*), Rhizoma Atractylodis Macrocephalae (*Bai Zhu*), Massa Medica Fermentata (*Shen Qu*), Radix Scutellariae Baicalensis (*Huang Qin*), Rhizoma Coptidis Chinensis (*Huang Lian*), Rhizoma Alismatis (*Ze Xie*), Sclerotium Poriae Cocos (*Fu Ling*)

435. *Zhi Shi Xiao Pi Wan* (Immature Citrus Disperse Glomus Pills): Fructus Immaturus Citri Seu Ponciri (*Zhi Shi*), Rhizoma Atractylodis Macrocephalae (*Bai Zhu*), Cortex Magnoliae Officinalis (*Hou Po*), Rhizoma Pinelliae Ternatae (*Ban Xia*), Fructus Germinatus Hordei Vulgaris (*Mai Ya*), mix-fried Radix Glycyrrhizae (*Zhi Gan Cao*), dry Rhizoma Zingiberis (*Gan Jiang*), Sclerotium Poriae Cocos (*Fu Ling*), Radix Panacis Ginseng (*Ren Shen*), Rhizoma Coptidis Chinensis (*Huang Lian*)

436. *Zhi Shi Xie Bai Gui Zhi Tang* (Immature Citrus, Allium Macrostemum & Cinnamon Twig Decoction): Bulbus Allii Macrostemi (*Xie Bai*), Ramulus Cinnamomi (*Gui Zhi*), Fructus Immaturus Citri Seu Ponciri (*Zhi Shi*), Semen Trichosanthis Kirlowii (*Gua Lou Ren*), Cortex Magnoliae Officinalis (*Hou Po*)

437. *Zhi Sou San* (Stop Cough Powder): Herba Schizonepetae Tenuifoliae (*Jing Jie*), Radix Cynanchi Stautonii (*Bai Qian*), Radix Platycodi Grandiflori (*Jie Geng*), Radix Stemonae (*Bai Bu*), Radix Asteris Tatarici (*Zi Wan*), Pericarpium Citri Reticulatae (*Chen Pi*), Radix Glycyrrhizae (*Gan Cao*)

438. *Zhi Xue Gui Pi Tang* (Stop Bleeding Return the Spleen Decoction): Radix Codonopsis Pilosulae (*Dang Shen*), Radix Astragali Membranacei (*Huang Qi*), Rhizoma Atractylodis Macrocephalae (*Bai Zhu*), Radix Angelicae Sinensis (*Dang Gui*), Folium Callicarpae Pediculantae (*Zi Zhu*), Herba Agrimoniae Pilosae (*He Xian Cao*), Radix Pseudoginseng (*San Qi*), Os Sepiae Seu Sepiellae (*Hai Piao Xiao*), Radix Saussureae Seu Vladimiriae (*Mu Xiang*), Radix Glycyrrhizae (*Gan Cao*)

439. ***Zhi Zhu Wan*** **(Citrus & Atractylodes Pills):** Fructus Immaturus Citri Seu Ponciri (*Zhi Shi*), Rhizoma Atractylodis Macrocephalae (*Bai Zhu*)

440. ***Zhi Zi Bai Pi Tang*** **(Gardenia & Phellodendron Decoction):** Fructus Gardeniae Jasminoidis (*Shan Zhi Zi*), Cortex Phellodendri (*Huang Bai*), Radix Glycyrrhizae (*Gan Cao*)

441. ***Zhi Zi Chi Tang*** **(Gardenia & Prepared Soybeans Decoction):** Fructus Gardeniae Jasminoidis (*Shan Zhi Zi*), Semen Praeparatum Sojae (*Dan Dou Chi*)

442. ***Zhi Zi Ren San*** **(Gardenia Powder):** Fructus Gardeniae Jasminoidis (*Shan Zhi Zi*), Semen Benincasae Hispidae (*Dong Gua Ren*), Rhizoma Imperatae Cylindricae (*Bai Mao Gen*), mix-fried Radix Glycyrrhizae (*Zhi Gan Cao*)

443. ***Zhi Zi Sheng Ji Tang*** **(Gardenia Overcome Accumulation Decoction):** Fructus Gardeniae Jasminoidis (*Shan Zhi Zi*), Periostracum Cicadae (*Chan Tui*), Semen Cassiae Torae (*Cao Jue Ming*), Radix Ligustici Wallichii (*Chuan Xiong*), Herba Schizonepetae Tenuifoliae (*Jing Jie*), Fructus Tribuli Terrestris (*Bai Ji Li*), Scapus Et Inflorescentia Eriocaulonis Buergeriani (*Gu Jing Cao*), Flos Chrysanthemi Morifolii (*Ju Hua*), Radix Ledebouriellae Sesloidis (*Fang Feng*), Radix Et Rhizoma Notopterygii (*Qiang Huo*), Flos Buddleiae Officinalis (*Mi Meng Hua*), mix-fried Radix Glycyrrhizae (*Zhi Gan Cao*), Fructus Viticis (*Man Jing Zi*), Herba Equiseti Hiemalis (*Mu Zei*), Radix Scutellariae Baicalensis (*Huang Qin*)

444. ***Zhou Che Wan*** **(Vessel & Vehicle Pills):** Semen Pharbitidis (*Qian Niu Zi*), Radix Et Rhizoma Rhei (*Da Huang*), Radix Euphorbiae Kansui (*Gan Sui*), Pericarpium Viridis Citri Reticulatae (*Qing Pi*), Radix Saussureae Seu Vladimiriae (*Mu Xiang*), Radix Euphorbiae Pekinensis (*Jing Da Ji*), Flos Daphnis Genkwae (*Yuan Hua*), Pericarpium Citri Reticulatae (*Chen Pi*), Semen Arecae Catechu (*Bing Lang*), Calomelas (*Qing Fen*)

445. ***Zhu Jing Wan*** **(Preserve Vistas Pills):** Prepared Radix Rehmanniae (*Shu Di Huang*), Semen Plantaginis (*Che Qian Zi*), Semen Cuscutae (*Tu Si Zi*)

446. ***Zhu Ye Liu Bang Tang*** **(Bamboo Leaf, Tamarisk & Arctium Decoction):** Periostracum Cicadae (*Chan Tui*), Folium Lophatheri Gracilis (*Dan Zhu Ye*), Fructus Arctii Lappae (*Niu Bang Zi*), Radix Puerariae (*Ge Gen*), Herba Menthae Haplocalycis (*Bo He*), Rhizoma Anemarrhenae (*Zhi Mu*), Radix Scrophulariae Ningpoensis (*Xuan Shen*), Tuber Ophiopogonis Japonicae (*Mai Men Dong*), Radix Glycyrrhizae (*Gan Cao*), Ramulus Et Folium Tamaricis (*Cheng Liu*)

447. ***Zi Shen Wan*** **(Enrich the Kidneys Pills):** Rhizoma Anemarrhenae (*Zhi Mu*), Cortex Cinnamomi (*Rou Gui*), Cortex Phellodendri (*Huang Bai*)

448. ***Zi Wan San*** **(Aster Powder [I]):** Radix Asteris Tatarici (*Zi Wan*), Flos Tussilaginis Farfarae (*Kuan Dong Hua*), Semen Pruni Armeniacae (*Xing Ren*), Herba Cum Radice Asari (*Xi Xin*)

449. ***Zi Wan San*** **(Aster Powder [II]):** Radix Asteris Tatarici (*Zi Wan*), Tuber Ophiopogonis Japonicae (*Mai Men Dong*), Gelatinum Corii Asini (*E Jiao*), Bulbus Fritillariae Cirrhosae

(*Chuan Bei Mu*), Radix Panacis Ginseng (*Ren Shen*), Sclerotium Poriae Cocos (*Fu Ling*), Radix Platycodi Grandiflori (*Jie Geng*), Fructus Schizandrae Chinensis (*Wu Wei Zi*), Radix Glycyrrhizae (*Gan Cao*)

450. *Zong Lu Bai Shao Tang* (General Collection Peony Decoction): Radix Albus Paeoniae Lactiflorae (*Bai Shao Yao*), Cacumen Biotae Orientalis (*Ce Bai Ye*)

451. *Zuo Gui Wan* (Restore the Left [Kidney] Pills): Prepared Radix Rehmanniae (*Shu Di Huang*), Radix Dioscoreae Oppositae (*Shan Yao*), Fructus Lycii Chinensis (*Gou Qi Zi*), Fructus Corni Officinalis (*Shan Zhu Yu*), Radix Achyranthis Bidentatae (*Huai Niu Xi*), Semen Cuscutae (*Tu Si Zi*), Gelatinum Cornu Cervi (*Lu Jiao Jiao*), Gelatinum Plastri Testudinis (*Gui Ban Jiao*)

452. *Zuo Jin Wan* (Left Gold Pills): Rhizoma Coptidis Chinensis (*Huang Lian*), Fructus Evodiae Rutecarpae (*Wu Zhu Yu*)

Symptom Index

chest pain and oppression 145, 180, 183
chest pain radiating to the back or left arm 177, 178
chest pain, severe 65
chest, sensation of heat in the 103, 176
chills 31-35, 48, 57, 69, 73, 81, 82, 103, 116, 119, 128, 166,
174, 177, 182, 184, 190, 193-195, 198, 258
chyluria 242
colds and flu 19, 20, 35-37, 73, 197
cold, aversion to 20, 21, 23, 25, 28, 33, 34, 36, 61, 71, 73-76,
106, 219, 221, 243, 284
common cold 21, 23, 28, 119, 184, 272
complexion, pale 23, 49, 73, 94, 103, 167, 191, 232, 257,
265, 267
complexion, pale, wan 196, 199, 207, 222
consciousness, loss of 27, 45, 54, 76, 122, 170, 173, 209
constipation 36, 39, 47, 49, 52, 54, 57, 61-63, 65, 66, 68, 74,
99, 100, 109, 110, 113, 114, 116, 120, 123, 138, 142,
179, 185, 195, 197, 201, 228, 243, 254, 255, 257, 259,
264, 269, 271, 292
constipation, alternating diarrhea and 254
constipation due to heat 36, 52, 123
constipation in the aged 292
convulsions 20, 34, 87, 165, 172, 173, 204, 206, 209, 212,
214, 215, 253, 268
convulsions, clonic 206, 209, 253, 268
convulsions, infantile 173
convulsions of the four limbs 165
cough 6, 11, 13, 20, 22-26, 28, 32, 36-38, 41, 44, 49, 55-58,
65, 68, 76, 82, 85, 91, 96, 102, 110, 113, 121, 122, 139,
141, 150, 152, 166-170, 172-186, 189-199, 209, 211,
220, 222-225, 228, 229, 232, 236, 247, 255, 258, 261,
263, 269, 272, 276, 282-285
cough, asthmatic 37
cough, barking 193
cough, chronic 276, 282-284
cough, dry 38, 58, 167, 176, 178, 179, 183, 185, 190-192,
194-196, 198, 199, 225, 258, 261, 272, 284, 285
cough due to dryness of the lungs 38
cough following measles 192
cough, incessant 166, 178, 190
cough, paroxysmal, spasmodic, like a cock's crow 190
cough with expectoration of clear, liquid mucus 22
cough which follows pain in the chest 178
cough with little mucus or mucus streaked with 56
cough with whitish mucus 177, 178
cries, piercing 202

D

dampness, excess of 22, 228
deafness 35, 202, 216, 239, 260, 266, 268, 271, 288
defecation, discharge of red blood before 21
delirium 45, 48, 51, 54, 62
desquamation 63
diaphragmatic oppression 119, 170, 203
diaphragm oppression 51, 78

diarrhea 6, 9-13, 21, 26, 33, 39, 46-48, 51, 62, 63, 69, 73,
76-83, 91, 94, 96, 97, 101, 103-106, 111, 113, 115, 119,
123, 138, 171, 205, 212, 219, 221-224, 227, 229, 233,
235, 236, 242, 245, 249, 254, 255, 273, 274, 277, 278,
282, 284-288
diarrhea and constipation, alternating 254
diarrhea, barely malodorous 235
diarrhea, bloody 48, 51, 63
diarrhea, bloody, with more blood than pus 51
diarrhea, chronic 39, 101, 115, 212, 223, 273, 274, 277, 282,
285, 286
diarrhea, chronic, incessant 205
diarrhea, cockcrow 284
diarrhea, daybreak 235, 236
diarrhea, painful 21, 254
diarrhea with undigested food 78
digestion, slow 102, 103, 114, 120, 171, 265
disorientation 72
dizziness 31, 94, 132, 220, 237, 244, 247, 253, 266
dream-disturbed sleep 207
dreams, abundant 201, 203, 207, 229, 261, 265
dreams, erotic 98, 205, 206, 208
drink cool liquids, desire to 58
dry heat 38
dysentery 11, 33, 44, 48, 50, 51, 62, 74, 83, 110, 115, 123,
131, 143, 155, 158, 162, 254, 273, 274, 277, 282, 285,
286, 288, 289
dysentery, bloody 51, 143, 277
dysentery, incessant 155, 285, 286
dysentery, incessant which will not heal 155
dysentery, resistent 273, 274, 277, 282
dysentery, slightly bloody 277
dysmenorrhea 22, 26, 43, 73, 85, 118, 119, 126, 130, 133,
140, 144, 145, 147, 149, 160, 161, 240, 254, 256
dysphagia 85, 113, 168
dyspnea 25, 68, 113, 117, 174, 177-179, 186, 189, 192, 193,
195, 197, 198, 202, 211, 213, 228, 229, 235, 236
dyspnea on exertion 113, 235, 236
dysuria 27, 41, 44, 59, 62, 65, 91, 92, 97, 100, 134, 160, 161,
175, 180, 185, 194

E

eczema 57, 77, 149, 165, 182
eczema, purulent 57
edema 22, 25, 27, 68, 73, 84, 86, 91, 94-97, 109, 151, 181,
185, 194, 220, 224, 225, 227
edema beginning in the eyelids 194, 227
edema, generalized 73, 109, 185, 194
edema of the limbs and body 181
edema, sudden in the eyelids and face 25
ejaculation, premature 91, 98, 235, 236, 238, 240-242, 244,
245, 247, 249, 250, 266
emaciation 63, 222, 226, 232, 262, 272, 278
enuresis 101, 118, 233, 236, 239, 244, 245, 249, 277, 279,
280

hematoma 54, 93, 136, 137, 140, 141, 145, 147, 160, 161, 248, 256
hematoma, traumatic injury with 140, 145, 160, 161
hematuria 41, 45, 50, 55, 60, 93, 120, 125, 134, 143, 151, 154, 155, 157, 159-163, 180, 242, 258
hemeralopia 216
hemiplegia 79, 89, 165, 166, 172, 212, 215, 227
hemoptysis 44, 50, 55, 63, 92, 150, 151, 154, 157, 159, 161-163, 166, 180, 181, 186, 191, 192, 195, 199, 212, 223, 242, 258, 261, 263-265
hemoptysis, chronic, incessant 159
hemorrhage 45, 55, 60, 120, 163, 202
hemorrhage due to traumatic injury 202
hemorrhoids 21, 157-159, 162, 192
hemorrhoids, bleeding 157-159, 192
hepatomegaly 139
hernia, inguinal 65, 72, 78, 79, 104, 110, 112, 114, 117-119, 146, 240, 249, 288
hips, rheumatic complaints localized especially in the 235
hot flashes 250, 253
hunger 228, 281
hydrothorax 185
hypersalivation 65, 249
hypochondrium 31
hypogalactia 142
hysteria 113, 130, 168

I

impotence 73, 226, 229, 235, 236, 238, 240-242, 244, 245, 247, 250, 269, 279, 280
indigestion 106, 114, 138, 224
indigestion of meat foods 138
infants, retarded growth in 87
infertility 22, 73, 210, 235, 244, 250
infertility, female 235
insomnia 19, 33, 47, 48, 50, 53, 59, 88, 93-95, 130, 170, 172, 187, 192, 201-204, 207, 209, 215, 216, 226, 229, 257, 261, 262, 265, 267, 268, 270, 283
insomnia with abundant dreams 203
intestinal parasites 109
irritability 31, 48, 49, 53, 88, 93, 117, 129, 194, 207, 216, 250, 254
itching, genital 157, 189

J, K

jaundice 25, 43, 48, 59, 62, 85, 88, 92, 97, 151
jaws, clenched 202
joint and sinew pain 247
joint stiffness 21
joint pains 20
joints, hot, swollen 21
joints, red, very painful, swollen, hot 263
knee and leg pain 240
knee, arthrosis of the 86
knees, atony of the feet and 44
knees, cold feet and 128
knees, swelling of the 125

L

lacrimation 35, 37, 47, 52
lateral costal distention and pain 47
lateral costal distention 47, 94, 128, 140, 240
lateral costal masses 262
lateral costal pain 48, 78, 114, 117, 119, 120, 128, 130, 140, 144, 146, 254, 280
legs, paralysis or atony of the 44
leprosy 79, 87
lethargy 76
lice 189
ligaments, torn 137, 239, 248
limbs and body, edema of the 181
limbs, cold 43, 47, 73-76, 103, 122, 221, 222, 273, 279
limbs, heavy 27, 152
limbs, pain in the four 145
lips, pale 267
lochia, retention of 63, 76, 104, 130, 137, 144, 147, 160, 161
low back and knees, soreness and weakness of the 41
low back pain 44, 79, 86, 98, 114, 128, 133, 235, 236, 238, 239, 241, 243, 244, 246, 248, 250, 260, 266, 269, 280, 287
low back weakness 225, 235, 236
lung abscess 96, 175, 184, 186
lungs and lateral costal region, pain in the 181
luxation with swelling, pain, hematoma 248

M

macules 53, 56, 129
macules, red, raised 53
malaria 31, 32, 109, 262, 289
malnutrition, infantile 278, 290
mammary nodules 102
mass, palpable 54
masses, abdominal 54, 85, 100, 116, 120, 122, 126, 127, 130, 132, 135, 137, 139, 141, 145, 262, 281
masses, fixed, palpable abdominal 120, 127, 141
masses in the breast 103
masses, palpable, fixed, painful 145
mastitis of the inflammatory and purulent stage 50, 53
mastitis 50, 53, 67, 103, 117, 126, 129, 140, 142, 168, 176, 177, 241, 247
measles 23, 33, 36, 38, 184, 192
measles (initial stage) 23, 33, 36, 38
melena 24, 120, 273, 286, 288
memory, poor 94, 95, 201, 203, 204, 207-209, 265, 268, 283
menopausal syndrome 250
menorrhagia 45, 50, 60, 76, 120, 150, 212, 257, 273, 280, 286
menses, clots in the 133
menstrual cycle, long 210

menstrual irregularity 22, 26, 31, 55, 119, 128, 130, 133, 147, 235, 253, 256, 267

menstruation, abundant or scanty 130

menstruation, scanty, dark colored with clots 143, 144

menstruation, scanty 43, 85, 140, 143, 254

mental agitation 208

mental and physical apathy 241

mental apathy 235, 280

mental confusion 50, 55, 59, 62, 65, 130, 208

mental troubles 62, 65

metrorrhagia 24, 45, 50, 55, 60, 76, 120, 141, 143, 147, 150, 154, 157, 161-163, 205, 206, 212, 217, 238, 242, 246, 248, 249, 254, 257, 259, 263-265, 267, 269, 273, 274, 276, 277, 282, 286, 288

metrorrhagia during pregnancy 150, 238, 246, 259

metrorrhagia, scanty 141

micturition, urgent, frequent 62

mobility, loss of 71-73, 80-82, 84-86, 88, 89, 96, 126, 132, 133, 137, 161, 181, 238, 256

mobility, restricted 21

mouth and throat, dry 37, 48, 57-59, 167, 191, 196, 198, 199, 206, 264, 269, 272, 285

mouth and eyes, deviated 72, 79, 89, 165, 166, 172, 212

mouth, bitter taste in the 31, 48, 49, 116, 117, 170, 187, 288

mouth, bland 106, 176

mouth, dry 25, 32, 33, 36-38, 41, 48, 54, 57-59, 66, 93, 150, 167, 186, 191, 195, 196, 198, 199, 206, 222, 229, 264, 269, 272, 283, 285

mouth, dry but without thirst 150

mouth, foaming 173

mouth, tasteless 71, 103

mouth, throat, and nose dry 195

mucus, abundant 26, 196, 197

mucus, excessive 22

mucus, expectoration of abundant, thick, sticky 167

mucus, difficult to expectorate 41, 183

mucus, thick, yellow 25, 49, 169, 223

mucus, thin, clear 184, 190, 196

mumps 36

muscular pain 132

muscular spasm 172

muscular spasms 87, 206, 224

mycoses, scabies with pruritus 72, 163

N

nails, pale 265, 267

nasal congestion 20, 28, 128, 184, 195

nausea 13, 26, 31, 46, 48, 49, 51, 69, 78, 81, 85, 92, 94, 99, 106, 111, 113, 116, 117, 119, 135-138, 168, 170-172, 174, 176, 187, 193, 197, 209, 211, 291

neck and nuchal region, pain of the 53

neck pain 128

neck, stiff 33

nightmares 207

night blindness 82

night-crying in infants 93

night sweats 44, 47, 56, 58, 176, 190-192, 201, 203, 205-207, 214, 227, 232, 253, 261-263, 266, 268, 272, 279, 283, 284

nodules, subcutaneous 53, 54, 70, 165, 172, 180, 181, 206, 213, 259, 281

nocturia 101, 236, 244, 247, 249, 277

nose, abundant runny 28

nose, dry 31, 33

nose, obstruction and congestion of the 28

numbness 81, 84, 96, 125, 133, 137, 172, 215, 256

numbness of the extremities 256

O

ocular distention 132

oligomenorrhea 73, 143

oliguria 22, 25, 27, 44, 58, 59, 62, 63, 68, 73, 91, 94, 95, 97, 109, 120, 174, 181, 185, 194, 220

optic atrophy 52, 82, 214

osteomylitis 242

P, Q

pain aggravated by pressure 54, 61, 63, 100, 104, 109, 137, 141, 145, 175

pain aggravated by stress or anger 140

pain ameliorated by heat and pressure 254

pain from traumatic injury 160

pain, generalized 25, 80, 169

pain, incessant 145

pain, pricking 41

palpitations 22, 47, 94, 95, 104, 130, 187, 201-203, 207, 209, 216, 220, 224, 229, 257, 261, 267, 268, 270, 283

paralysis 44, 71

paralysis or atony of the legs 44

parasites, intestinal 109

paresthesia of the hands and feet 172

periumbilical pain 78, 112, 288

perspiration 19, 21, 23, 26, 53-55, 57, 81, 113, 176, 196, 198, 199, 201, 205-207, 220, 227-229, 253, 272, 279, 283-285

perspiration, no 21

perspiration, profuse 55, 57

perspiration, slight 53

perspiration, spontaneous 26, 113, 176, 191, 196, 198, 199, 205-207, 220, 227, 229, 253, 272, 279, 284, 285

pertussis 190

phlegmon 242

phlegm, abundant 25, 37, 110, 121, 170, 195, 198, 226

phlegm cold 69, 113, 165, 167, 168, 172, 174, 175, 183, 189, 191, 196-198, 224

phlegm, expectoration of blood-streaked 151

phlegm, expectoration of purulent, malodorous 175

phlegm, purulent, bloody 183

phlegm, scanty 178, 179

phlegm, scanty, dry, which is difficult to expectorate 167

phlegm streaked with blood 161, 178, 180, 190, 191, 194, 199, 261

phlegm, thin, abundant 195

phlegm which is difficult to expectorate, thick, yellow166

phlegm which is difficult to expectorate 37, 58, 166, 167, 176, 180, 183

phlegm which is thick and pasty 37

photophobia 42, 47, 52, 59, 91, 271

pinworms 189

placenta, retention of the 126, 133, 147, 160

pleural effusion 185

plum pit qi 113, 168

postpartum abdominal pain 76, 104, 130, 137, 256

postpartum vertigo 248

pregnancy, vomiting during 46, 187

premenstrual syndrome 26

pruritus 44, 66, 72, 77, 129, 163, 165, 212, 217, 259, 275

psychoses 203, 204

ptosis of the internal organs 32

pus 1, 42, 51, 57, 96, 126, 135, 137, 142, 175, 183, 186, 216, 226, 227, 242

pus, production of 42

pyogenic infection 64

pyogenic inflammation 126, 161

qi, disharmony of the 26

R

rectal prolapse 122, 227, 277

rectal or uterine prolapse 39

retardation in learning to walk 87

rheumatic complaints 21, 25, 36, 55, 56, 70-73, 79-89, 96, 125, 126, 128, 133, 139, 161, 169, 172, 215, 220, 227, 235, 237, 238, 246, 247, 250, 256, 263

rheumatic complaints localized especially in the hips 235

rhinitis 28. 81

rhinorrhea 37 80, 184

rhinorrhea, abundant 37

rhinorrhea, clear 184

S

saliva, thick, sticky 122

scabies 72, 79, 87, 163

scabies with pruritus, mycoses 72, 163

scarlatina 36

scrofula 53, 54, 70, 79, 80, 165, 172, 180, 181, 206, 213, 259, 281

scrotum or testicles, maladies of the 72, 104, 110, 114, 117, 146, 240, 249, 288

sinew contracture 79, 135, 137, 237

sinew pain 71, 247

sinews and bones, pain of the 285

sinusitis 28, 80, 81

skin, dry 63

skin eruptions, ruby red 55

skin infections, purulent 57

skin inflammation 42, 44, 50, 134, 135, 137, 146, 156, 223, 241, 259

skin inflammation with ulceration 134

skin lesions spreading, diffuse, deeply subcutaneous 242

skin, shiny 194

skin ulcers 182

sleep, agitated 93, 95, 129, 203

sleep, dream-disturbed 207

sleep, disturbed 43, 207

sleep, restless 208

sores, bleeding 275

sores, oozing, with pruritus 217

sores, purulent 275

sound, impossibility of expressing the slightest 213

spermatorrhea 41, 58, 91, 98, 205, 206, 208, 226, 236, 242, 244, 249, 266, 269, 273, 276, 277, 279, 280, 284

splenomegaly 117

stomach acidity and pain 182, 206, 223, 275, 281

stomach, clamoring 281

stomach heat 28, 33, 46, 50, 150, 170, 180, 272, 281

stomach, sensation of malaise and of heat in the 59

stomach troubles 51

stools accompanied by fresh blood, purple and pussy 51

stools, blackish 63

stools, bloody 21, 44-46, 55, 62, 105, 153, 155-159, 161, 162, 258, 282, 288

stools, dry 52, 228, 243

stools dry, hard 57, 66, 114, 123, 179, 197

stools, loose 26, 71, 73, 99, 105, 106, 111, 113, 168, 170, 171, 179, 196, 220, 223, 224, 226, 227, 233, 235, 242, 255, 265, 284

stools, loose, containing undigested food 235, 242

stools, loose or liquid 288

stools, pussy, bloody 44, 46, 62, 105

stools streaked with blood 265

strangury 41, 59, 62, 92, 95, 100, 125, 126, 134, 143, 151, 155, 159, 163, 176, 180, 236, 242, 243, 249, 258, 277, 278, 287

strangury with chyluria 242

strangury with hematuria 41, 143, 159, 163, 180, 258

swallows, sensation of obstruction when the patient 85

sweating, no 23, 25, 33, 119

sweating on slight exertion 207, 227, 279, 283

sweating, slight 23, 26

sweats, night 32

swelling of the abdomen 61

swelling of the hands and feet 20

swelling of the knees 125

syncope 122

syphilis 79

T

taste, loss of 71, 105, 111, 176

tearing 59, 91, 212

tendonomuscular spasms 237

tenesmus 46, 48, 51, 62, 110, 115, 131, 158

Pinyin Index of Medicinals

This index contains only medicinals whose processing instruction are described in this book and only give the pages on which these descriptions appear.

Latin Index of Medicinals

This index contains only medicinals whose processing instructions are described in this book and only gives the pages on which these descriptions appear.

Radix Sophorae Flavescentis 288
Radix Stellariae Dichotomae 290
Radix Stemonae 189-190
Radix Trichosanthis Kirlowii 180
Ramulus Cinnamomi 21-23
Ramulus Mori Albi 83-84
Ramus Loranthi Seu Visci 289
Realgar 290
Resina Myrrhae 134-136
Resina Olibani 136-138
Rhizoma Acori Graminei 289
Rhizoma Alismatis 97-98
Rhizoma Alpiniae Officinari 287
Rhizoma Anemarrhenae 57-58
Rhizoma Arisaematis 172-173
Rhizoma Atractylodis Macrocephalae 220-221
Rhizoma Atractylodis 81-82
Rhizoma Belamcandae 289
Rhizoma Cibotii Barometz 238-239
Rhizoma Cimicifugae 38-39
Rhizoma Coptidis Chinensis 45-48
Rhizoma Corydalis Yanhusuo 145-146
Rhizoma Curculiginis Orchiodis 246-247
Rhizoma Curcumae Zedoariae 131-132
Rhizoma Cyperi Rotundi 119-120
Rhizoma Dioscoreae Hypoglaucae 287
Rhizoma Drynariae 239-240
Rhizoma Gastrodiae Elatae 215-216
Rhizoma Imperatae Cylindricae 150-152
Rhizoma Pinelliae Ternatae 168-171
Rhizoma Polygonati 225-226
Rhizoma Polygonati Odorati 272
Rhizoma Sparganii 138-139
Rhizoma Typhonii 165-166
Rhizoma Zingiberis 26-27
Rhizoma Zingiberis, dry 75-76

S

Sclerotium Album Poriae Cocos 95
Sclerotium Pararadicis Poriae Cocos 95
Sclerotium Poriae Cocos 94-95
Sclerotium Rubrum Poriae Cocos 95
Scolopendra Subspinipes 292
Semen Astragali 244-245
Semen Alpiniae Katsumadai 287
Semen Arecae Catechu 109-110
Semen Benincasae Hispidae 175-176
Semen Biotae Orientalis 201-202

Semen Cannabis Sativae 291
Semen Cassiae Torae 52
Semen Citri Reticulatae 288
Semen Coicis Lachryma-jobi 95-96
Semen Crotonis Tiglii 291
Semen Cuscutae 245-246
Semen Dolichoris Lablab 219-220
Semen Euphorbiae Lathyridis 292
Semen Euryalis Ferocis 277-278
Semen Ginkgonis Bilobae 291
Semen Lepidii 185-187
Semen Litchi Chinensis 288
Semen Myristicae Fragrantis 289
Semen Nelumbinis Nuciferae 288
Semen Pharbitidis 67
Semen Plantaginis 91-92
Semen Praeparatum Sojae 19-20
Semen Pruni 292
Semen Pruni Armeniacae 141-142
Semen Pruni Persicae 141-143
Semen Raphani Sativi 102
Semen Sinapis Albae 179-180
Semen Trichosanthis Kirlowii 179-181
Semen Trigonellae Foeni-graecae 240-241
Semen Vaccariae Segetalis 142-143
Semen Zizyphi Spinosae 207-208
Smithsonitum 288
Squama Manitis Pentadactylis 126-127
Sulfur 289

T

Talcum 288
Tuber Asparagi Cochinensis 290
Tuber Curcumae 288
Tuber Ophiopogonis Japonicae 269-270

Z

Zaocys Dhumnades 87-88

ACUPOINT POCKET REFERENCE
by Bob Flaws
ISBN 0-936185-93-7

ACUPUNCTURE & IVF
by Lifang Liang
ISBN 0-891845-24-1

ACUPUNCTURE AND MOXIBUSTION
FORMULAS & TREATMENTS
by Cheng Dan-an, trans. by Wu Ming
ISBN 0-936185-68-6

ACUPUNCTURE FOR STROKE
REHABILITATION
Three Decades of Information from China
by Hoy Ping Yee Chan, et al.
ISBN 1-891845-35-7

ACUPUNCTURE PHYSICAL MEDICINE:
An Acupuncture Touchpoint Approach to the
Treatment of Chronic Pain, Fatigue, and Stress
Disorders
by Mark Seem
ISBN 1-891845-13-6

AGING & BLOOD STASIS:
A New Approach to TCM Geriatrics
by Yan De-xin
ISBN 0-936185-63-5

A NEW AMERICAN ACUPUNTURE
By Mark Seem
ISBN 0-936185-44-9

BETTER BREAST HEALTH NATURALLY
with CHINESE MEDICINE
by Honora Lee Wolfe & Bob Flaws
ISBN 0-936185-90-2

BIOMEDICINE: A Textbook for Practitioners of
Acupuncture and Oriental Medicine
by Bruce H. Robinson, MD
ISBN 1-891845-38-1

THE BOOK OF JOOK:
Chinese Medicinal Porridges
by B. Flaws
ISBN 0-936185-60-0

CHANNEL DIVERGENCES
Deeper Pathways of the Web
by Miki Shima and Charles Chase
ISBN 1-891845-15-2

CHINESE MEDICAL OBSTETRICS
by Bob Flaws
ISBN 1-891845-30-6

CHINESE MEDICAL PALMISTRY:
Your Health in Your Hand
by Zong Xiao-fan & Gary Liscum
ISBN 0-936185-64-3

CHINESE MEDICAL PSYCHIATRY
A Textbook and Clinical Manual
by Bob Flaws and James Lake, MD
ISBN 1-845891-17-9

CHINESE MEDICINAL TEAS:
Simple, Proven, Folk Formulas for
Common Diseases & Promoting Health
by Zong Xiao-fan & Gary Liscum
ISBN 0-936185-76-7

CHINESE MEDICINAL WINES & ELIXIRS
by Bob Flaws
ISBN 0-936185-58-9

CHINESE MEDICINE & HEALTHY WEIGHT
MANAGEMENT
An Evidence-based Integrated Approach
by Juliette Aiyana, L. Ac.
ISBN 1-891845-44-6

CHINESE PEDIATRIC MASSAGE THERAPY: A
Parent's & Practitioner's Guide to the
Prevention & Treatment of Childhood Illness
by Fan Ya-li
ISBN 0-936185-54-6

CHINESE SELF-MASSAGE THERAPY:
The Easy Way to Health
by Fan Ya-li
ISBN 0-936185-74-0

THE CLASSIC OF DIFFICULTIES:
A Translation of the Nan Jing
translation by Bob Flaws
ISBN 1-891845-07-1

A COMPENDIUM OF CHINESE MEDICAL
MENSTRUAL DISEASES
by Bob Flaws
ISBN 1-891845-31-4

CONTROLLING DIABETES NATURALLY
WITH CHINESE MEDICINE
by Lynn Kuchinski
ISBN 0-936185-06-3

CURING ARTHRITIS NATURALLY WITH
CHINESE MEDICINE
by Douglas Frank & Bob Flaws
ISBN 0-936185-87-2

CURING DEPRESSION NATURALLY WITH
CHINESE MEDICINE
by Rosa Schnyer & Bob Flaws
ISBN 0-936185-94-5

CURING FIBROMYALGIA NATURALLY WITH
CHINESE MEDICINE
by Bob Flaws
ISBN 1-891845-09-8

CURING HAY FEVER NATURALLY WITH
CHINESE MEDICINE
by Bob Flaws
ISBN 0-936185-91-0

CURING HEADACHES NATURALLY WITH
CHINESE MEDICINE
by Bob Flaws
ISBN 0-936185-95-3

CURING IBS NATURALLY WITH CHINESE
MEDICINE
by Jane Bean Oberski
ISBN 1-891845-11-X

CURING INSOMNIA NATURALLY WITH
CHINESE MEDICINE
by Bob Flaws
ISBN 0-936185-86-4

CURING PMS NATURALLY WITH
CHINESE MEDICINE
by Bob Flaws
ISBN 0-936185-85-6

DISEASES OF THE KIDNEY & BLADDER
by Hoy Ping Yee Chan, *et al.*
ISBN 1-891845-35-7

THE DIVINE FARMER'S MATERIA MEDICA
A Translation of the Shen Nong Ben Cao
translation by Yang Shouz-zhong
ISBN 0-936185-96-1

DUI YAO: THE ART OF COMBINING
CHINESE HERBAL MEDICINALS
by Philippe Sionneau
ISBN 0-936185-81-3

ENDOMETRIOSIS, INFERTILITY AND
TRADITIONAL CHINESE MEDICINE:
A Laywoman's Guide
by Bob Flaws
ISBN 0-936185-14-7

THE ESSENCE OF LIU FENG-WU'S
GYNECOLOGY
by Liu Feng-wu, translated by Yang Shou-zhong
ISBN 0-936185-88-0

EXTRA TREATISES BASED ON
INVESTIGATION & INQUIRY:
A Translation of Zhu Dan-xi's Ge Zhi Yu Lun
translation by Yang Shou-zhong
ISBN 0-936185-53-8

FIRE IN THE VALLEY: TCM Diagnosis &
Treatment of Vaginal Diseases
by Bob Flaws
ISBN 0-936185-25-2

FU QING-ZHU'S GYNECOLOGY
trans. by Yang Shou-zhong and Liu Da-wei
ISBN 0-936185-35-X

FULFILLING THE ESSENCE:
A Handbook of Traditional & Contemporary
Treatments for Female Infertility
by Bob Flaws
ISBN 0-936185-48-1

GOLDEN NEEDLE WANG LE-TING: A 20th
Century Master's Approach to Acupuncture
by Yu Hui-chan and Han Fu-ru, trans. by Shuai Xue-
zhong
ISBN 0-936185-789-3

A GUIDE TO GYNECOLOGY
by Ye Heng-yin,
trans. by Bob Flaws and Shuai Xue-zhong
ISBN 1-891845-19-5

A HANDBOOK OF TCM PATTERNS
& TREATMENTS
by Bob Flaws & Daniel Finney
ISBN 0-936185-70-8

A HANDBOOK OF TRADITIONAL
CHINESE DERMATOLOGY
by Liang Jian-hui, trans. by Zhang Ting-liang
& Bob Flaws
ISBN 0-936185-07-4

A HANDBOOK OF TRADITIONAL
CHINESE GYNECOLOGY

by Zhejiang College of TCM, trans. by Zhang
Ting-liang & Bob Flaws
ISBN 0-936185-06-6 (4th edit.)

A HANDBOOK OF CHINESE HEMATOLOGY
by Simon Becker
ISBN 1-891845-16-0

A HANDBOOK OF MENSTRUAL DISEASES
IN CHINESE MEDICINE
by Bob Flaws
ISBN 0-936185-82-1

A HANDBOOK of TCM PEDIATRICS
by Bob Flaws
ISBN 0-936185-72-4

THE HEART & ESSENCE OF DAN-XI'S
METHODS OF TREATMENT
by Xu Dan-xi, trans. by Yang Shou-zhong
ISBN 0-926185-49-X

HERB TOXICITIES & DRUG INTERACTIONS:
A Formula Approach
by Fred Jennes with Bob Flaws
ISBN 1-891845-26-8

IMPERIAL SECRETS OF HEALTH
& LONGEVITY
by Bob Flaws
ISBN 0-936185-51-1

THE TREATMENT OF DISEASE IN TCM, Vol.
II: Diseases of the Eyes, Ears, Nose, & Throat
by Sionneau & Lü
ISBN 0-936185-69-4

THE TREATMENT OF DISEASE, Vol. III:
Diseases of the Mouth, Lips, Tongue,
Teeth & Gums
by Sionneau & Lü
ISBN 0-936185-79-1

THE TREATMENT OF DISEASE, Vol IV:
Diseases of the Neck, Shoulders,
Back, & Limbs
by Philippe Sionneau & Lü Gang
ISBN 0-936185-89-9

THE TREATMENT OF DISEASE, Vol V:
Diseases of the Chest & Abdomen
by Philippe Sionneau & Lü Gang
ISBN 1-891845-02-0

THE TREATMENT OF DISEASE, Vol VI:
Diseases of the Urogential System
& Proctology
by Philippe Sionneau & Lü Gang
ISBN 1-891845-05-5

THE TREATMENT OF DISEASE, Vol VII:
General Symptoms
by Philippe Sionneau & Lü Gang
ISBN 1-891845-14-4

THE TREATMENT OF EXTERNAL
DISEASES WITH ACUPUNCTURE
& MOXIBUSTION
by Yan Cui-lan and Zhu Yun-long, trans. by Yang Shou-
zhong
ISBN 0-936185-80-5

THE TREATMENT OF MODERN
WESTERN MEDICAL DISEASES
WITH CHINESE MEDICINE
by Bob Flaws & Philippe Sionneau
ISBN 1-891845-20-9

THE TREATMENT OF DIABETES
MELLITUS WITH CHINESE MEDICINE
by Bob Flaws, Lynn Kuchinski
& Robert Casañas, MD
ISBN 1-891845-21-7

UNDERSTANDING THE DIFFICULT
PATIENT: A Guide for Practitioners of Oriental
Medicine
by Nancy Bilello, RN, L.ac.
ISBN 1-891845-32-2

YI LIN GAI CUO (Correcting the Errors in the
Forest of Medicine)
by Wang Qing-ren
ISBN 1-891845-39-X

70 ESSENTIAL CHINESE
HERBAL FORMULAS
by Bob Flaws
ISBN 0-936185-59-7

160 ESSENTIAL CHINESE HERBAL PATENT
MEDICINES
by Bob Flaws
ISBN 1-891945-12-8

630 QUESTIONS & ANSWERS ABOUT CHI-
NESE HERBAL MEDICINE:
A Workbook & Study Guide
by Bob Flaws
ISBN 1-891845-04-7

230 ESSENTIAL CHINESE MEDICINALS
by Bob Flaws
ISBN 1-891845-03-9

750 QUESTIONS & ANSWERS ABOUT
ACUPUNCTURE
Exam Preparation & Study Guide
by Fred Jennes
ISBN 1-891845-22-5